Evidence-Guided Practice

A Framework for Clinical Decision Making in Athletic Training

Evidence-Guided Practice

A Framework for Clinical Decision Making in Athletic Training

Bonnie L. Van Lunen, PhD, ATC, FNATA
Professor and Chair
Director, Athletic Training Program
School of Physical Therapy and Athletic Training
Norfolk, Virginia

Dorice A. Hankemeier, PhD, ATC
Clinical Education Coordinator
Assistant Professor
Ball State University
School of Physical Education, Sport & Exercise Science
Muncie, Indiana

Cailee E. Welch, PhD, ATC
Assistant Professor, Athletic Training Program
Department of Interdisciplinary Health Sciences
A.T. Still University
Mesa, Arizona

Routledge
Taylor & Francis Group
NEW YORK AND LONDON

First published in hardback 2024

First published in 2015 by SLACK Incorporated

Published 2024 by Routledge
605 Third Avenue, New York, NY 10158

and by Routledge
4 Park Square, Milton Park, Abingdon, Oxon OX14 4RN

Routledge is an imprint of the Taylor & Francis Group, an informa business

Publisher's Note
The publisher has gone to great lengths to ensure the quality of this reprint but points out that some imperfections in the original copies may be apparent.

Library of Congress Cataloging-in-Publication Data
Van Lunen, Bonnie, author.
Evidence-guided practice : a framework for clinical decision making in athletic training / Bonnie Van Lunen, Dorice A. Hankemeier, Cailee E. Welch.
p. ; cm.
Includes bibliographical references and index.
(paperback : alk. paper)
I. Hankemeier, Dorice A., author. II. Welch, Cailee E., author. III. Title.
[DNLM: 1. Sports Medicine--methods. 2. Athletes. 3. Athletic Performance. 4. Evidence-Based Medicine. QT 261]
RC1211
617.1'027--dc23
2014046920

ISBN: 978-1-03-295251-2 (hbk)
ISBN: 978-1-61711-603-2 (pbk)
ISBN: 978-1-003-52411-3 (ebk)

DOI: 10.4324/9781003524113

Additional resources can be found at
www.routledge.com/9781032952512

Dedication

To my entire family: all of you make my world go round.
Bonnie L. Van Lunen, PhD, ATC, FNATA

To my family and all of my students past and present: you make all of this worth it.
Dorice A. Hankemeier, PhD, ATC

To my family, friends, colleagues, and students: you inspire me each and every day.
Cailee E. Welch, PhD, ATC

Contents

Acknowledgments

Many individuals assisted with the formulation and review of this text, and we are grateful for their time and expertise.

Taylor Arman, North Central College
Mandi Baldwin, Ball State University
R. Curtis Bay, A.T. Still University
Julie Cavallario, Old Dominion University
Jennifer Cuchna, Old Dominion University
Lucas Dargo, Ball State University
Christine Feldbauer, Old Dominion University
Leah Ginn, Ball State University
Matthew Hoch, Old Dominion University
Megan Houston, Old Dominion University
Melissa Kay, A.T. Still University
Sarah Manspeaker, Duquesne University
Jordan Matchett, Ball State University
Tamara Valovich McLeod, A.T. Still University
William Perkins, Old Dominion University
Kelsey Picha, A.T. Still University
Jennifer Popp, Ball State University
Cameron Powden, Old Dominion University
Christine Schultz, Ball State University
Lisa Stobierski, A.T. Still University
Ashley Thrasher, Arkansas State University
Jessica Trcka, Ball State University
Alison Snyder Valier, A.T. Still University
Jessica Walter, Old Dominion University
Michelle Weber, A.T. Still University
Shelby Welsh, Ball State University

About the Authors

Bonnie L. Van Lunen, PhD, ATC, FNATA serves as the Director of the Commission on Accreditation of Athletic Training Education Accredited Post-Professional Athletic Training Program and is the Chair of the School of Physical Therapy and Athletic Training at Old Dominion University (Norfolk, Virginia). She received her bachelor of science degree in physical education with a specialization in athletic training from Castleton State College (Castleton, Vermont) in 1990 and her master of education degree in athletic training from the University of Virginia (Charlottesville, Virginia) in 1991. In addition, she received her doctor of philosophy degree in sports medicine from the University of Virginia in 1998. Her primary area of research interest is in outcomes related to competency development and implementation. Dr. Van Lunen has served in various capacities on committees for the National Athletic Trainers' Association (NATA) and the Commission on Accreditation of Athletic Training Education throughout her career. She serves on numerous editorial boards, publishes frequently in athletic training and sports medicine journals, and is a NATA Fellow. She was awarded the NATA Distinguished Educator Award in 2014 and the NATA Service Award in 2012. She resides in the Outer Banks of North Carolina with her husband, John, daughter, Alivian, and sons, Brady and Cameron.

Dorice A. Hankemeier, PhD, ATC is an Assistant Professor of Athletic Training in the School of Physical Education and Exercise Science at Ball State University (Muncie, Indiana). Dr. Hankemeier earned her bachelor of arts degree in exercise science with a concentration in athletic training from Central College (Pella, Iowa), and her master of science degree in education with an emphasis in athletic training from Old Dominion University (Norfolk, Virginia). After obtaining her degree, she served as an Athletic Trainer and Clinical Education Coordinator at Anderson University (Anderson, Indiana). Dr. Hankemeier then returned to Old Dominion University to obtain her doctorate in human movement science with an emphasis in athletic training curriculum and instruction. Her research focused on the implementation of evidence-based practice in the clinical education setting. Currently, Dr. Hankemeier serves as the Clinical Education Coordinator at Ball State University. She serves as a Site Visitor for the Commission on Accreditation of Athletic Training Education, is a manuscript reviewer for several journals, and is a member of the Great Lakes Athletic Trainers Association Education Committee. She was awarded the National Athletic Trainers' Association Research & Educational Foundation Doctoral Dissertation Award in 2013. Dr. Hankemeier's research interests focus on promoting evidence-based practice in athletic training and investigating educational outcomes of athletic training programs.

Cailee E. Welch, PhD, ATC is an Assistant Professor of Athletic Training within the Department of Interdisciplinary Health Sciences at A.T. Still University (Mesa, Arizona). Dr. Welch earned her bachelor of science degree in Athletic Training from Boston University (Boston, Massachusetts), followed by a master of science in education degree in athletic training from Old Dominion University (Norfolk, Virginia). She also earned her doctorate in human movement science with a special focus in athletic training curriculum and instruction from Old Dominion University, where she investigated the effectiveness of educational techniques to aid athletic trainers in learning the fundamentals of evidence-based practice. While at Old Dominion University, Dr. Welch served as an instructor for several undergraduate courses within the Health and Physical Education and Exercise Science Departments and was a teaching fellow for numerous courses with the Post-Professional Athletic Training Program. Recently, Dr. Welch completed a postdoctoral research fellowship in the Center for Clinical Outcome Studies at A.T. Still University. As a part of her postdoctoral fellowship, Dr. Welch assisted with clinical outcomes and evidence-based practice courses within the Post-Professional Athletic Training Program. Currently, she serves as the Clinical Practice Site Coordinator within the Athletic Training Practice-Based Research Network, which includes conducting the education and training for athletic trainers across the country. Additionally, Dr. Welch currently serves on the Commission on Accreditation of Athletic Training Education Post-Professional Annual Report Committee and the Board of Certification Evidence-Based Practice Review Panel and is the Managing Editor for the Clinical Bottom Line in the National Athletic Trainers' Association News. Dr. Welch's research agenda focuses on health care professional education and practice interventions to enhance clinical practice behaviors. Specifically, she is interested in assessing athletic training educational outcomes and identifying interventions to promote concussion education and enhance concussion management practices.

Contributing Authors

Johanna Hoch, PhD, ATC (Chapter 15)
Assistant Professor
Director of Clinical Education, Post-Professional Athletic Training Program
School of Physical Therapy and Athletic Training
Old Dominion University
Norfolk, Virginia

Matthew Hoch, PhD, ATC (Chapter 14)
Assistant Professor
Director of Research, Post-Professional Athletic Training Program
School of Physical Therapy and Athletic Training
Old Dominion University
Norfolk, Virginia

Kenneth Lam, ScD, ATC (Chapter 18)
Assistant Professor of Clinical Research
Department of Interdisciplinary Health Sciences
A.T. Still University
Mesa, Arizona

Jennifer McKeon, PhD, ATC (Chapter 14)
Assistant Professor
Department of Exercise and Sport Sciences
Ithaca College
Ithaca, New York

Alison Snyder Valier, PhD, ATC (Chapters 16, 17)
Associate Professor, Post-Professional Athletic Training Program
Department of Interdisciplinary Health Sciences
A.T. Still University
Mesa, Arizona

Drs. Van Lunen, Hankemeier, and Welch contributed to every chapter in the book.

Introduction

As we have delved into research regarding evidence-based practice concepts within educational programming in athletic training, it became evident that there were limited inclusive sources for athletic trainers to access. Athletic trainers are health care professionals who must have a foundation in the concepts of evidence-based practice to deliver patient care in an effective way; therefore, providing a resource for all of you was paramount. It is our hope that athletic training educators and preceptors use this text as a resource for students to formulate clinical plans that will be effective for individual patients.

Evidence-based practice should be habitual for every health care professional. Over the years, many of us have consulted the available evidence as we decided the plan of care for our patients. Unfortunately, this practice is not uniform among all health care providers. Now that the Board of Certification has mandated evidence-based practice continuing education units as part of athletic training certification maintenance requirements, it appears that we are heading in the right direction. Athletic trainers will be seeking out opportunities for evidence-based practice education and, therefore, will begin to automatically stay up to date on advances in the health care profession. We hope our textbook will also serve as a resource for every athletic trainer to use because they may need assistance with the interpretation of what the available evidence means for them and how they can effectively apply the evidence in daily patient care.

1

Construction of Clinical Questions

A typical day within the athletic training clinic consists of various patients and clients approaching you concerning the next steps that should be taken to progress toward a favorable outcome. All of these individuals seek your advice because they consider you to be the expert within the discipline. To provide information that is current and within the realm of supported decision making, you find that you need to devise an appropriate clinical question to formulate an answer that will encompass the possibilities associated with a desired outcome. The art and science of formulating a well-thought-out clinical question begins with deciphering the direction that you intend to go. Many of us start by asking a basic question, such as, "*What treatment approach will be most effective for this individual with patellofemoral pain?*" or "*What evaluation special tissue test will help me to decide whether this patient may have a meniscal injury?*" You will often find that this broad type of question does not assist you with narrowing down the possibilities and clinical decisions that are in front of you. These broad questions often lead to the inclusion of many special tissue tests that may not be relevant to the condition or to inclusion of many kinds of modalities to cover all things that could be happening within the injured tissue.

Formulating Clinical Questions

The process of finding evidence to assist with clinical decision making depends upon how the question is formulated. Using a **background question** similar to the ones mentioned previously only allows us to explore broader issues and obtain general knowledge concerning the issue we are investigating. A **foreground question**, however, is much more specific to the case at hand and assists with identifying pieces of the clinical problem that will lead to a clinical decision particular to the patient. We can utilize the background question of "*What treatment approach will be most effective for this individual with patellofemoral pain?*" and make it more specific. The specific question could be "*For an individual with patellofemoral pain, would the implementation of an orthosis compared with a taping application produce greater reductions in pain within 1 week?*" This type

Van Lunen BL, Hankemeier DA, Welch CE.
Evidence-Guided Practice: A Framework for Clinical Decision Making in Athletic Training (pp 1-9).

of question specifies what you would like to focus on and will allow you to address the condition in a targeted approach. The question can be formulated in a variety of ways, but you can use the **PIO**, **PICO**, **PIOT**, or **PICOT** approach (explained in the following section) depending upon the information you are seeking. The construction of questions using one of these approaches will be defined in the next section.

Constructing the Clinical Question With the PICOT Format

The **patient population** (P) or disease of interest should include an explicit description of the population (eg, age range, sport played, sex, ethnicity) or targeted disorder/disease (eg, diabetes, sickle cell anemia) to assist you with a targeted focus. The P can also be broad in the event little evidence may be available for your narrowed population.

The **intervention** (I), or issue of interest, is characterized by an intervention, prognosis or predictor, diagnosis or diagnostic test, etiology, or condition in which you are interested. This intervention can also be as broad (eg, exercise, cryotherapy, manual therapy) as you intend it to be or more focused (eg, stabilization exercises, ice massage, joint mobilizations) so that your search strategy will yield results within the focus you desire.

The **comparison** (C) is what you want to contrast the intervention or issue of interest against and includes things such as no intervention, placebo intervention, alternative therapies, no disease, a prognostic factor, or absence of a risk factor. The comparison is an optional piece of the question and is not included in every clinical question. Sometimes, the comparison is just the standard of care, which would be considered the control group, and, therefore, is truly not a comparison intervention.

The **outcome** (O) relates to what you are interested in examining concerning the effects of the intervention, diagnostic test, or prognosis you are seeking. These may be outcomes from a therapy that you implemented (eg, pain, patient-reported outcome score, range of motion), the risk of a disease, the accuracy of the diagnosis (eg, likelihood ratios, predictive value), or rate of occurrence of adverse outcomes (eg, ankle injuries, number of concussions). Often, there are many outcomes of interest that are associated with your question, and it is suggested to utilize broad terms rather than specific ones when constructing the question (ankle range of motion vs seated dorsiflexion, weighted dorsiflexion, supine dorsiflexion, prone knee bent dorsiflexion).

A **time** (T) component may be appropriate in your clinical question if your outcome of interest has a specific time period of observation. For example, questions examining a precise block of time (a 2-week joint mobilizations intervention or 6 weeks following anterior cruciate ligament reconstruction) would benefit from including the relevant time in addition to the PICO. A time (T) frame may not be appropriate to include in every clinical question; it all depends on whether you decide to narrow down your question.

The description and example in Table 1-1 demonstrate a fully developed clinical question using the PICOT format. You can further define the clinical question that is presented within the table by inquiring about a specific type of tape or brace application or by limiting the age group of the patient population to include only high school–aged individuals. Given these adjustments, your question from Table 1-1 would now read as: *"In high school–aged patients with anterior knee pain (P), how does a McConnell taping application (I) compared with neoprene open patella bracing (C) affect pain and function within 2 weeks?"* Utilization of the PICOT format for clinical questions is further demonstrated within Table 1-2.

Types of Clinical Questions

Many different types of clinical questions can be formulated, and the makeup of the question depends upon the information that you are seeking. **Intervention or therapy questions** will assist you with determining the efficacy of what you have chosen for treatment to address your patients'

Table 1-1.
PICOT Format for Clinical Questions

ACRONYM LETTER	DEFINITION	EXAMPLE
P	Patient population	Adolescents with anterior knee pain
I	Intervention of interest	Taping
C	Comparison intervention or issue of interest	Bracing
O	Outcome(s) of interest	Reduction in pain, increase in function
T	Time of interest	Immediate (within 2 weeks)
Intervention Clinical Question: In adolescents with anterior knee pain, how does taping compared with bracing affect pain and function within 2 weeks?		

needs and will lead you to determine what factors may be important for immediate results, as well as long-term outcomes based upon the condition. **Etiology questions** refer to the examination of the cause or causes associated with a condition and are utilized to determine which factors may be the primary elements that are associated with the greatest risk for the condition. A **diagnosis or diagnostic test–framed question** is appropriate to construct when you are interested in determining whether one test is better at assessing if an individual has a certain condition. **Prognostic or prediction questions** are utilized when you want to determine the factors that may complicate the clinical plan of treatment over time and if you can then incorporate this information to better assist the patient with a favorable outcome. Lastly, a **meaning-phrased question** assists you with understanding the meaning of an experience for a particular individual, group, or community and often deals with obtaining perceptual information from the patients.

For example, if you are seeking whether a diagnostic tissue test is more effective at identifying the existence of a condition over another tissue test, then you develop a diagnostic test–framed question which may or may not include a time frame. The question would be formulated something like this: "*In patients who have shoulder pain, is the Neer impingement test better at identifying impingement syndrome as compared with the Hawkins impingement test?*" If you are seeking information regarding the prediction of an outcome, then you would develop a prediction question that may be worded like this: "*In patients with carpal tunnel syndrome, how does incorporation of a night splint compared with no night splint influence pain and function over 4 weeks?*" Table 1-3 provides examples of types of clinical questions that you might ask over the course of an evaluation or treatment plan. Formulating your question in this manner allows you to effectively and efficiently search for evidence that will assist with answering the type of question that you have.

Table 1-2.
Question Types That Formulate Clinical Questions

QUESTION TYPE	DEFINITION	TEMPLATE	EXAMPLE
Intervention or therapy	To determine which treatment leads to the best outcome	In ________ (P), how does ________ (I) compared with ______ (C) affect ________ (O) within ________ (T)?	In recreationally active college students with chronic ankle instability (P), how do joint mobilizations in combination with standardized treatment (I) compared with standardized treatment alone (C) affect range of motion and functional scores (O) within a 2-week treatment period (T)?
Etiology	To determine the greatest risk factors or causes of a condition	Are ________ (P) who have ________ (I), compared with those with/without ______ (C), at ____ risk for ______ (O) over ________ (T)?	Are military recruits (P) who have pes planus foot types (I) compared with those with "normal" foot types (C) at greater risk for developing fibular stress fractures (O) over the initial training period (T)?
Diagnosis or diagnostic test	To determine which test is more accurate and precise in diagnosing a condition	In ________ (P), are/is ________ (I) compared with ______ (C) more accurate in diagnosing ______ (O)?	In acute knee injured patients (P), is the Thessaly test (I) compared with the McMurray test (C) more accurate in diagnosing a meniscal injury (O)?

(continued)

Table 1-2. (continued)

Question Types That Formulate Clinical Questions

QUESTION TYPE	DEFINITION	TEMPLATE	EXAMPLE
Prognosis or prediction	To determine the clinical course over time and likely complications of a condition	In ______ (P), how does ______ (I) compared with ______ (C) influence ______ (O) over ______ (T)?	In patients with acute low back pain (P), how does incorporation of spinal manipulations (I) compared with a home exercise program (C) influence pain and function (O) over 2 weeks (T)?
Meaning	To understand the meaning of an experience for a particular individual, group, or community	How do ______ (P) with ______ (I) perceive ______ (O) during ______ (T)?	How do collegiate patients (P) with anterior cruciate ligament reconstruction (I) perceive the care provided by the athletic trainer (O) during the initial 6 weeks of the rehabilitation process (T)?

Engaging Athletic Trainers in the Clinical Question Process

Evidence-based practice (EBP) is a term that athletic trainers (ATs) are hearing in everyday clinical practice and within educational programming. Although the term is recognized, the infrastructure for creating an environment in which there is support for a process to raise and address relevant clinical issues is lacking. To monitor quality improvement (ie, validation or changes made based upon evaluation of patient care practices) within your clinical practice setting, you need to be able to include a mechanism and process for addressing clinical questions that are important to your clinical staff.

The opportunities for generating clinical questions within your practice setting are numerous. A whiteboard could be placed within your clinic, and you could pose a question of the week that would be addressed during a clinical staff meeting. Additionally, a clinical question box could be placed within the clinic, and your peers could be required to place a clinical question within the box on a weekly basis, one of which would be discussed within the staff meeting. If your clinical practice setting is one in which you are the only provider, you could create a group (interested ATs, ATs within the conference, ATs within other clinics) that would be interested in participating in

Table 1-3. Clinical Questions Associated With Scenarios

QUESTION TYPE	SCENARIO EXAMPLE	CLINICAL QUESTION
Intervention or therapy	A former collegiate soccer player has been diagnosed with postconcussion syndrome. She has been having significant trouble with her balance, and it is affecting her daily activities. Although she can no longer play contact sports, she wants to be recreationally active. You are curious as to what type of therapy would be beneficial for her.	In physically active individuals (P), how does vestibular rehabilitation therapy (I) compared with a pharmacological intervention (C) affect balance and activities of daily living (O) within 1 month time period (T)?
	One of your patients, who is a softball player at the high school, has been diagnosed with shoulder impingement syndrome, and you are seeking to address her immediate issues concerning pain and discomfort.	In a high school softball player with impingement syndrome (P), how does ice massage (I) compared with nonsteroidal anti-inflammatory drug medication (C) affect pain perception (O) within the first 24 hours (T)?
Diagnosis or diagnostic test	A local factory worker has been referred to you for a shoulder evaluation. He has been experiencing pain with overhead movements and with internal and external rotation of the glenohumeral joint. You suspect that he may be suffering from impingement of the supraspinatus tendon and would like to know information about the diagnostic accuracy of tests for this condition.	In patients with shoulder pain (P), is the Neer shoulder impingement test (I) more accurate at diagnosing supraspinatus impingement (O) than the Hawkins shoulder impingement test (C)?
	An ice hockey player reports having medial joint line knee pain that is sporadic in nature but seems to be occurring on a more frequent basis over the past month. He does not recall a mechanism of injury related to the condition but does report that pushing off of that leg can cause a sharp, pinching feeling on the inside of his knee. You would like to determine which special tissue test is better at determining the possibility of a meniscal tear.	In a male ice hockey player with knee pain (P), is the Thessaly Test (I) better at diagnosing a meniscal tear (O) than the McMurray test (C)?

(continued)

Table 1-3. (continued)
Clinical Questions Associated With Scenarios

QUESTION TYPE	SCENARIO EXAMPLE	CLINICAL QUESTION
Etiology	You recently started working with the women's cross country team at your institution. The members of the team have been working with a sports psychologist over the course of the season on issues related to self-esteem. Based on some of the information that has been gained through these sports psychology sessions, you begin to wonder how low self-esteem could affect the health of these patients.	Are female endurance athletes (P) with low self-esteem (I) compared with those that have higher self-esteem (C) at greater risk for developing an eating disorder (O) over the course of the season (T)?
	You are assigned to examine the incidence of distal fibular stress fractures in the military recruits that have occurred during boot camp training. The female military recruits have developed significantly more stress fractures within the training period and are lacking in physical readiness for participating.	Are female military recruits (P) with high body mass indexes (I) compared with those with low body mass indexes (C) at greater risk for developing fibular stress fractures (O) within the first few weeks of basic training (T)?
Prognosis or prediction	Your patient, who is a high school freshman basketball player, has recently torn her anterior cruciate ligament and will require reconstructive surgery. Their surgeon has given her the option of choosing a patellar tendon autograft or a cadaver patellar tendon allograft. Your patient is concerned about the rehabilitation differences between the 2 grafts and the longevity of the graft choice given her young age.	In young adolescent females (P), how does a patellar tendon autograft (I) compare with a cadaver patellar tendon allograft (C) when assessing the 3- to 5-year (T) success rate of anterior cruciate ligament reconstructive surgery (O)?
	Within the physician clinical practice in which you work, everyone is considering the implementation of tests for the preparticipation examination, which will potentially assist with the prediction of the incidence of lower extremity injuries to the ankle. You need to decide which test would be a better predictor of future injury to the ankle so that you can then implement the appropriate prevention strategy for individuals who perform poorly.	In high school–aged patients (P), how does the weighted dorsiflexion test (I) compare with the single leg hop test (C) when predicting an ankle injury (O) over the course of an athletic season (T)?

(continued)

TABLE 1-3. (CONTINUED)
CLINICAL QUESTIONS ASSOCIATED WITH SCENARIOS

QUESTION TYPE	SCENARIO EXAMPLE	CLINICAL QUESTION
Meaning	As a high school athletic trainer, you often become the liaison between the parents and several health care team members as you coordinate the care for many patients. You are curious as to how the parents perceive the interdisciplinary collaboration.	How do parents (P) of high school patients (I) perceive the interdisciplinary collaboration between health care providers (O) during the first 2 weeks after an injury during the diagnosis and treatment phase (T)?
	The head athletic trainer has asked you to develop the emergency action plan for your new football facility. Before you begin, however, you decide to inquire about how other athletic training facilities structure their emergency action plans so that you can ensure your plan includes all the necessary information.	How do athletic trainers (P) develop emergency action plans (I) to ensure efficient procedures occur during all situations that may occur in a football facility (O)?

the endeavor. This group could be formulated through an online mechanism, and questions would be uploaded to a wiki or similar service. Discussion of the clinical question may lead to creating or revising a policy or procedure currently in use, educating staff on the issue, the need to make an administrative decision, further inquiry into the research and literature, or an on-the-spot problem resolution or decision.

An example of implementing a process for clinical question development within your practice would be to utilize a clinical question that has been posed by your peers concerning whether you should continue the use of hydroculator packs in the treatment of musculotendinous injuries. You would take this question and put it into the PICOT format for an interventional approach, and the question could be formulated as, *"In patients with musculotendinous injuries (P), how does a hydroculator pack (I) as compared with the use of X treatment (C) affect tissue temperature (O) within the application time of 15 minutes (T)?"* This question could be further defined if needed to be associated with deep musculotendinous injuries or those that are superficial. You could also choose to examine different patient populations (eg, elderly, adolescent). Another potential way to ask this clinical question would be to use the meaning approach so that you could examine the perceptions of your patients on the effectiveness of the hydroculator pack for musculotendinous injuries. The potential peer discussion as a result of this question could lead to determining whether additional evidence should be sought to make a sound clinical decision. Furthermore, this decision could transfer into an administrative conclusion regarding the appropriateness of this modality in treating patients (or conditions). It would also generate discussion as to what would replace this modality choice in achieving the desired outcome for which the hydroculator pack was used in the first place.

The incorporation of each staff member presents an avenue for everyone who is interested in making a difference in his or her practice and patient care. The quality of care will also increase, as the questions will be answered with supporting evidence and then implemented or validated within the practice setting. The ability to write an effective clinical question will assist you in finding the best possible evidence to support your practice while also engaging fellow practitioners in shared decision-making processes concerning patient care. Understanding how to write a clinical question is the first step in engaging in the EBP process.

Summary

Construction of a clinical question is the foundational step in using evidence to guide your clinical practice. Clinical questions can be broad, to allow more evidence to be found, or more specific, so that you are able to directly answer a question for a particular patient. In the end, ATs must use well-formulated clinical questions on a regular basis to generate clinical discussions and to foster clinical decision making.

Key Points

- Understanding how to write a clinical question is the first step in engaging in the EBP process.
- Clinical questions can be formulated in a variety of ways, but you can use the PIO, PICO, PIOT, or PICOT approach depending upon the information you are seeking.
- The ability to write an effective clinical question will assist you in finding the best possible evidence to support your practice while also engaging fellow practitioners in shared decision-making processes concerning patient care.

Bibliography

Cross NB, Craig JC, Webster AC. Asking the right question and finding the right answers. *Nephrology (Carlton)*. 2010;15(1):8-11.

Melnyk BM, Fineout-Overholt E, Stillwell SB, Williamson KM. Evidence-based practice: igniting a spirit of inquiry: an essential foundation for evidence-based practice. *Am J Nurs*. 2009;109(11):49-52.

Melnyk BM, Fineout-Overholt E. *Evidence-Based Practice in Nursing & Healthcare: A Guide to Best Practice*. 2nd ed. Philadelphia, PA: Lippincott Williams & Wilkins; 2011.

Miller SA, Forrest JL. Enhancing your practice through evidence-based decision making: PICO, learning how to ask good questions. *J Evid Base Dent Pract*. 2001;1(2):136-141.

Pangarakis S, Graner T. Engage nurses in EBP with the nursing clinical question process. *Nurs Manage*. 2010;41(6):15-17.

Staunton M. Evidence-based radiology: steps 1 and 2–asking answerable questions and searching for evidence. *Radiology*. 2007;242(1):23-31.

Stillwell SB, Fineout-Overholt E, Melynk BM, Williamson KM. Evidence-based practice, step by step: asking the clinical question: a key step in evidence-based practice. *Am J Nurs*. 2010;110(3):58-61.

2

Types of Research Design

You will encounter several research study designs as you search for available evidence, and it is imperative that you understand the level of scientific rigor associated with each design and what type of clinical question the design is intended to address (Figure 2-1). Research study designs can be simple to investigate foundational information (eg, how long do cryotherapy effects last, what stretching program is most effective for increasing flexibility of the hamstrings) or sophisticated and complex to answer questions that have multiple layers (eg, randomized, clinical trial of treatments for low back pain; a prediction model for lower extremity injury patterns). The important aspect to remember is that you can only use the information from the study design for the clinical question that was asked, and you should not expand information from the study to address other questions not directly investigated. We often try to imply more from the study findings than we should, and that is not recommended because what we are trying to imply was not examined; therefore, it cannot be answered within the context of the study's results. Another piece to consider within this context is that one study does not equate to a defined answer to the problem. Most clinical problems are usually multifaceted and, therefore, need to be supported by additional findings that may have incorporated a different population, different parameters, or measured different variables. For example, let us consider a study that focused on the effects of a 1-week intervention of talocrural joint mobilizations for the treatment of dorsiflexion deficits in individuals who have a history of ankle sprains. The outcome was that the mobilizations increased dorsiflexion range of motion. You would not be able to deduct that (1) joint mobilizations increase range of motion for all joints within the body, (2) the joint mobilization treatments had lasting effects beyond the first week, and (3) joint mobilizations also increased the functional abilities of the individuals because the researchers did not measure those parameters. You should always go into a question with your eyes wide open so that you are aware of what other factors may have had an effect on the results. The first step in this process is to understand what each type of study design is able to provide. That is the purpose of this chapter.

Oftentimes, research study designs are determined based upon the time frame of interest (Figure 2-2). Studies that examine data that have already been collected (eg, preparticipation

Van Lunen BL, Hankemeier DA, Welch CE.
Evidence-Guided Practice: A Framework for Clinical Decision Making in Athletic Training (pp 11-21).

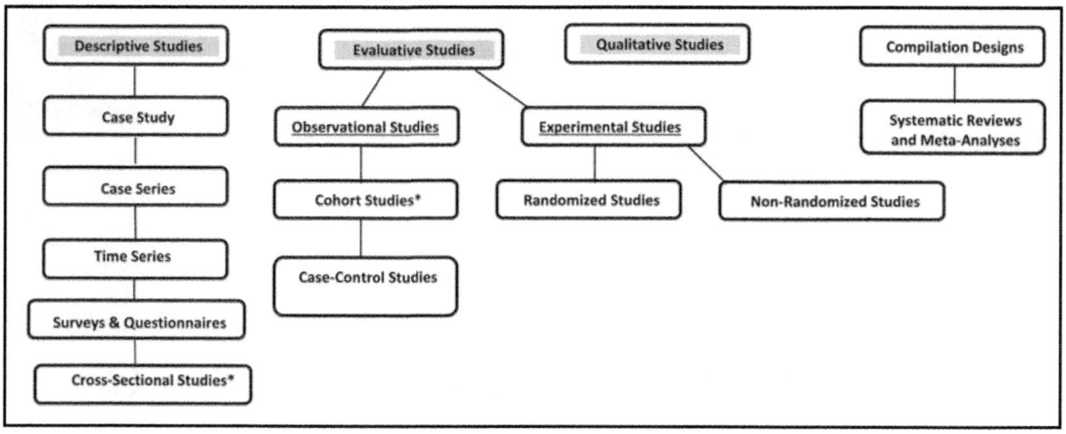

Figure 2-1. Types of research flowchart. *This type of research design can be prospective and retrospective.

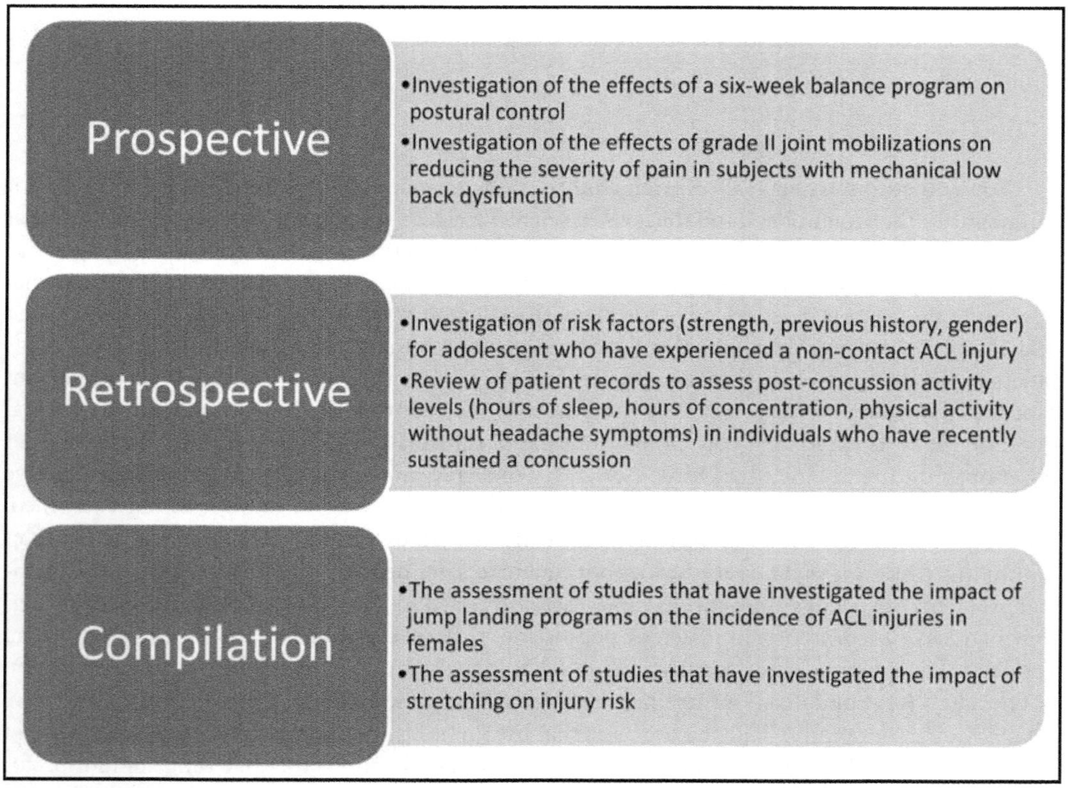

Figure 2-2. Time frames associated with study design. Abbreviation: ACL, anterior cruciate ligament.

information, electronic medical record information) or for which data on subjects who already have the condition of interest (eg, ankle sprain, concussion) and who are compared with a control group that has not had the condition would be considered **retrospective**, or ***ex post facto***. This could include examination of an individual's or group's current condition and the examination of factors or events in the past that could affect the condition, such as examining individuals with a fibular stress fracture and examining training habits, functional performance measures, and anatomical measures taken at the preparticipation examination. This could also include the examination of individuals with chronic ankle instability and those without and the comparison of factors that may be different between the groups. **Prospective study designs** examine the current condition (eg, concussion, hamstring injury) and follow the individuals over a designated period of time. Prospective research also can examine a group of individuals; you wait until a patient presents with the injury under study to predict the factors that contributed to the condition. When there is enough information and data concerning a topic area, you will be able to locate **compilation research**, which involves the aggregation of a large pool of data from multiple studies in an attempt to answer a clinical question that may not be answerable with a single research study. Assembling the information into a review or analysis (ie, systematic review or meta-analysis) entails the ability to identify enough usable findings to be able to formulate an outcome statement. If there is not enough information for this to occur, then you may find a brief summary statement on the clinical question of interest within a critically appraised topic. All of these types of research designs are incorporated into other design components that will be discussed within the next section of the text.

Research study designs are often categorized into groupings based upon the type of data collected or the questions that are being asked. The designs within the next section are categorized into (1) descriptive studies, (2) evaluative studies, or (3) qualitative studies; however, designs often cross over into more than one category because there may be a combination of methods used. For example, a mixed-methods approach (descriptive and qualitative) could be used to examine the perspectives of professional level athletic training students on how they believe their program prepared them within the competencies associated with evidence-based practice.

Descriptive Study Designs

The aim of **descriptive studies** (Table 2-1) is to examine something at a point in time and provide information concerning the findings. Descriptive studies often combine elements of quantitative (numeric findings) and qualitative methodologies within the design to answer the question of "what is" and to describe events. Since there are numerous scenarios in which you can examine something at a point in time, descriptive studies are further divided into 5 subcategories: case reports, case series, time series, surveys and questionnaires, and cross-sectional studies. These types of designs are considered a lower level of evidence because they require minimal scientific rigor.

A **case report**, also referred to as a **case study**, is a useful descriptive study design when you are seeking to conduct an in-depth examination of a patient and to help to develop and design larger studies or provide knowledge of a phenomenon to be studied further based on the information collected. Case reports vary depending on the type and focus of the clinical question; therefore, when you locate one within a peer-reviewed journal, it may look different and be composed of different components (eg, differential diagnosis, rehabilitation plan, clinical outcomes). These reports are often related to unique conditions or outcomes and are useful when you need to locate distinctive information for which there are not enough larger study outcomes available. Unfortunately, a case report can only be related to the patient involved in the process because many extraneous variables are not controlled for and may have contributed to the outcome. Therefore, application of the findings to all patients with a similar condition is not feasible.

A **case series** is a descriptive study that follows a group of patients who have a similar diagnosis or who are undergoing the same procedure over a certain period of time. Case series designs are also beneficial to describe outcomes of novel treatments (eg, low level laser therapy, instrument-assisted soft tissue mobilization), and the information can be used to generate questions that lead to focused studies with stronger and more robust designs. This type of design is easy to conduct and requires less time and financial resources than other types of studies. A limitation would be that they cannot be used to draw causal inferences regarding the efficacy of the treatment because there are inherent limitations within the design, such as lack of a control group, limited subjects, and other outside constraints.

Table 2-1.
Descriptive Studies

CLINICAL QUESTION EXAMPLE	BEST RESEARCH DESIGN	PUBLISHED ARTICLE EXAMPLE
How was exertional rhabdomyolysis recognized and treated in a 15-year-old male high school football player with no prior medical history?	Case study	Felton SD, Heinemann D, Craddock J. Exertional rhabdomyolysis in a high school athlete: a case review. *Athl Train Sport Health Care.* 2011;3(5):230-234.
Do thermal 3-MHz ultrasound and joint mobilization increase range of motion in the wrist in patients with decreased range of motion due to trauma?	Case series	Draper DO. Ultrasound and joint mobilizations for achieving normal wrist range of motion after injury or surgery: a case series. *J Athl Train.* 2010;45(5):486-491.
Are patients with low back pain more vulnerable to quadriceps inhibition after isometric, fatiguing lumbar extension exercises than healthy patients over time?	Time series	Hart JM, Fritz JM, Kerrigan DC, Saliba EN, Gansneder BM, Ingersoll CD. Quadriceps inhibition after repetitive lumbar extension exercise in persons with a history of low back pain. *J Athl Train.* 2006;41(3):264-269.
How do athletic training students perceive the importance and effectiveness of psychological skills in the rehabilitation of sport injury?	Survey/ questionnaire	Kamphoff CS, Hamson-Utley JJ, Antoine B, Knutson R, Thomae J, Hoenig C. Athletic training students' perceptions of an academic preparation in the use of psychological skills in sport injury rehabilitation. *Athl Train Educ J.* 2010;5(3):109-116.
How do athletic trainers perceive professional commitment and maintain commitment while working in a challenging environment?	Qualitative study	Pitney WA. A qualitative examination of professional role commitment among athletic trainers working in the secondary school setting. *J Athl Train.* 2010;45(2):198-204.

A **time series** involves the observation of a participant or a group of participants (also known as a sample) over multiple time instances, and measurements are compared with prior time instances that are of interest to you. Each participant or sample serves as their own control, and the outcome is repeatedly measured during one or more baseline and treatment periods. The data that you can obtain through this approach allow you to examine trends and fluctuations within the course of the treatment or intervention. The advantage of this design is that you are able to examine the full course of events throughout the time frame you are interested in, therefore bringing a real-life factor into your question. These type of designs can be referred to as single-subject designs because they focus on the individual and use of multiple measures over a designated time period rather than just using a large sample and collecting pre- and postintervention information only. However, single-subject designs often include more than one participant within the study so that comparisons can be made and are used to examine trends and variability within the data collected. This type of design is similar to what happens in your clinical practice on a daily basis because you track the progress of your patient multiple times throughout the course of your treatment plan.

Cross-sectional studies are considered snapshots in time, as exposure and outcome are simultaneously assessed. These types of studies are used to determine the prevalence of the condition or the total number of cases of a condition in a given population at a specific point in time; therefore, no causal relationships can be drawn from the reported results. For example, a cross-sectional study might report the prevalence of previous concussions in high school–aged football players or the prevalence of sickle cell trait in collegiate basketball players. You would be able to get an understanding of the number of cases within your interested group at the time you asked the survey questions; however, you would have limited information to be able to link it to any causal component.

Surveys and **questionnaires** are some of the most commonly used methods for collecting information about a group and can range from being purely descriptive to assessing relationships and cause and effect outcomes. The first thing that you need to decide on when using this type of approach is whether to utilize an existing survey instrument or create one of your own. Existing survey instruments often have already been assessed for reliability and validity, making them the preferred choice; however, you need to be able to locate an instrument that matches your research question, which may not be feasible. Your next option is to create your own instrument. This sounds like an achievable task until you realize that you need to create the questions, organize the questions into themes or areas to ensure that all aspects are covered, choose the type of quantitative outcome scoring mode (eg, Likert scale, open-ended response), assess reliability and validity components, and choose the mode of delivery. All of these factors, and others, must be considered when deciding to utilize this design because, without careful planning and consideration to detail, the information obtained through data collection will not be useful for understanding the sample. For example, if you are interested in examining burnout in faculty members who are primarily working within professional level educational programs, you may decide to use the Maslach Burnout Inventory–Educators edition because this instrument has already gone through the rigors of reliability and validity assessment. However, if you would like to examine knowledge levels in pharmacology for clinicians who have been practicing within athletic training for the past 10 years, then you would have to create your own instrument to assess knowledge as one does not currently exist. The development of the instrument would take a significant amount of time and have to undergo all levels of scrutiny before being implemented within your study.

Evaluative Study Designs

Evaluative study designs are used to determine the existence and strength of a possible association between an intervention and an outcome (Tables 2-2 and 2-3) and are associated with higher levels of evidence due to the rigor of the research design. The main focus of evaluative studies is to reach a conclusion based upon comparisons of groups and findings. Since there are numerous scenarios in which you can determine the effect of an intervention on a particular outcome, evaluative study designs can be further divided into 2 subcategories: **observational** and **experimental**.

Table 2-2.
Observational Studies

CLINICAL QUESTION EXAMPLE	BEST RESEARCH DESIGN	PUBLISHED ARTICLE EXAMPLE
Are high school–aged athletes who have an eating disorder, menstrual dysfunction, and low bone mineral density at higher risk for musculoskeletal injury?	Prospective cohort	Rauh MJ, Nichols JF, Barrack MT. Relationship among injury and disordered eating, menstrual dysfunction, and low bone mineral density in high school athletes: a prospective study. *J Athl Train.* 2010;45(3):243-252.
What role does postinjury activity level play in postconcussive symptoms and performance on neurocognitive tests in student athletes?	Retrospective cohort	Majerske CW, Mihalik JP, Ren D, et al. Concussions in sports: postconcussive activity levels, symptoms, and neurocognitive performance. *J Athl Train.* 2008;43(3):265-274.
Does knowledge, sex, or institutional level of athletic trainers affect reported incidence of methicillin-resistant *Staphylococcus aureus*?	Cross-sectional	Kahanov L, Gilmore EJ, Eberman LE, Roberts J, Semerjian T, Baldwin L. Certified athletic trainers' knowledge of methicillin-resistant *Staphylococcus aureus* and common disinfectants. *J Athl Train.* 2011;46(4):415-423.
Is pitching performance in Major League Baseball players who need operative treatment of rotator cuff tears different than in healthy pitchers?	Case control	Namdari S, Baldwin K, Ahn A, Huffman GR, Sennett BJ. Performance after rotator cuff tear and operative treatment: a case-control study of major league baseball pitchers. *J Athl Train.* 2011;46(3):296-302.

Observational Study Designs

Cohort studies are used for determining the incidence (number of new cases within a defined time period) and natural history of a condition and can be prospective or retrospective. In a **prospective cohort study**, a group of people are studied who do not have the condition (eg, ankle sprain, anterior cruciate ligament injury, shoulder impingement, concussion), and investigators measure several variables that may be linked to the condition. For example, if you are interested in ankle sprains within the high school–aged individual, then you would prescreen those who fit the inclusion criteria. The prescreening could include assessing potential predictors or risk factors for incurring an ankle injury and may include testing, such as weighted ankle dorsiflexion, single leg hop for distance, the Landing Error Scoring System, or history of ankle injury. All of the variables that you collect are usually thought to contribute to the injury you are interested in,

Table 2-3.
Experimental Studies

CLINICAL QUESTION EXAMPLE	BEST RESEARCH DESIGN	PUBLISHED ARTICLE EXAMPLE
In industrial workers with nonspecific neck and shoulder pain, does a high-intensity strength training program compared with normal physical activity change self-reported neck and shoulder pain intensity?	Randomized study	Zebis MK, Andersen LL, Pedersen MT, et al. Implementation of neck/shoulder exercises for pain relief among industrial workers: a randomized controlled trial. *BMC Musculoskelet Disord.* 2011;12:205.
How does exposure to a sport psychology workshop compare to not having exposure to a workshop impact athletic training students' use of sport psychology behaviors?	Nonrandomized study	Clement D, Shannon V. The impact of a workshop on athletic training students' sport psychology behaviors. *Sport Psychol.* 2009;23:504-522.
In healthy athletic individuals, can balance training be effective at enhancing performance and changing neuromuscular control?	Systematic review	Zech A, Hüubscher M, Vogt L, Banzer W, Hänsel F, Pfeifer K. Balance traning for neuromuscular control and performance enhancement; a systematic review. *J Athl Train.* 2010;45(4):392-403.
How effective are various concussion assessment techniques in detecting the effects of concussion on cognition, balance, and symptoms in athletic patients?	Meta-analysis	Broglio SP, Puetz TW. The effect of sport concussion on neurocognitive function, self-report symptoms, and postural control: a meta-analysis. *Sports Med.* 2008;38(1):53-67.

and, oftentimes, other clinicians may be asked to participate in these types of studies if you are examining large numbers of individuals. The participants in the study are then followed over a defined period of time to see if they incur the condition, and then the groups are compared (those with the condition and those without the condition). Therefore, within the high school ankle injury study described previously, you would examine individuals who incurred an ankle sprain compared with those who did not incur a sprain by reviewing the prescreening factors that were collected at the start of the season. This information will then assist you in determining if there are preexisting factors that may contribute to the susceptibility to incur an ankle sprain, and you would implement a prevention strategy based on this information. In a **retrospective cohort study**, data that have been collected from other resources (ie, electronic medical records, administrative data) are used to assemble the cohort or groups. For example, you could examine your electronic medical records database for individuals who were treated for shoulder instability and compare the outcomes of those who had surgical intervention and those who did not. To do this properly, you would have to ensure that you had a predetermined set of outcome variables that were collected from each of the participants to make appropriate comparisons. Cohort designs allow you to examine the natural course of a disease or condition, determine the risk factors for a condition, clarify the outcome of an intervention, and usually have a high degree of quality control. However, you need to be aware that this type of design can be expensive, time-consuming, and difficult in terms of controlling the extraneous variables (individual, organizational, or environmental characteristics other than the factor of interest); require strict inclusion and exclusion criteria; and include subjects that must adhere to strict standardized time frames.

Case-control studies are the opposite of cohort studies because the outcome has already occurred and individuals are chosen for the study based on whether they have the condition of interest (ie, ankle sprain, no ankle sprain). Therefore, case-control studies are usually considered retrospective. The aim of case-control studies is to identify predictors of an outcome through examination of exposures that may have contributed to one group incurring the condition of interest (cases) and the other not (controls). For example, you may be interested in examining which factors may be different between individuals with patellofemoral pain and those without. The limitation is that those factors may be a byproduct of having the condition and were not present prior to developing the condition; therefore, it is difficult to determine a cause and effect relationship with this type of design.

Experimental Designs

Experimental study designs involve the prospective investigation of groups over time and the manipulation of subjects and are used to determine causal relationships. You may be interested in the examination of a treatment approach or intervention strategy for a particular condition. You would need to investigate variables at the beginning and end of the time period of interest to determine if one approach is more effective than the other. You will need to make a decision as to whether to randomly assign individuals to your groups; therefore, you need to decide the most effective approach for your clinical question. These types of designs adhere to strict protocols that make it difficult to identify subjects and retain them within the studies. The methods are often time-consuming and expensive; however, the information obtained from the outcomes is considered to be some of the highest-quality evidence available.

Randomized, experimental designs are considered to be one of the most robust types of research designs. The main component of these designs is the randomization of individuals into the predetermined groupings, such as an experimental treatment group or control group. Random assignment means that each subject has an equal chance of being assigned to any of the groups, and all personal judgment or bias is removed from assigning individuals to groups. The act of randomly assigning subjects to groups creates a balance of subjects within each of the groups and assists with the elimination of other factors contributing to the outcome that you did not intend to be factors (ie, age, mass, height). An additional feature that can be utilized with this design occurs when all of the individuals have the condition of interest (eg, patellofemoral pain), and you would like to randomly assign them into an experimental treatment of exercise or a control group that receives no treatment. These studies are often called randomized, controlled trials and are considered to be the gold standard of research study designs; however, due to the fact that these designs are generally expensive, time consuming, and require a high level of rigor, they are often not easy to institute. Additionally, it may be difficult to utilize an intercollegiate patient because we seldom withhold treatment or place the individual into a group that we believe may not have desired outcomes. It is important to realize that although these types of designs are at the higher end of the level of evidence paradigm, they may not be appropriate for all clinical questions.

Nonrandomized experimental designs, or quasiexperimental designs, involve no randomization procedures when placing individuals into groups. This may be the only choice for the experimental design due to examination of an intervention or prevention strategy in use at one clinical site and not at another. For example, you may be interested in comparing the outcomes of 2 surgical techniques for the treatment of multidirectional instability at the glenohumeral joint. One surgeon who performs technique A refers all of his patients to a particular clinic, while the other surgeon who performs technique B refers her patients to a different clinic. You are unable to randomly assign patients to the surgeons, and you are unable to randomly assign patients to clinics. The question you would like to investigate is viable; therefore, you perform a quasiexperimental study, or nonrandomized study, to answer the question because your groups are already predetermined. The 2 groups are prospectively followed over time, and comparisons are made between them.

Experimental research designs are further strengthened within compilation research in which you can examine multiple findings from similar studies that examine a similar clinical question within a systematic review and combine data for analysis within a meta-analysis. **Systematic reviews** are narratives of the critical evaluation of the research question through an exhaustive search of the available evidence, followed by the appraisal, selection, and synthesis of many sources for a clinical question that is relevant. Systematic reviews are developed through the following steps: (1) defining an appropriate health care question, (2) searching the literature, (3) assessing the studies, (4) combining the results, and (5) placing the findings in context. Systematic reviews have become more readily available due to the explosion of research within certain areas and the need for clinicians, health care managers, policy makers, and consumers to access good quality information on the effectiveness, meaningfulness, feasibility, and appropriateness of interventions. Systematic reviews are considered to be one of the highest levels of evidence that inform evidence-guided practice; however, you must still critically evaluate the process in which the review was conducted and the quality of the evidence that is included to utilize the information in clinical practice.

A **meta-analysis** provides a quantitative assessment of the pooled statistical results from studies that have met the inclusion criteria within the systematic review. For example, once the systematic review is conducted, the investigators would then utilize the available data from each study (obtained through the manuscript or from the authors directly) and conduct statistical analyses with all of the data from all of the studies combined. Meta-analyses are considered to be one of the highest levels of evidence because they take into account multiple pieces of information that are examined critically before they can even be included in the process. Meta-analyses can be completed on most types of study designs but are considered to be more relevant if the design includes randomized, clinical trials because more of the variables were controlled for within the study. The product of the meta-analysis is a consensus, based on the available evidence, for best practice for the condition that was examined.

Qualitative Study Designs

Qualitative studies aim to develop concepts that help us to understand social phenomena in natural settings, giving emphasis to the meanings, experiences, and views of the participants. Qualitative research focuses on a deeper understanding of a phenomenon through narrative descriptions that are derived via open-ended questions, interviews, and observations. These types of designs are concerned with why something is happening; how it works; and what people think, perceive, and believe about the issue at hand using observations, interviews, focus groups, and consensus methods. The primary objective is to obtain a more in-depth understanding of the individual's perspective within a certain context by using the person's own words rather than quantitative data. This approach emphasizes an understanding of the human experience and is the best approach to gain an appreciation of the experiences individuals have with themselves, others, and their surroundings. Qualitative study designs are useful in the exploration of patients'

Table 2-4.
Qualitative Research Examples

RESEARCH QUESTION	ASSOCIATED ARTICLE
What strategies are used by approved clinical instructors (preceptors) to implement evidence-based practice in clinical education of athletic training students?	Hankemeier DA, Van Lunen BL. Approved clinical instructors' perspectives on implementation strategies in evidence-based practice for athletic training students. *J Athl Train.* 2011;46(6):655-664.
How do potential athletic training students perceive the roles and responsibilities of athletic trainers?	Mensch J, Mitchell M. Choosing a career in athletic training: exploring the perceptions of potential recruits. *J Athl Train.* 2008;43(1):70-79.

preferences, as practitioners are able to understand several concepts (ie, health, illness, disability) from the direct perspective of the individual who experiences it on a daily basis. Triangulation of data is a process often used to confirm that concepts are evident and linked between different sources (ie, more than one source of data, more than one data collection method, more than one set of researchers). Triangulating data allows you to support your findings due to the fact that you are cross-checking the information for accuracy amongst multiple sources. Additionally, qualitative and quantitative approaches are often combined (mixed-methods design) to measure certain components of behavior, thereby increasing the validity of the findings because the quantitative piece provides specific information about variables of interest. Two examples of different qualitative questions along with the associated manuscripts are presented in Table 2-4.

Summary

Research study designs are chosen based upon the question that is being asked and the information that you are interested in seeking. The research paradigms were presented within 1 of 3 groupings (descriptive, evaluative, qualitative); however, you need to remember that the designs can be mixed and can cross over into other paradigms. Several journals require that the authors provide the type of design for the study within the abstract; this will assist you with understanding the context of a study as you begin to assess its value.

Key Points

- You can only use information from the study design for the clinical question that was asked, and you should not expand information from the study to address other questions not directly investigated.
- Research designs are often classified as descriptive, evaluative, or qualitative; however, crossover exists, and these studies are often classified as mixed methods.
- Descriptive studies examine something at a point in time and provide information concerning the findings.

- Evaluative study designs are used to determine the existence and strength of a possible association between an intervention and an outcome.
- Qualitative research studies aim to develop concepts that help us to understand social phenomena in natural settings, with emphasis on the meanings, experiences, and views of the participants.

Bibliography

Backman CL, Harris SR. Case studies, single-subject research, and N of 1 randomized trials: comparisons and contrasts. *Am J Phys Med Rehabil.* 1999;78(2):170-176.

Clancy MJ. Overview of research designs. *Emerg Med J.* 2002;19(6):546-549.

Grimes DA, Schulz KF. An overview of clinical research: the lay of the land. *Lancet.* 2002;359(9300):57-61.

Grimes DA, Schulz KF. Cohort studies: marching towards outcomes. *Lancet.* 2002;359(9303):341-345.

Hartung DM, Touchette D. Overview of clinical research design. *Am J Health Syst Pharm.* 2009;66(4):398-408.

Healy P, Devane D. Methodological considerations in cohort study designs. *Nurse Res.* 2011;18(3):32-36.

Hemingway P, Brereton N. What is a systematic review? www.whatisseries.co.uk. Accessed March 10, 2013.

Kendall JM. Designing a research project: randomised controlled trials and their principles. *Emerg Med J.* 2003;20(2):164-168.

Klassen TP, Jadad AR, Moher D. Guides for reading and interpreting systematic reviews: I. Getting started. *Arch Pediatr Adolesc Med.* 1998;152(7):700-704.

Mann CJ. Observational research methods. Research design II: cohort, cross sectional, and case-control studies. *Emerg Med J.* 2003;20(1):54-60.

Maslach C, Jackson SE, Leiter MP. *Maslach Burnout Inventory: Manual.* 3rd ed. Palo Alto, CA: Consulting Psychologists Press; 1996.

McKeon PO, Medina JM, Hertel J. Hierarchy of research design in evidence-based medicine. *Athl Ther Today.* 2006;11(4):42-45.

3

Searching the Literature for Evidence

Once you have a well-defined clinical question, the next step in the evidence-based practice (EBP) process is to search for the best available evidence. Fortunately, rapid technological advancements over the years have allowed easy access to electronic formats and bibliographic databases via the Internet. Clinicians now have several mechanisms they can utilize to search for relevant literature related to their clinical question. Additionally, the ease and accessibility of the Internet provides clinicians with the availability to search for evidence from almost anywhere. This chapter highlights various databases that may be available to you as you conduct your literature search and discusses some helpful search strategies (eg, controlled vocabulary, Boolean operators, truncation) to help enhance your search process. Once you have a good understanding of the different aspects of conducting a literature search, you will be able to utilize your clinical question to determine which online databases are most appropriate to search as well as which specific keywords will be most influential in obtaining accurate and useful information.

Although developing the clinical question may be the most crucial step to guide you through the EBP process, searching for accurate literature and narrowing it down to a manageable amount of information may be considered the most time intensive. Knowing how to search through numerous resources and locate the most relevant information related to your clinical question is important to comprehend. One of the benefits of a well-defined clinical question is that it makes the search for quality evidence more straightforward. The clinical question allows you to combine appropriate words and phrases that will suit the specific query (ie, search) language of many online search databases. Developing a literature search strategy that works best for you will help you stay on track and reduce your feelings of being overwhelmed by the amount of research literature that is available.

Databases

There are many different types of resources that provide us with the evidence we may be seeking. Textbooks and journals are often the first 2 resources we consider, but if a textbook is not

Van Lunen BL, Hankemeier DA, Welch CE.
Evidence-Guided Practice: A Framework for Clinical Decision Making in Athletic Training (pp 23-40).

updated regularly, it may contain old or outdated information. Therefore, with the rapid evolution of technology, online literature searching via a database has become the most efficient and timely way to find the information you are seeking. A **database** is an organized online collection of scholarly journal articles, periodicals, or books that provides a variety of information that will be helpful to you during your literature search. Although each database is unique, a majority of online databases contain references to articles, full article citations, abstracts, and full-text articles for free or for purchase. Most databases require a subscription to access the articles, so you should check with your school, employer, state government, or public library to see if you can gain access.

Because there are numerous databases available through the Internet, it is important to have a good understanding of which database can help you find the evidence you are seeking. While the type of database is directly dependent of the topic of information (eg, education, biological science, government, health care) for which you are searching, the next section of this text focuses on databases that are most commonly accessed among health care professionals. Specifically, this chapter focuses on the following databases:

- Google Scholar
- Cochrane Databases
- Cumulative Index to Nursing and Allied Health Literature (CINAHL)
- MEDLINE and PubMed
- Physiotherapy Evidence Database (PEDro)

Google Scholar

Clinicians often debate whether Google Scholar should be considered a scholarly database for conducting a literature search. Regardless of your point of view, it is important to have a good understanding of the benefits and limitations to this resource. **Google Scholar** is a free-access search engine that indexes resources from numerous scholarly publishers, and it is most often the top choice for clinicians searching for information. While Google Scholar is known for its simplicity and ease of access, the search engine has some limitations that must be considered. The article retrieval process of Google Scholar is illogical, meaning that articles retrieved from a general search are not listed by how current they are but instead by how relevant the article is to the search words used and how often the article has been cited in other scholarly literature. In addition to scholarly articles, Google Scholar retrieves theses, textbooks, abstracts, and other academic resources during the search process. Furthermore, you may not be able to access the full article retrieved during the Google Scholar search and will need to go to another database to download it.

Google Scholar continues to advance its search engine, and capabilities to conduct advanced searches are now available. More specifically, while using Google Scholar, you have the ability to search by date or relevance, establish custom ranges for the dates for which you want to retrieve articles, and/or search by author name if you choose. Although new information is added weekly, it may take anywhere from 6 months to longer than a year for Google Scholar to update current records, so the most recent literature may not be available during your search. Thus, while Google Scholar may be a convenient mechanism to conduct a general literature search, you must be aware that you may not be acquiring the most essential information to answer your clinical question. Google Scholar can be accessed at http://scholar.google.com.

Cochrane Databases

The **Cochrane Collaboration** is an international nonprofit organization established in 1993 that aims to assist health care professionals, policy makers, and patients to make informed decisions about health care. The Collaboration manages the 6 databases (Table 3-1) included in the Cochrane Library, but for this chapter the primary focus is on the Cochrane Database of

Table 3-1.
Databases of the Cochrane Library

Cochrane Database of Systematic Reviews	Database of Abstracts of Review of Effects
Cochrane Central Register of Controlled Trials	Health Technology Assessment Database
Cochrane Methodology Register	NHS Economic Evaluation Database

Systematic Reviews (CDSR). The CDSR consists of more than 5000 systematic reviews, providing health care professionals with the most up-to-date evidence on health care treatments, interventions, and diagnostic tests. Since the CDSR is a database solely comprised of literature that is the highest level of evidence (ie, systematic reviews), it is considered to be the gold standard of databases. However, unlike other databases that will be discussed, the CDSR only contains systematic reviews. The CDSR and the other databases managed by the Cochrane Collaboration are available at http://www.cochrane.org.

Cumulative Index to Nursing and Allied Health Literature

The **Cumulative Index to Nursing and Allied Health Literature (CINAHL)** database includes a collection of literature from nursing, biomedicine, health science librarianship, alternative medicine, consumer health, and numerous other health care professions, including athletic training. This database is privately owned by EBSCO Publishing and provides a comprehensive index of full-text articles from more than 760 journals and 275 books. The CINAHL database has several features, which include extensive assistance with search formulation and search strategy hints, subject vs keyword searching, and the availability to limit or modify searches. However, access to CINAHL requires a subscription, so you will have to check with your institution, state government, or public library to see if you can access this database. The CINAHL database is available at http://www.ebscohost.com/cinahl.

MEDLINE and PubMed

MEDLINE is the National Library of Medicine's (NLM's) bibliographical database and includes more than 19 million journal article references from numerous health fields, including medicine, dentistry, nursing, and other health care fields. While MEDLINE does include publications from newspapers, magazines, and newsletters, the majority of items included are articles from refereed scholarly journals. MEDLINE is constantly updated, with approximately 2000 to 4000 citations added daily. Similar to other databases, this database has several search features, but the most commonly recognized feature of MEDLINE is its inclusion of the NLM's **controlled vocabulary** (ie, **Medical Subject Headings [MeSH]**), which will be discussed further in the next section of this chapter. One unique feature of MEDLINE is that the database is accessible throughout various interfaces. More specifically, the NLM leases the database to vendors, who then integrate it through their specific system. If you are familiar with EBSCOhost or Ovid, you are actually accessing the MEDLINE database. Therefore, these interfaces will also have the same features that are available through MEDLINE.

Although you may not be as familiar with MEDLINE, you most likely have heard of or accessed PubMed. **PubMed** is a freely accessible online database maintained by the National Center for Biotechnology Information (NCBI) at the NLM. Essentially, PubMed provides health care professionals with free access to article citations that are indexed in MEDLINE. This database is user friendly and allows you to conduct literature searches utilizing several of the same search features available in MEDLINE (eg, MeSH). Thus, PubMed has become one of the most popular online databases utilized by health care professionals not only because it is free, but because when available, it provides you with links to access the full text of a journal article via PubMed Central or through publisher websites. The PubMed database is available at http://www.ncbi.nlm.nih.gov/pubmed.

Physiotherapy Evidence Database

The **Physiotherapy Evidence Database (PEDro)** is a free database managed by the Centre for Evidence-Based Physiotherapy at The George Institute for Global Health in Australia. This database provides you with access to more than 22,000 randomized, controlled trials, systematic reviews, and physiotherapy clinical practice guidelines. Each article included in the PEDro database is given a quality score via the PEDro appraisal scale, which provides readers with a numeric value (ie, 0 to 10) assessing the methodological quality of the article. The higher the score, the better the methodological quality of the trial. The PEDro database has individual search options, which allow you to conduct a simple or advanced search. Additionally, you have the ability to conduct an Allied Health Evidence search, which searches 4 databases (ie, PEDro, OTSeeker, PsycBITE, SpeechBITE) simultaneously. One limitation to this database, however, is the number of full-text articles that are available for download. While citations for articles always appear from a literature search, you may need to access another database to retrieve the full text of the article you are interested in. The PEDro database is available at www.pedro.org.au.

As you can see, each database that has been discussed has strengths and weaknesses when it comes to helping you retrieve the best available literature to answer your clinical question. Additionally, there are several other databases available that contain useful information. To ensure you are thoroughly searching all of the available literature, best practice should include the use of multiple databases because each database may provide you with different results. Finally, as technology continues to advance, it is likely that the features of these databases will improve as well. Therefore, you should access the database tutorials on an annual basis to check if any updates or new features become available to help you refine your literature searches.

Strategies for Searching Databases

Regardless of the database being used, the key to literature searching is to locate applicable articles while simultaneously eliminating irrelevant ones. Fortunately, there are various search techniques, such as MeSH searching, Boolean operators, exploding, and truncation, that can help you expedite the process.

Keywords vs Controlled Vocabulary

When you begin your literature search, it is important to have a solid understanding of the differences between keyword searching and controlled vocabulary searching. **Keyword searching**, also referred to as text word searching, is the type you may naturally think of when conducting a literature search, and it can provide you with a good starting point. More specifically, keyword searching involves the use of simple terms from everyday vocabulary. Keywords can be derived from the components of your clinical question and may often be the same terms used in your PICO chart, if one was utilized. For example, let us consider the following clinical question:

Can lower extremity injury prevention programs effectively reduce anterior cruciate ligament injury rates in adolescent athletes?

For this clinical question, our literature search may include the use of any of the following keywords:

- Adolescent athlete
- Youth
- Lower extremity injury prevention program
- Knee injury prevention
- Anterior cruciate ligament (ACL) injury rate
- Knee injury incidence
- Knee injury risk

Although using keywords seems to be the easiest approach to searching for literature, an inherent challenge with keyword searching is that it will only search for the term used. Therefore, if the synonyms of a keyword are not included in the search (eg, adolescent, youth, child, pubescent), key articles may be missed. For example, if you enter the term *walker* into a search engine, you may retrieve articles pertaining to an individual who is exercising along with articles relating the ambulatory device.

To help ensure that you do not miss any relevant research articles during the search process, you may consider utilizing MeSH. Medical Subject Headings are a controlled vocabulary managed by the NLM (http://www.nlm.nih.gov/mesh/meshhome.html). Terms included in the MeSH database are indexed in a controlled vocabulary hierarchy to help you become more efficient in your search when utilizing a MEDLINE-affiliated database. Furthermore, utilizing MeSH terms in your search process allows you to retrieve relevant articles even though the author may not have used the same term for that topic or concept. MeSH terms lower on the hierarchy are more narrow and specific than MeSH terms toward the top of the hierarchy (Figure 3-1). For example, the first branch of the hierarchy includes 16 terms, such as *anatomy* or *diseases*. If we were to select *anatomy*, we would go to the next level of the hierarchy, which includes terms such as *body region* or *musculoskeletal system*. This selection process can continue through more hierarchical levels until the specific term you are looking for is reached. Figure 3-2 provides you with an example of the MeSH hierarchical levels you may encounter when searching for *anterior cruciate ligament*.

Choosing to use keywords vs MeSH terms is dependent on your goals for the literature search. Utilizing keywords can result in searches that are more sensitive, in which you are able to retrieve a larger number of article citations, whereas a search using MeSH terms may be more specific and retrieve fewer article citations. However, even though a search from MeSH terms may retrieve fewer article citations, these citations may be of higher relevance since they will most likely relate directly to the information you are seeking. Therefore, in a situation where your clinical question focuses on an intervention that is commonly utilized in practice, you may benefit from using MeSH terms to conduct your literature search. Conversely, when you are seeking information on a topic that is new or innovative (eg, low-level laser therapy, kinesiotaping, instrumented soft tissue mobilizations), using keywords may be beneficial to help retrieve articles that would include those terms. Fortunately, some databases (eg, MEDLINE, PubMed) utilize a **mapping** feature in which the database will automatically attempt to match a keyword entered in the search box to a MeSH term that already exists.

Enhancing Your Literature Search

Along with understanding how using keywords and MeSH terms can benefit you throughout the literature search process, there are additional features available to enhance your search. These

Branch 1	**Branch 2**	**Branch 3**	**Branch 4**	**Branch 5**
1. Anatomy				
	• **Body Regions**			
		– Body Regions		
		– Anatomic Landmarks		
		– Breast		
		– **Extremities**		
			○ Amputation Stumps	
			○ **Lower Extremity**	
				■ Buttocks
				■ Foot
				■ Hip
				■ Knee
				■ Leg
				■ Thigh
			○ Upper Extremity	
		– Head		
		– Neck		
		– Organs at Risk		
		– Perineum		
		– Torso		
		– Transplant Donor Site		
		– Trigger Points		
		– Viscera		
	• Musculoskeletal System			
	• Digestive System			
	• Respiratory System			
	• Urogenital System			
	• Endocrine System			
	• Cardiovascular System			
	• Nervous System			
	• Sense Organs			
	• Tissues			
	• Cells			
	• Fluids and Secretions			
	• Animal Structures			
	• Stomatognathic System			
	• Hemic and Immune System			
	• Embryonic Structures			
	• Integumentary System			
	• Plant Structure			
	• Fungal Structure			

Figure 3-1. Medical Subject Headings hierarchy. *(continued)*

- Bacterial Structure
- Viral Structure

2. Organisms
3. Diseases
4. Chemicals and Drugs
5. Analytical, Diagnostic and Therapeutic Techniques and Equipment
6. Psychiatry and Psychology
7. Phenomena and Processes
8. Disciplines and Occupations
9. Anthropology, Education, Sociology and Social Phenomena
10. Technology, Industry, Agriculture
11. Humanities
12. Information Science
13. Named Groups
14. Health Care
15. Publication Characteristics
16. Geographicals

Figure 3-1 *(continued)*. Medical Subject Headings hierarchy. (Adapted from National Institutes of Health. MeSH tree structures – 2014. http://www.nlm.nih.gov/mesh/2014/mesh_browser/MeSHtree.html. Accessed November 12, 2014.)

features are useful to minimize the amount of literature retrieved during your search and, if used correctly, will help you locate the most relevant literature to help you answer your clinical question.

Boolean Operators

It is natural during the literature search process that you will identify more than one keyword or MeSH term that is relevant to your clinical question. Conveniently, we can use Boolean operators to help us refine our search. A **Boolean operator** is a logical word or symbol that is used to connect 2 or more words or phrases. The 3 most common Boolean operators used for literature searching are "AND," "OR," and "NOT." The operator term "AND" is used to help reduce the number of potential article citations when you want to include 2 unrelated concepts in 1 search. For example, if we search PubMed for *chronic ankle instability* and *balance program* separately, search results may yield 680 and 4836 article citations, respectively. However, if we use the operator term "AND" to combine the search terms (ie, *chronic ankle instability* AND *balance program*) together, our search results may yield 9 article citations. The operator term "AND" is a restrictive term, meaning that both keywords or controlled vocabulary terms must appear in the article for the citation to be listed in the search results.

In contrast to "AND," you also have the option to use the operator term "OR," which allows you to search for related material using one term or another. The operator term "OR" is most often

Branch 1	Branch 2	Branch 3	Branch 4	Branch 5
1. Anatomy				
	• Body Regions			
	• **Musculoskeletal System**			
		– Musculoskeletal System		
		– Cartilage		
		– Fascia		
		– **Ligaments**		
			○ Broad Ligaments	
			○ **Ligaments, Articular**	
				▪ **Anterior Cruciate Ligament**
				▪ Collateral Ligaments
				▪ Ligamentum Flavum
				▪ Longitudinal Ligaments
				▪ Patellar Ligament
				▪ Posterior Cruciate Ligament
			○ Round Ligaments	
		– Muscles		
		– Skeleton		
		– Tendons		
	• Digestive System			
	• Respiratory System			
	• Urogenital System			
	• Endocrine System			
	• Cardiovascular System			
	• Nervous System			
	• Sense Organs			
	• Tissues			
	• Cells			
	• Fluids and Secretions			
	• Animal Structures			
	• Stomatognathic System			
	• Hemic and Immune System			
	• Embryonic Structures			
	• Integumentary System			

Figure 3-2. Anterior cruciate ligament Medical Subject Headings hierarchy. *(continued)*

- Plant Structure
- Fungal Structure
- Bacterial Structure
- Viral Structure

2. Organisms
3. Diseases
4. Chemicals and Drugs
5. Analytical, Diagnostic and Therapeutic Techniques and Equipment
6. Psychiatry and Psychology
7. Phenomena and Processes
8. Disciplines and Occupations
9. Anthropology, Education, Sociology and Social Phenomena
10. Technology, Industry, Agriculture
11. Humanities
12. Information Science
13. Named Groups
14. Health Care
15. Publication Characteristics
16. Geographicals

Figure 3-2 *(continued)*. Anterior cruciate ligament Medical Subject Headings hierarchy. (Adapted from National Institutes of Health. MeSH tree structures – 2014. http://www.nlm.nih.gov/mesh/2014/mesh_browser/MeSHtree.html. Accessed November 12, 2014.)

used when searching for synonymous terms. Let us consider the following clinical question as an example:

Can lower extremity injury balance training programs effectively reduce reinjury rates of adolescent athletes with chronic ankle instability?

If you wanted to search for research articles to help you answer this clinical question, you may begin by searching for *adolescent* OR *youth* OR *children*. The operator term "OR" is also beneficial when you are exploring to see which literature is available for a topic.

Thirdly, the operator term "NOT" may also be used. This term is helpful when you know you are looking for something more specific during your search or when you would like to exclude a particular term that regularly appears during a particular search. For example, if you were conducting a literature search to retrieve information on isolated ACL injuries, you may choose to search for *ACL injury* NOT *meniscal injury*. Since a meniscal injury is often associated with ACL injuries, it is likely that a general search of *ACL injury* would include literature on meniscal injuries as well. However, if you know you only want to focus on isolated ACL injuries, using the "NOT" operator will help reduce the amount of citations retrieved. While the operator "NOT" can be helpful to narrow down your literature search, you should use this Boolean operator with caution. In our example above, using the operator "NOT" to eliminate articles that focus on meniscal injury may be beneficial to narrow our search findings; however, it may also exclude articles that discuss isolated ACL injuries in addition to other topics. Therefore, this operator term may potentially exclude articles that could be useful to help you answer your clinical question.

To further enhance your literature search, in some instances you may choose to combine any of the operator terms to narrow down your findings. However, using more than 1 operator term simultaneously may make your search too narrow, resulting in no related article citations. For example, to help us find literature for the clinical question previously discussed (*Can lower extremity injury balance training programs effectively reduce reinjury rates of adolescent athletes with chronic ankle instability?*), we may choose to conduct a search using the following combination of terms: *chronic ankle instability* AND *balance program* AND *adolescent* OR *youth* OR *children*. In PubMed, this combination of terms may result in only 2 article citations. Therefore, if you were only looking for literature specifically related to these terms, your search may be complete. However, if you want to check what other literature related to the topic is available, you may choose to broaden your search to see if any other relevant article citations are located. For example, conducting a literature search for *ankle instability* AND *prevention* AND *adolescent* will most likely broaden your search to retrieve more than 2 article citations.

Exploding and Truncation

Along with Boolean operators, you may choose to explode or truncate a keyword during the search process. During the mapping process, **exploding** a term means that the search engine will not only retrieve article citations that include the keyword entered, but will also retrieve article citations that fall into the subheadings of the controlled vocabulary term with which the keyword is matched. For example, if you enter *ankle joint* as your keyword and select the exploding feature, the database may also reveal subheadings related to *ankle joint*, such as *abnormalities*, *analysis*, *pathology*, or *radiography*. Since the clinical question focuses on chronic ankle instability, you may choose to select the *analysis* and *pathology* subheadings for your literature search.

Truncation is another search strategy that can be used to help locate related article citations. **Truncating** a term allows you to search for all terms that are associated with a word stem. To truncate a term, you will need to enter the root of the word into the search box followed by an asterisk (*). For example, if you type *nutrition** into the search box, your search will retrieve article citations that include the words *nutritional* and *nutritionist*. Truncating a term may be beneficial when multiple variations of a word are often used. However, truncating terms may also retrieve an abundance of article citations that are not relevant to your clinical question. For example, if your clinical question is related to walking, truncating *walk** may be beneficial because it allows us to retrieve citations that include the words *walking*, *walks*, *walker*, and *walked*. However, since this search can produce article citations related to *walker*, it will not distinguish between the description of a person who walks and the stabilization tool.

Filters

In addition to using Boolean operators, explodes, and truncation, most databases also allow you to select certain limiting variables, known as **filters**, to help refine your literature search. While each database may vary regarding the type of filters it offers, the most common filters you will come across are as follows:

- Article type
- Text availability
- Publication dates

- Species
- Languages
- Sex
- Subjects
- Journal categories
- Ages
- Search fields

Using filters is a quick and easy way to help reduce an overload of literature that may not be useful to answer your clinical question. At a minimum, you should use a language filter for each literature search you conduct to eliminate any citations that may only be available in another language.

Using Your Clinical Question to Conduct a Literature Search

Similar to most new skills you will learn as an athletic trainer (AT), being able to conduct an efficient literature search takes time and practice. Understanding which databases will provide you with the right type of information you are seeking and using the various search features offered in most databases will help you to enhance your literature searches, but you must remember that your efficiency in literature searching will improve with time. One of the most difficult tasks ATs who are new to literature searching struggle with is how to turn their well-developed clinical question into a literature search. More specifically, you have likely spent time formulating a solid clinical question using the PICOT format but now may be unsure how to translate that question into an effective literature search. Therefore, to be efficient at the task, it will be beneficial for you to develop a systematic approach to literature searching that works for you. Keep in mind that the systematic approach that may work best for you may not be the best approach for your peers. There are several different ways you can conduct a good literature search to retrieve information to help answer your clinical question, so it is important to identify which method works best for you.

Although each AT's literature searching strategy may differ slightly depending on the type of information they are seeking or their own personal preferences, in general, you should follow 3 universal steps as you begin the literature search process. Once you have developed an answerable clinical question, you should:

1. Determine which database(s) will be most useful
2. Execute your literature search strategy
3. Examine the evidence retrieved from your literature search

To help us discuss each of these steps, we will use our previously developed clinical question as our example:

Can lower extremity injury balance training programs effectively reduce reinjury rates of adolescent athletes with chronic ankle instability?

Determine Which Database(s) Will Be Most Useful

Before you can determine which database(s) will be most helpful in retrieving information to help you answer your clinical question, it is important to take a step back and identify whether your question is a background clinical question or a foreground clinical question. Remember, a background clinical question allows you to explore broader issues and obtain general knowledge

Table 3-2.
PICOT Format for the Clinical Question Example

ACRONYM LETTER	KEYWORD OR PHRASE
P	*Adolescent athletes with chronic ankle instability*
I	*Lower extremity balance training*
C	None
O	*Reduction in reinjury rate*
T	None
Clinical Question: *Can lower extremity injury balance training programs effectively reduce reinjury rates of adolescent athletes with chronic ankle instability?*	

concerning the issue you are investigating. These types of questions are more theoretical in nature, and their answers may be best found in standard textbooks. Foreground questions are much more specific and assist with identifying pieces of the clinical problem that will lead you to a clinical decision particular to the patient. Typically, when you are planning to conduct a thorough literature search, it is likely you are aiming to answer a foreground question, such as our example clinical question. Therefore, locating information to help you answer a foreground question will likely be available through various databases.

As we discussed previously, each database is dependent on the topic of information for which you are searching and may provide different types of evidence. As you begin to seek information to help you answer your clinical question, it is important to identify which databases will be most helpful. Although there are a variety of databases available, we have already provided you with a list of 5 databases that includes research literature related to patient care. Therefore, any one of these databases should be a good stepping stone to help you conduct your literature search. If you have access, however, it is recommended to begin your literature search by using the CDSR. Remember, systematic reviews, which are considered the highest level of evidence, are narratives of the critical evaluation of a research question through an exhaustive search of the available evidence, followed by the appraisal, selection, and synthesis of many sources for a clinical question that is relevant. Since this database only contains systematic reviews and is considered to be the gold standard of databases, it is a great place to start. But regardless of the database you choose to begin your literature search, you should always consider searching more than one database. As we previously discussed, databases may not contain the same available research literature or may be updated at different intervals of time. Therefore, conducting your literature search in more than one database will help ensure you are thoroughly searching for the most relevant and available information to answer your clinical question.

Execute Your Literature Search Strategy

Once you have decided on a database to begin your search, it is now time to determine which keywords or phrases you will use to conduct the literature search. Choosing the best terms will be easier if you have developed your clinical question using the PICOT format. More specifically, the phrases used to develop the PICOT clinical question will be a great starting point to begin the search (Table 3-2). There are a variety of different ways you can combine keywords or phrases as you begin your literature search. There is no one best way, so it is useful to develop a systematic approach that works for you. One option is to enter all of the keywords or phrases you identified in your PICOT table at the same time. For example, using the keywords and phrases from the PICOT example in Table 3-2, you could combine all the keywords and phrases and enter the following into the database search box: *adolescent athletes with chronic ankle instability lower extremity balance training reduction in reinjury rate* (Figure 3-3).

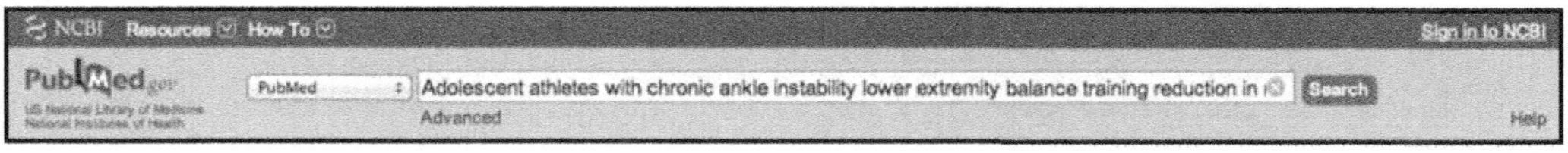

Figure 3-3. PubMed screenshot.

Entering all the terms together may produce a very small number of citations that are extremely closely related to your clinical question. If you are lucky to have 1 or 2 citations retrieved by simultaneously entering all the terms, it is likely that this very specific search will have excluded additional citations that may have been useful to help you answer your clinical question. However, it is more likely that entering all the terms at once will result in a message indicating, "No items were found." Therefore, it is often more feasible to enter 1 to 2 keywords or phrases at a time and then combine your individual searches together.

Using the PubMed database, let us walk through how we can conduct individual searches for our keywords and then combine the searches together. To begin, we will start broadly and enter only our first phrase, *adolescent athlete,* into the search box (Figure 3-4).

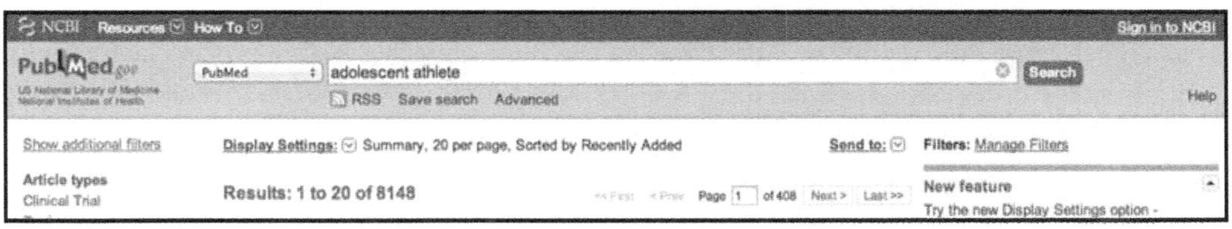

Figure 3-4. PubMed screenshot.

This broad search returned more than 8000 citations that may be of relevance. Moving on, we will now conduct a new search and enter our second phrase, *chronic ankle instability,* into the search box (Figure 3-5).

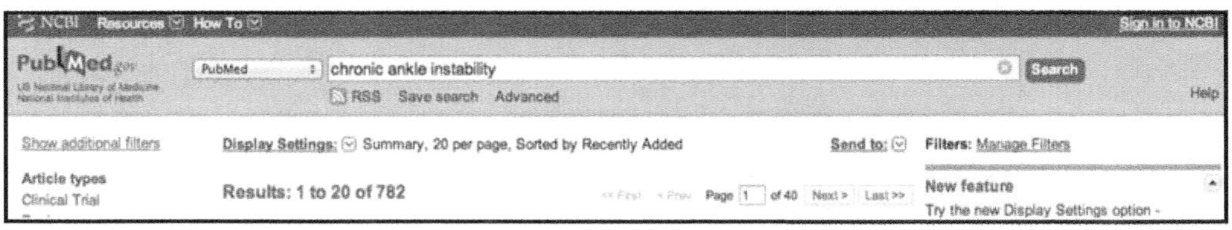

Figure 3-5. PubMed screenshot.

This search was narrower than our *adolescent athlete* search but still retrieved more than 700 articles that may be useful. It is not feasible to go through all 8000 *adolescent athlete* citations and 700 *chronic ankle instability* citations to determine which ones are relevant. Fortunately, we have the ability to combine these 2 searches together to help reduce the number of possible citations. Under the *Advanced* feature, we can combine our 2 searches using the Boolean operator term "AND" so that it reads *adolescent athlete* AND *chronic ankle instability* (Figure 3-6).

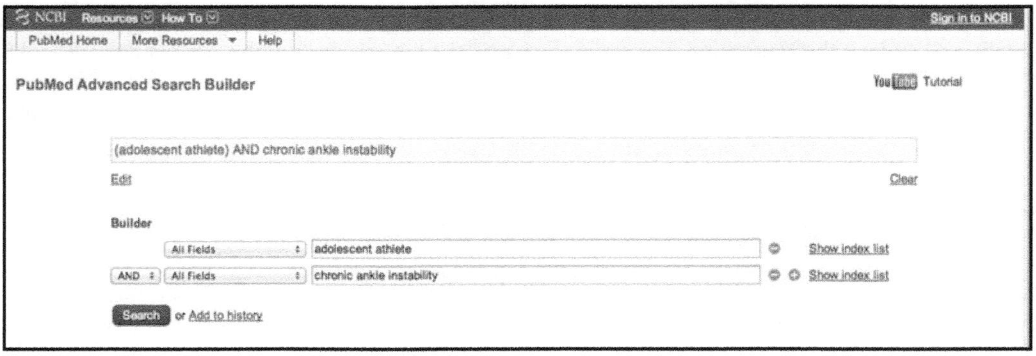

Figure 3-6. PubMed screenshot.

By combining the 2 searches, we now have 23 potential citations that may be useful (Figure 3-7).

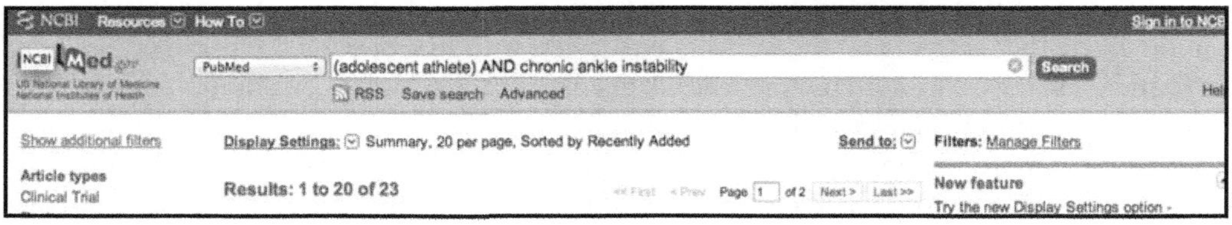

Figure 3-7. PubMed screenshot.

As you can see, combining individual searches can help reduce the potential number of citations to a much more manageable number. You can then continue your search process by individually searching the other phrases from your PICO table and combine searches as needed to help you locate the best available research literature to help you answer your clinical question.

As you conduct your literature search using individual searches and the combined search feature, keep in mind that literature searching can often be a trial and error process. More specifically, it is useful to conduct several individual searches for your keywords and phrases and then mix and match the combined searches to see what type of citations are retrieved. From our example, we noted that 23 citations were retrieved when we combined the 2 individuals searches *adolescent athlete* AND *chronic ankle instability*. However, if we were to search *adolescent athlete with chronic ankle instability* as 1 search, we retrieve 22 citations instead of 23 (Figure 3-8).

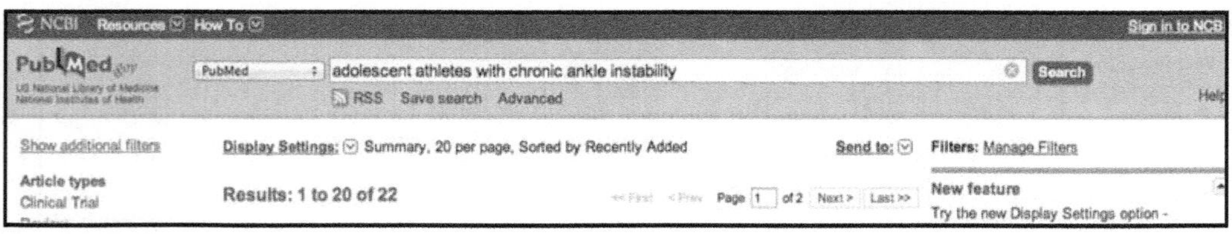

Figure 3-8. PubMed screenshot.

While the difference in this example is minute, it is important to note that different combinations of searches may yield different results. Therefore, it is important to remember to use the additional search features that will help you enhance your literature search (eg, truncation, exploding, filters) and reduce the number of citations retrieved. Additionally, it is essential to develop a systematic literature searching approach that works best for you (eg, conducting individual searches and then combining vs combining multiple keywords or phrases in 1 search) so that you do not get lost in the abundance of literature available. It is often helpful to keep track of the search terms you use, single or combined searches you have conducted, and databases you have searched. As we will discuss in the Managing Your Literature Search section, some databases automatically record your recent activity and searches, while other databases may require that you take notes on which terms you have used and searches you have conducted.

Examine the Evidence Retrieved From Your Literature Search

Once you have conducted your literature search in one or several databases, the next step will be to review the information you retrieved and examine whether it will be useful to help you answer your clinical question. To do so, you must critically assess the information and appraise whether the information will be useful to your particular clinical question or patient case. In our combined search example of *adolescent athlete* AND *chronic ankle instability*, we were able to retrieve a manageable number of citations. We must now take it one step further and determine if these citations are useful and/or relevant to our topic of interest. It is not uncommon for citations to be retrieved that may contain the keywords or phrases you have entered in the search box but do not relate to the clinical question you are seeking to answer. The process of critical appraisal and the various concepts involved will be thoroughly discussed in the upcoming chapters. However, before you proceed into the critical appraisal phase of EBP, we must first discuss the importance of managing your literature search once it has been conducted.

Managing Your Literature Search

Once you have begun your literature search, it will be important to remain organized. Filtering through hundreds of research citations and articles can be daunting and time consuming. Along with using the available features to help refine your literature search, it is also important to know how to manage your searches. Managing your literature search will help ensure you are not conducting redundant searches as you seek information to help you answer your clinical question. Fortunately, almost every database you will access offers options to help you manage your literature searches. In fact, several databases allow you to create a free account so that you can save previous searches, bookmark specific citations of interest, and create notifications and alerts. Thus, while each database may differ slightly in the options available for managing literature searches, for the purposes of this chapter, we will only discuss the management features available on PubMed since it is free to the public and one of the most commonly utilized databases.

Within the PubMed database, you are able to create a free literature management account, known as My NCBI. Registering for a My NCBI account is easy, and it is accessible by clicking the "Sign in to NCBI" link on the top right corner of the PubMed website (http://www.ncbi.nlm.nih.gov/pubmed). This account includes several features that allow you to customize your literature searches to be as specific or general as you would like. We will discuss 2 of the most commonly utilized features available in a My NCBI account: saving literature searches and setting up automatic email alerts.

Saving Literature Searches

The ability to save your literature searches is a great feature that can reduce frustration and redundancy during the searching process. Saving your recent activity, an automatic feature in My NCBI, allows you to repeat a search if needed, as well as remember which search terms were used and which citations were excluded or included in a previous search. For example, let us say you are interested in searching the literature for information to help you develop a rehabilitation protocol for adolescent athletes following ACL reconstruction surgery. During your initial search, you retrieve several articles you believe will be useful to you; however, you have to step away from this task and are unable to return to the search process for a few days. If the save literature searches feature were not available, you would have to start from scratch to relocate the original articles you found, as well as continue to search for new information you may not have previously accessed during your initial search. This process would require more of your time, as your previous search efforts may have been wasted. Fortunately, using the save literature search feature eliminates the possibility of having to repeat previous searches. Therefore, when you return to your search to locate information to develop a post-ACL reconstruction rehabilitation protocol, you can easily review your initial search that was conducted a few days ago and then continue to search for new information you may not have accessed yet.

Setting Up Automatic Alerts

Another great feature available in My NCBI, as well as most other databases, is the ability to set up automatic email alerts. More specifically, this feature allows you to store keywords that will automatically be checked against the PubMed database on a regular basis. Once the database retrieves a new article that matches your keyword(s), you will receive an email alert notifying you that a new citation has been located. For example, let us say you have conducted a thorough literature search and retrieved several articles relating to rehabilitation protocols for adolescent athletes following ACL reconstruction surgery. However, you are still interested in this topic and would like to know when new information becomes available. Using the automatic alerts feature in My NCBI, you decide to save *ACL reconstruction rehabilitation* and *knee rehabilitation* as keywords in your account. Now, any time a new citation becomes available on PubMed, you will automatically receive an email alert notifying you. Setting up automatic citation alerts is a fantastic way to stay current with available citations for a topic of interest without having to routinely search the database yourself. However, it is important to note that this automatic feature will alert you any time your saved keyword appears in a citation. Therefore, if you save a keyword (eg, *ACL reconstruction*) that may be used in a variety of contexts (eg, surgical technique, rehabilitation), you will likely need to filter through the notifications to eliminate any citations that are not of interest to you. Additionally, new articles may become available that you are interested in but do not include your saved keywords. To combat this issue, it is still helpful to conduct a new search with different keywords every once in a while to double-check if new citations have become available about which you were not notified.

Using Citation Management Software

In addition to managing your literature searches, it is also important to stay organized once you have retrieved useful articles to help you answer your particular clinical question. Saving relevant evidence in an organized manner allows you to quickly access it when you it need later. Fortunately, there are several citation management software programs, also referred to as bibliographic management software, available to help you store and organize articles and citations. Some of the more common citation management software you may come across are EndNote (Thomson Reuters), RefWorks (RefWorks), Mendeley (Mendeley Ltd), and Zotero (Roy Rosenzweig Center for History and New Media). While they all differ slightly in available features, these programs generally allow you to save and sort citations and/or full-text articles. Additionally, some of the software programs (eg, EndNote) also allow you search databases and automatically store citations directly in the software program. Similar to the availability of databases, some of the citation management software programs require you to purchase an individual license (eg, EndNote, RefWorks), while others offer free access (eg, Mendeley, Zotero).

While the use of citation management software can be very beneficial to help keep your evidence organized, it is not necessary to use this software. However, regardless of how you choose to organize articles you have retrieved, you should always save them similarly so it is easier to locate them when you need the information. With the abundant amount of research literature that is available via the Internet, it is necessary to develop your own systematic approach to saving and organizing your articles so that you will not have to repeat the process of literature searching if you need to access a particular article in the future.

Summary

While the majority of search strategies discussed in this chapter can be used across all databases, each individual database may offer different features. Additionally, as technology continues to advance, databases will likely enhance searching capabilities and available features. Most databases include free tutorials that discuss the various features included; it is recommended that you view that tutorial before you begin to incorporate that database in your literature search routine. Furthermore, each database typically has a help feature, which provides answers to frequently asked questions about that database. As previously discussed, literature searching is necessary to help you retrieve resources to answer your clinical question, but it is often the most time consuming part of the EBP process. Fortunately, the more you practice searching for literature, the better you will become at quickly retrieving relevant information.

Key Points

- Literature searching is necessary to help you retrieve resources to answer your clinical question, but it is often the most time consuming part of the EBP process.
- Before you can determine which database(s) will be most helpful in retrieving information to help you answer your clinical question, it is important to take a step back and identify whether your question is a background clinical question or a foreground clinical question.
- Once you have conducted your literature search in one or several databases, the next step will be to review the information you retrieved and examine whether it will be useful to help you answer your clinical question.
- Saving your recent activity, an automatic feature in My NCBI, allows you to repeat a search if needed as well as remember which search terms were used and which citations were excluded or included in a previous search.
- Setting up automatic alerts allows you to store keywords that will automatically be checked against the PubMed database on a regular basis. Once the database retrieves a new article that matches your keyword(s), you will receive an email alert notifying you that a new citation has been located.

Bibliography

Bigby M. Evidence-based medicine in a nutshell. A guide to finding and using the best evidence in caring for patients. *Arch Dermatol.* 1998;134(12):1609-1618.

Cochrane Database of Systematic Reviews. http://www.cochrane.org. Accessed November 15, 2014.

Cumulative Index to Nursing and Allied Health Literature. http://www.ebscohost.com/cinahl. Accessed November 15, 2014.

Fineout-Overholt E, Melynk BM, Shultz A. Transforming health care from the inside out: advancing evidence-based practice in the 21st century. *J Prof Nurs.* 2005;21(6):335-344.

Google Scholar. http://scholar.google.com/. Accessed November 15, 2014.

Giustini D, Barsky E. A look at Google Scholar, PubMed, and Scirus: comparisons and recommendations. *JCHLA/JABSC.* 2005;26:85-89.

Lawrence JC. Techniques for searching the CINAHL database using the EBSCO interface. *AORN J.* 2007;85(4):779-791.

Physiotherapy Evidence Database (PEDro). www.pedro.org.au. Accessed November 15, 2014.

PubMed. http://www.ncbi.nlm.nih.gov/pubmed. Accessed November 15, 2014.

Schlonsky, A., & Gibbs, L. Will the real evidence-based practice please stand up? Teaching the process of evidence-based practice to the helping professions. *Brief Treatment and Crisis Intervention*. 2004;4(2):137-153.

Shariff SZ, Bejaimal SA, Sontrop JM, et al. Retrieving clinical evidence: a comparison of PubMed and Google Scholar for quick clinical searches. *J Med Internet Res*. 2013;15(8):e164.

4

Foundations of Research and Statistics

Before you can begin to critically appraise the research literature to help you during the clinical decision-making process, it is essential that you understand certain basic terms and concepts commonly encountered in journal publications. While you may not need to fully understand these topics, you will not be able to accurately appraise the literature without an appreciation of their purpose and meaning. Therefore, as a clinician, it is your responsibility to comprehend the foundations and terminology of research and statistics that are used as a part of every research study.

Data Measurement Scales

Fundamentally, you must become familiar with the different types of data routinely collected during a research study. Athletic trainers (ATs) collect data through several different mechanisms during routine clinical practice. Whether the data reflect demographic characteristics of the patient or are obtained through patient-oriented outcome instruments, clinician-oriented measures, clinician observations, or a thorough history during an evaluation, the information is valuable and necessary to help you make informed clinical decisions with your patient. Therefore, it is important to understand what types of data are being collected so that they can be analyzed (or were analyzed by the manuscript's authors) appropriately.

Data are classified as *nominal*, *ordinal*, *interval*, or *ratio*. Each type of scale provides different information and is defined by how it is collected. The **nominal scale** is the simplest level of measurement. Nominal data are classified into predetermined categories, such as sex, leg dominance, blood type, or highest educational degree. Nominal data are mutually exclusive and exhaustive. **Mutually exclusive** means that a subject (or characteristic) fits into only one category. If you consider the example of blood type, it is impossible for a person to be type O- and type A+. To be **exhaustive**, nominal categories must include all values potentially encountered. If you were assessing the highest educational degree, you would want to include all possibilities instead of just high school and college. There are multiple levels of college degrees, and the researcher must determine

Van Lunen BL, Hankemeier DA, & Welch CE.
Evidence-Guided Practice: A Framework for Clinical Decision Making in Athletic Training (pp 41-57).

how finely he or she wants to discriminate among the possible categories (eg, associate, bachelors, masters, doctoral, or postsecondary), but all possible responses must fit into a category (and only one category). For purposes of analysis, nominal data are assigned a number that corresponds to each category (eg, male = 1, female = 2). Assigning numbers to the variables allows you to analyze the data but does not change the qualitative meaning of the value.

The **ordinal scale** is used for data that have a rank order or hierarchy of meaning. In the ordinal scale, data are often assigned a numeric value, but unlike nominal data, this value signifies that there is an order to the data. Ordinal data are commonly collected using Likert scales. Likert scales ask individuals to rate their experience or perceptions based on a set scale (eg, strongly agree, agree, neutral, disagree, strongly disagree). Each response in the scale is assigned a number (eg, 5 = strongly agree to 1 = strongly disagree). These numbers typically reflect a degree of change in the magnitude of the **construct** being measured: a score of 1 is less than a score of 5, and a score of 3 is somewhere in between. However, it is important to understand that in an ordinal scale, the distance between adjoining numbers is not necessarily equal. The interval between a 5 (strongly agree) and a 4 (agree) may be very small for one person, while another individual subjectively thinks that there is a much larger difference between the two. Because of this variability in interpretation, ordinal data points are labels and not necessarily a representation of quantity. The absence of equal interval scaling in ordinal data makes mathematical manipulation of these numbers (eg, addition, division, calculating an average) problematic.

A scale that incorporates an ordinal characteristic and equal distance between adjoining data points is the **interval scale**. However, in the interval scale, there is no true zero point because zero is an arbitrary number on the scale. For example, if you are assessing the outdoor temperature using the Fahrenheit scale, a temperature of 0°F does not indicate that there is no temperature, but instead, a point on a scale of numbers. The range in temperature between 15°F and 30°F is the same as the temperature range between 60°F and 75°F; however, 60° is not "twice as cold" as 30°F because you have no true anchor value.

A **ratio scale** is the highest level of measurement and is very similar to an interval scale with one key distinction. A ratio scale includes an absolute zero point (eg, temperature expressed on a Kelvin scale). A zero on the ratio scale indicates that there is a total absence of what is being measured. Height is an example of ratio data because if you had 0 cm of height, there would be an absence of height. Negative values in the ratio scale are not possible because they would go beyond the absolute zero point. With ratio data, you are able to accurately quantify and express the quantity that is actually being measured. For example, if someone weighs 60 lb, you can safely assume that someone who weighs a third of that would weigh 20 lb. Ratio data can also be converted between units of measurements (eg, 1 kg = 2.20 lb) because statistical and mathematical functions are permissible with ratio data.

As you continue through the remainder of this chapter, it is crucial for you to be familiar with the differences between nominal, ordinal, interval, and ratio data. Table 4-1 provides some common examples to help you remember the distinguishing features of each type of data. Understanding the differences between the types of data will be particularly important when we discuss descriptive and inferential statistics because the type of statistical test you choose to use depends on the type of data you are analyzing. However, before we discuss descriptive and inferential statistics, it is important to highlight some components that are commonly included in a research study.

Components of a Research Study

Although each research study can differ greatly in how the methodology is designed and conducted, there are several components that are staples. To accurately appraise a research study, it is essential to be comfortable with these concepts so that you can easily identify them. As you may

Table 4-1.
Types of Data

DATA TYPE	EXAMPLES OF DATA
Nominal	Sex, race, blood type, dominant limb
Ordinal	Numeric pain rating scale (no pain to extreme pain), Likert scales (strongly agree to strongly disagree)
Interval	Temperature (Fahrenheit scale), range of motion
Ratio	Height, weight, strength output, age, distance

	Pain (Dependent Variable)	
Treatment (Independent Variable)	*Treatment A*	X
	Treatment B	X

Figure 4-1. Basic study design layout.

know, a research study is conducted to determine the answer to a specific question. Along with the research question, a researcher may identify specific variables that will be manipulated (**independent variables**) and measured (**dependent variables**), as well as hypotheses indicating what he or she anticipates the data will reveal. These concepts are the foundation of any research study and serve as the building blocks upon which a researcher should design the investigation.

Independent and Dependent Variables

An independent variable is a variable that is manipulated or influenced by the researcher and may include various levels, which are determined by the research question. In its most basic form, the aim of a research study may be to compare the effectiveness of an experimental treatment (eg, treatment A) against a control treatment (eg, treatment B) relative to a specific outcome (eg, pain) (Figure 4-1).

In this simple design, the independent variable would be "treatment" with 2 levels (A and B). In a more complicated study, the investigator could compare 5 different types of cryotherapy to reduce pain in males vs females. The independent variables for this design would be "types of cryotherapy," with 5 levels, and "sex," with 2 levels (Figure 4-2). Let us look at a third research study that includes 3 independent variables (Figure 4-3). This study aims to compare the effectiveness of 3 types of stretching interventions to increase hamstring flexibility in males vs females over time. To determine which stretching technique is most effective, we will need to measure the participants' hamstring flexibility prior to the intervention. Additionally, since we want to know if stretching influences hamstring flexibility immediately and over the long term, we will measure the participants' hamstring flexibility immediately following the intervention, as well as 1 and 2 weeks postintervention. Based on this study design, you can see that it includes 3 independent variables: type of stretching intervention with 3 levels, sex with 2 levels, and time with 4 levels. Depending on the research question, a study may include one independent variable or several (eg, time and sex). Furthermore, the more independent variables you attempt to incorporate in a study, the more complex the study layout becomes.

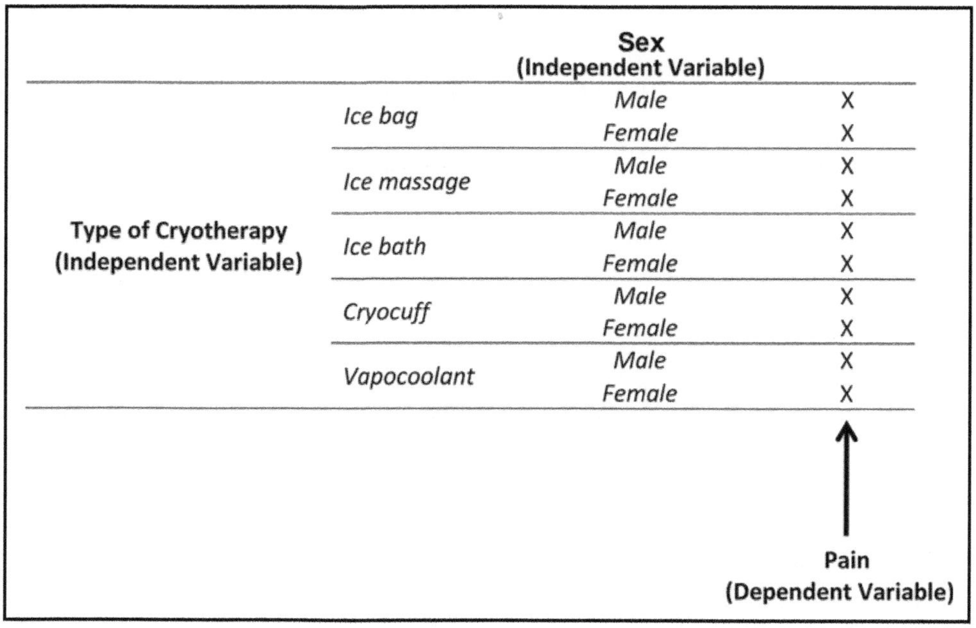

Figure 4-2. Study #1 research design layout.

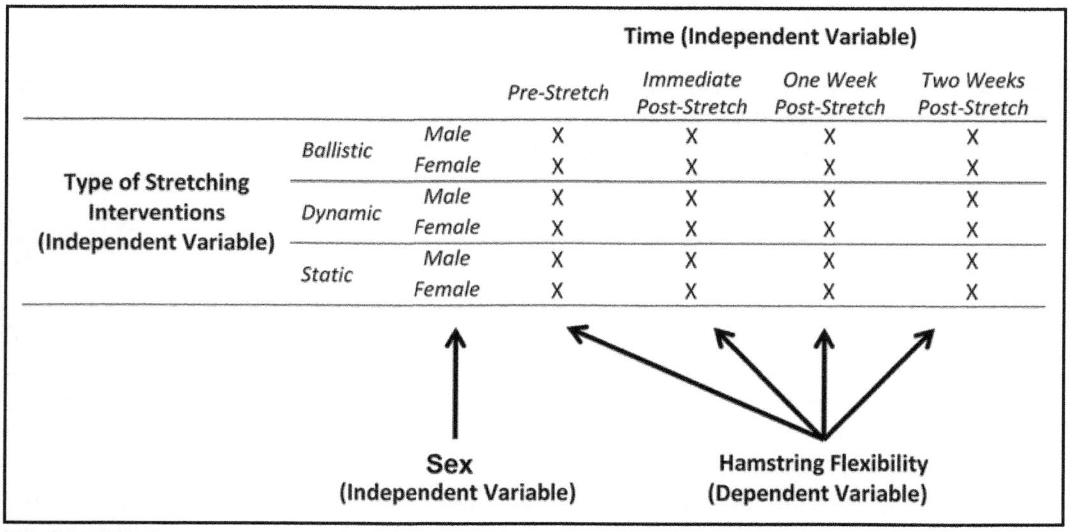

Figure 4-3. Study #2 research design layout.

A dependent variable, also referred to as an outcome variable, is a variable that will be measured by the investigator. More specifically, the dependent variable is the variable, or outcome, that is hypothesized to be affected by the independent variable and, therefore, the variable that is measured. More simply, the dependent variable is the measure that determines if a difference or relationship between the independent and dependent variables exists. Examples of dependent variables include the following:

- Scores on a knowledge assessment
- Degrees of range of motion
- Level of function
- Patient-oriented outcome scores

- Balance Error Scoring System score
- Peak torque strength measurement

If we take a look at the study layouts in Figures 4-2 and 4-3, we can now highlight the dependent variables for the study. In Study #1, the independent variables are type of cryotherapy and sex. Because the study aims to determine if the cryotherapy treatments reduce pain, our dependent variable will be the participants' responses to a numeric pain rating scale (indicated by X in the figure). Because we also want to determine if sex affects the participants' pain rating for the type of cryotherapy, we can optimize the design by having approximately the same number of males and females for each type of cryotherapy. In Study #2, the independent variables are type of stretching intervention, sex, and time. For this study, the aim is to determine if the different stretching interventions increase hamstring flexibility differentially for males and females over time. Therefore, the dependent variable will be hamstring flexibility, as measured by the 90/90 active knee extension test.

Hypotheses

After a researcher has identified the research question, he or she will likely develop hypotheses. A **hypothesis** is a proposed explanation of if a phenomenon may occur. In the simplest scenario, there are 2 types of hypotheses about which we are concerned: a null hypothesis and a research hypothesis. A **null hypothesis** is a statement made by the researcher indicating there is no difference or relationship between the variables being investigated. More simply, the null hypothesis indicates that no change will occur during the study. Using our study examples, we could create the following null hypotheses:

- Study #1: There will be no difference in pain scores between males and females regardless of the type of cryotherapy administered.
- Study #2: There will be no difference in hamstring flexibility between males and females at any time point regardless of the type of stretching intervention implemented.

It is important to identify the null hypothesis for each research question because this hypothesis will be what the investigator is trying to test. In Study #1, the investigator will test whether pain scores will differ between males and females following a cryotherapy treatment. If the investigator determines that there *is a difference* in scores between males and females, he or she would *reject* the null hypothesis. By rejecting the null hypothesis, the investigator is claiming that the null hypothesis (ie, no difference between groups) is false since there is a difference between groups. However, if the investigator determines that there *is no difference* in scores between males and females, he or she would *accept* the null hypothesis. An investigator accepts the null hypothesis when it is true, which indicates that there is no difference between groups.

Unlike a null hypothesis, a **research hypothesis** is a statement made by the investigator indicating his or her expectations about the differences or relationships among the variables being investigated. Research hypotheses should be directional (eg, an increase, a decrease), meaning the researcher has formulated an educated guess as to what they think they will find. In our study examples, you may choose to hypothesize the following:

- Study #1: Males will report significantly lower pain scores than females following a Cryo/Cuff intervention.
- Study #1: Females who received a vapocoolant will report significantly higher pain scores than females who received an ice massage.
- Study #2: Prior to a dynamic stretching intervention, there will be no significant differences between males and females regarding hamstring flexibility.
- Study #2: Females will have significantly greater hamstring flexibility immediately following a dynamic stretching intervention compared with a static stretching intervention.

- Study #2: There will be a significant positive relationship between time and hamstring flexibility for participants who received the dynamic stretching intervention.

As you may have noticed, the third research hypothesis listed (ie, *prior to a dynamic stretching intervention, there will be no significant differences between males and females regarding hamstring flexibility*) is similar to the null hypothesis that was previously identified. Sometimes, the null hypothesis and research hypothesis are the same because, while the null hypothesis *always* indicates there will be no difference between groups, the investigators may also believe that there will be no difference in the outcomes. Thus, since the independent and dependent variables and the types of hypotheses are used to guide a research study, it is important to have a solid grasp on each component. Understanding the components of a research study is not only important for ATs planning to conduct a research study, but it also allows you, as a clinician, to understand the research literature you appraise to help you make informed clinical decisions.

Descriptive and Inferential Statistics

In addition to setting up a strong research design, the components of a research study are also crucial to help ATs identify which type of statistics are appropriate to analyze the data once they have been collected. Although there are a variety of statistical procedures, we typically separate them into 2 major categories: descriptive and inferential.

Descriptive statistics, also referred to as summary statistics, provide you with a summary of the main characteristics about the data collected during a study. As you read through a research article, the authors will always include descriptive statistics to provide basic information about the sample group and the overall findings from the study. For example, it is not uncommon for a research article to include a table that provides you with demographic information about the participants who were included in the study. This information allows you to understand the characteristics of the sample group (eg, age, sex, weight, height) and may help you to interpret the findings from the study in a clinically relevant manner. Additionally, descriptive statistics are also commonly used to show if groups are equal prior to the start of data collection. One important consideration to remember is that descriptive statistics cannot be used to draw conclusions about the hypothesis; this type of information can only provide what the label suggests: a description of the data. The most commonly reported descriptive statistics include means, standard deviations (SDs), frequencies, and confidence intervals (Table 4-2).

Inferential statistics are used to draw conclusions about the hypotheses posed. More specifically, inferential statistics often involve the use of statistical tests to analyze the data and deduce, or infer, how the findings could potentially represent what may occur in a given patient population. For example, by using an appropriately selected statistical test, an AT may estimate the efficacy of a preseason lower extremity balance protocol on the rate of future lower extremity injuries in the adolescent athletic population using a sample of 50 male and female adolescent soccer athletes. Inferential statistics may be used to assess the probability that an observed difference between 2 groups is due to an intervention or simply a function of chance. If a clinician is interested in assessing whether sex impacts the effectiveness of the preseason lower extremity balance program, he or she may include a variable in the analysis indicating the sex of the participant and conduct statistical analyses to determine if such differences existed.

Statistical Tests and Procedures

Unless you are planning to conduct a research study, it is not essential to comprehend the details about how each statistical test is conducted. However, to be able to critically appraise all

Table 4-2.
Commonly Reported Descriptive Statistics

DESCRIPTIVE STATISTIC	DEFINITION	EXAMPLE[a]
Median	The "middle" value in a distribution of values; also defined as the midpoint in which 50% of the values fall on either side of the value	The midpoint test score was 53.0.
Mode	The value that most commonly occurs in a group of values	The most commonly occurring score was 57.
Mean (M)	The average of a group of values, calculated by summing the values and then dividing by the number of values included	The average test score was 51.94.
Standard deviation (SD)	A value that reflects the variability of observations around the M	The SD for this test was 7.63.
Range	The difference between the largest and smallest values in a group of values	The range of test scores was 29.50 to 60.
Frequency (%)	A count (eg, percentage) of the number of times each value occurs	Of the students, 50% scored greater than 53 points on the examination.
Confidence interval (CI)[b]	A range of values (minimum to maximum) that estimates where the population value is likely to fall	We are 95% confident that the population average test score will fall between 50.33 and 55.67.

[a]This example is based on a test with a maximum of 60 possible points.
[b]Confidence intervals may also be considered as inferential statistics.

aspects of the research literature, it is important to understand the logic underlying the statistical tests most commonly presented in the literature. Generally, to be able to draw conclusions from data, it is necessary to use inferential statistical tests. Although the number of statistical tests that can be used to analyze data is large, these tests are typically divided into 2 groups: parametric tests and nonparametric tests.

Parametric statistical tests are utilized to draw conclusions about particular parameters (ie, variables) in the population from which the sample was selected via mathematical calculations and require that 3 general assumptions be met:

1. **Quantitative data**: To conduct a parametric test, the data must be numeric (ie, they must be mathematically quantitative). Of the 4 types of data discussed previously, only interval and ratio data fit this criterion. Interval and ratio data consist of measurable data points, and only the presence of an absolute zero point for ratio data distinguishes the 2 types.

Figure 4-4. Normal distribution of data.

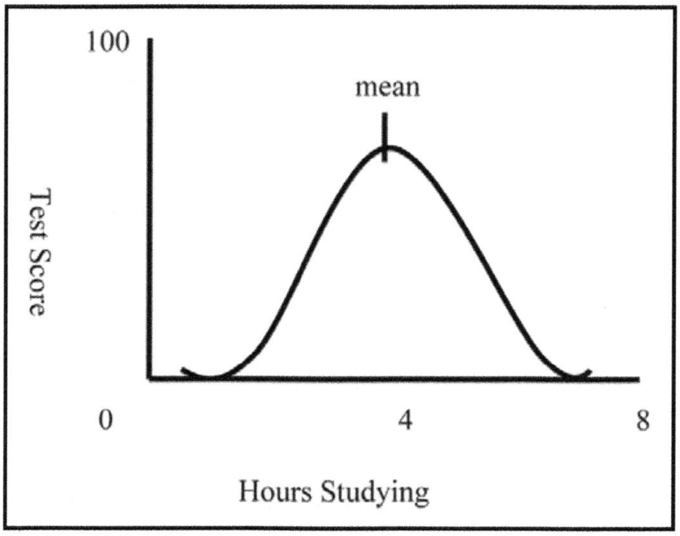

2. **Normal distribution**: A normal distribution involves data that are continuous and primarily cluster around a central value (the mean or arithmetic average). Normally distributed data may be displayed in a bell curve, where the mean value is the highest point of the curve and the remaining data fall on either side of that point. For example, let us consider the relationship between the number of hours a student spends studying and scores achieved on a test (Figure 4-4). As you can see from the figure, on average, students achieved the highest test scores when they studied for approximately 4 hours. From this distribution, you may also note that studying for more than 4 hours seems to have a negative effect on students' test scores. Thus, to achieve the bell curve, approximately 50% of the data should be greater than the mean while 50% of the data are less than the mean. Additionally, in a perfect normal distribution, the mean equals the median (ie, the midpoint value), which equals the mode (ie, the most frequently reported value).
3. **Homogeneity of variance**: Also referred to as the equality of variance, homogeneity of variance occurs when there is no discrepancy in the average dispersion of values for the dependent variable among the groups.

For example, an AT wants to determine the effects of a joint mobilization technique for increased dorsiflexion range of motion in adolescent females with chronic ankle instability and an identified limitation in dorsiflexion range of motion. To assess the clinical significance of this treatment technique, the AT finds 50 adolescent females who have chronic ankle instability. The participants are randomly divided into 2 groups: 25 adolescent females in the experimental group who will receive the treatment and 25 adolescent females in the control group who will not receive the treatment. If these 2 groups are similar at the inception of the study with regard to any variables that might, ultimately, impact the outcome and the only way they are treated differently during the study is the level of intervention to which they were assigned, the AT is able to estimate the true effects of the joint mobilization technique.

If the data are not normally distributed, they may be skewed. **Skewness** is a measure of the amount of asymmetry of a distribution and often occurs when there are **outliers** (data points that are numerically distant from the rest of the data). The distribution is considered to have a *negative skew* if the left side (also referred to as a tail) of the distribution curve is longer, indicating that outliers exist on the left side of the distribution. However, the distribution is considered to have a *positive skew* if the right tail of the distribution curve is longer (ie, outliers are on the right side of the distribution). Let us look at our hours of studying example used to discuss normal

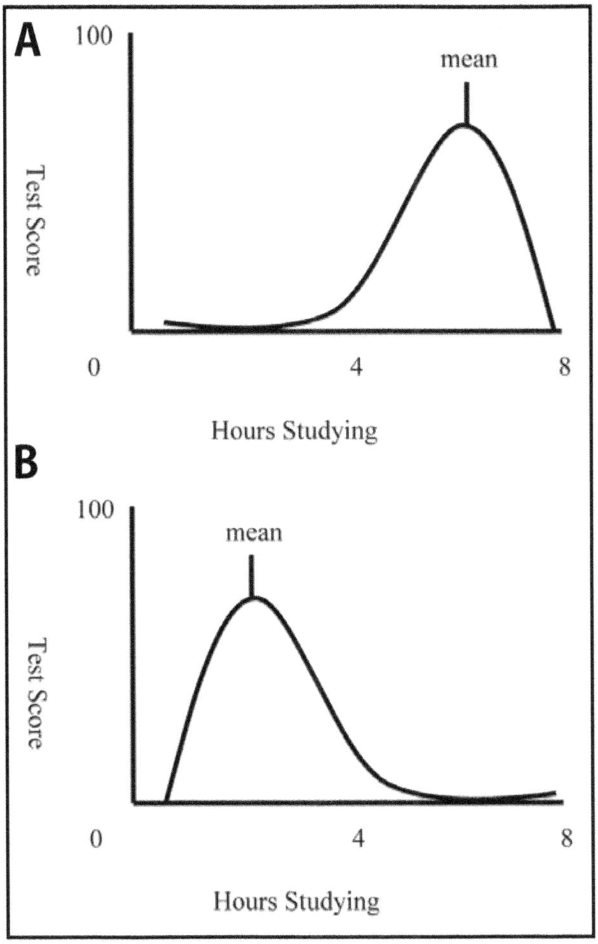

Figure 4-5. (A) Negative skewness of the data. (B) Positive skewness of the data.

distribution. In this example, we identified that, on average, students received the highest scores when they studied for approximately 4 hours. If there were a few individuals who received high scores while studying for 6 hours, their data points would shift the distribution of the mean to the right, creating a longer tail on the left side of the distribution curve. In this case, the data would create a negative skew (Figure 4-5A). However, if there were a few individuals who received high scores while only studying for 2 hours, their data points would shift the mean of the distribution toward the left, creating a longer tail on the right side. In this case, the distribution would have a positive skew (Figure 4-5B).

If even 1 of the 3 assumptions for parametric tests is not met, we should use a **nonparametric test** to conduct our statistical analyses. Nonparametric tests do not require data to have a normal distribution, nor is the variance of the outcome variable required to be equal (homogeneous) across groups. Nonparametric tests are often utilized when the research study has a small sample size or when the data being analyzed are collected on a nominal or ordinal scale. For example, if you were interested in determining whether males or females had lower pain scores following a cryotherapy treatment, as we discussed in Study #1 (see Figure 4-2), you may likely choose to collect data using the numeric pain rating scale. The numeric pain rating scale, which ranges from 0 = no pain to 10 = extreme pain, provides you with ordinal data; therefore, you must use a nonparametric statistical test to assess whether differences between males and females exist.

As you become more familiar with critically appraising the research literature, you will see many types of statistical tests used to analyze data. While it is not necessary to understand the

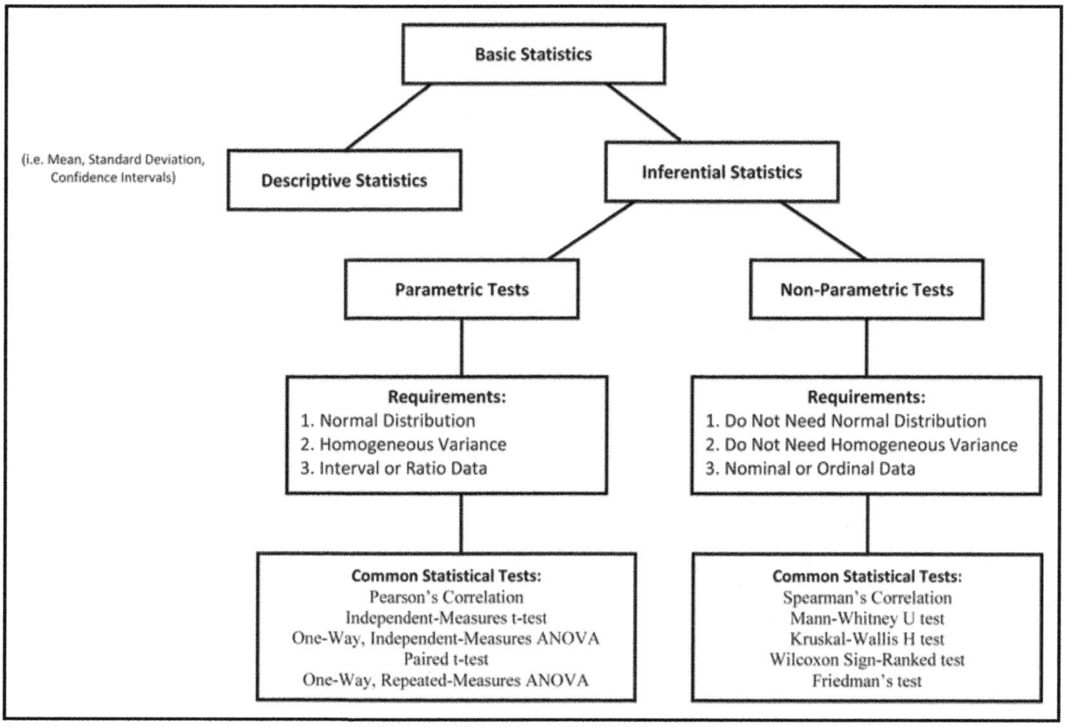

Figure 4-6. Breakdown of statistics. Abbreviation: ANOVA, analysis of variance.

specifics of these statistical tests unless you are planning to conduct a research study, it is helpful to be familiar with whether these tests are categorized as parametric or nonparametric. Depending on the research question, parametric and nonparametric tests can be used to assess differences between variables or relationships between variables. Figure 4-6 provides you with a breakdown of the different types of statistical tests used for parametric and nonparametric data.

Considerations for Interpreting Research Findings

Regardless of the type of statistical test that is chosen to analyze the data, it is necessary to attempt to identify whether any observed differences are real or may be due to chance. Statisticians have calculated the *P* value to estimate the probability that outcomes are due to chance. The *P* is an abbreviation for probability, and a *P* value is properly interpreted, in a test of differences, as the probability that a difference as large as that found is simply due to chance and is not real. Researchers use statistical tests to assess the probability that observed differences in the research study were not caused by chance. Going back to our cryotherapy example in Study #1, you use a nonparametric statistical test to compare the observed differences in pain scores between the 2 groups (ie, males and females), and it yields a probability value of $P = .30$. This *P* value indicates that there is a 30% probability that the observed differences in pain scores between males and females may have occurred by chance.

To estimate that findings are not due to chance, researchers should identify a threshold value, also referred to as the **significance level**, to determine whether results are significant. Typically, a significance level, denoted alpha (α), is assigned by the investigator to represent a threshold value at which the results of the statistical test will be declared significant or nonsignificant. Conventionally, alpha is set **a priori**, meaning that the level is determined prior to data collection. Alpha is typically 0.05, or 5%. This value is the maximal acceptable level of estimated error in the conclusion as to whether the difference was determined merely by chance. An alpha of .05 indicates that the researcher is willing to accept a 5% probability that a difference as large as that reported was caused by chance. A *P* value of .06 would result in a nonsignificant result (ie, the researcher would fail to conclude that the difference he or she found was real). A *P* value of .04 would result in the declaration of statistical significance ($P < .05$). If an appropriately applied statistical test yields a *P* value smaller than .05, the researcher can conclude that there is less than a 5% probability that the differences found were caused by chance. In some instances, a researcher may choose to use an alpha smaller than .05 (eg, .01, .001), which indicates that they want to be more stringent about the amount of probability they are willing to accept. For example, a researcher may use an alpha of .001, indicating they are willing to only accept a .1% probability that a difference is caused by chance when they are investigating a new drug that is intended to prevent heart attacks in individuals with heart disease.

To help bring together some of the concepts we have discussed, let us consider the following scenario as an example:

Dr. Academy is conducting a randomized, controlled trial to determine the effects of a lower extremity stretching protocol on ankle range of motion, as measured by a goniometer, among male collegiate soccer players with limited dorsiflexion. Dr. Academy randomly assigns 64 male collegiate soccer players into 2 groups: 32 individuals will compose group 1 (the experimental group) and will receive the lower extremity stretching protocol, while 32 individuals in group 2 (the control group) will not receive the lower extremity stretching protocol. For the purposes of this scenario, we will assume that the groups are homogenous prior to data collection (ie, the groups are the same) and that the data collected follow a normal distribution.

Based on the information provided in the scenario so far, we can identify the following:

- The independent variable of this study is the lower extremity stretching protocol group and has 2 levels (experimental stretch group, control nonstretch group).
- The dependent variable of this study is ankle dorsiflexion range of motion, which will be measured using a standard goniometer.
- Because 0 degrees of range of motion does not necessarily indicate a true absence of motion, but simply a neutral joint position, the type of data that will be collected is interval data.
- A plausible null hypothesis for this study could be:
    - There will be no group differences in ankle dorsiflexion range of motion following a joint mobilization protocol.
- A plausible research hypothesis for this study could be the following:
    - Participants in the experimental group will have a significantly greater increase in ankle dorsiflexion range of motion following the lower extremity stretching protocol than participants in the control group.
- Because the data are interval data, normally distributed, and the variance was homogenous, parametric tests will be used during inferential statistical analyses.

Before he begins to conduct statistical analysis, Dr. Academy predetermines his a priori significance level (alpha) to be .05. Once he has collected the data, Dr. Academy conducts a statistical analysis to determine if there is an observed difference in ankle dorsiflexion range of motion between the experimental group (15.6 degrees ± 2.3 degrees) and control group (11.2 degrees ± 1.7 degrees) following their assigned treatment protocols; the analysis yields a P *value of .013.*

In this example, statistical analysis has revealed a *P* value of .013. This finding indicates that there is no more than a 1.3% probability that the observed differences between groups regarding ankle dorsiflexion range of motion occurred by chance. Since Dr. Academy set an a priori significance level of $P = .05$, and the *P* value from the study was smaller than .05 (ie, .013), you can determine that the observed difference between groups was statistically significant. Therefore,

Table 4-3.
Confidence Interval Example Values

CONFIDENCE INTERVAL	RANGE OF VALUES[a]
85%	53.04 to 56.96 degrees
90%	52.76 to 57.24 degrees
95%	52.33 to 57.67 degrees
99%	51.50 to 58.50 degrees

[a]These ranges of values are based on a mean of 55 degrees.

Dr. Academy can reject the null hypothesis (ie, *there are no group differences in ankle dorsiflexion range of motion following a lower extremity stretching protocol*), and have evidence to believe that the observed differences between the 2 groups are real (ie, the result of the lower extremity stretching protocol) and are *not* due to chance.

Because data gathered in a research study are typically only collected on a sample of participants, you cannot be certain that the findings from the study are representative of what might be found in the larger population. As was discussed previously, using *P* values allows you to estimate the probability that observed differences may have been caused by chance in one study, and this finding may not translate to the population at large. In Dr. Academy's study, he specifically collected data on male collegiate soccer players. While the findings from this investigation were significant, indicating that ankle dorsiflexion range of motion was greater in the experimental group following the lower extremity stretching protocol, we cannot be certain that these same findings would occur in a different sample group (eg, recreational adults, adolescent female field hockey players). Therefore, you cannot be completely confident that the observed differences from the sample group would also occur in the target population.

Confidence Intervals

The **confidence interval** (CI) serves this purpose nicely. Many researchers incorporate CIs for their statistical estimates of population values. Many peer-reviewed journals require or strongly recommend researchers to report CIs along with *P* values. A CI is a range of values (minimum to maximum) that tells us how our estimates of sample statistics (eg, the mean value) are distributed in the population from which the sample was drawn. Similar to *P* values, a researcher designates their level of confidence about the calculated values (typically 95%). Setting the CI at 95% indicates that the researcher is 95% confident that the population mean will fall within the calculated confidence range. Specifically, the 95% CI for a statistic provides a range of values around the sample statistic within which we are 95% confident that the population value lies. Confidence intervals are used as descriptive and inferential statistics; however, because these statistics are inferring something about the population distribution, they are commonly considered inferential. Other common CIs range from 85% to 99%; however, it is important to understand that the higher percentage you set, the larger the minimum to maximum range is going to be.

The calculation of CIs is beyond the scope of this textbook, but we will consider the following example to better understand the different range of values based on the CI selected (Table 4-3). An AT investigating knee flexion range of motion in a random sample of 42 individuals determined an average of 55 degrees knee flexion range of motion, with an SD of 8.8 degrees. The AT now wants to know the probable range of these values (sample means) in the population. As you can see in Table 4-3, the higher the CI, the larger the range of values becomes. If the AT decided to set the CI at 99%, she could conclude that she can be 99% confident that the *true* mean value for knee flexion range of motion would fall between 51.50 degrees and 58.50 degrees for the target population. However, if she chose a CI of 90%, she would be 90% confident that the true mean value for knee flexion range of motion would fall between 52.76 degrees and 57.24 degrees.

Effect Size

In addition to determining if any observed differences from a research study are significant, it is also important to estimate how large the differences are. To estimate the size of the difference, researchers often calculate the effect size. An effect size is the magnitude of difference or relationship between 2 variables presented in a standardized fashion so that the results of similar studies can be compared. To help you understand effect size, let us go back to the research study conducted by Dr. Academy. Previously, we determined that there was a significant difference in ankle joint range of motion between participants in the experimental group (ie, received the lower extremity stretching protocol) and participants in the control group. The *P* value was reported at .013, which allows us to reject the null hypothesis. However, while we know there is a significant difference between groups, we are unsure just how effective the lower extremity stretching protocol is for increasing ankle joint range of motion compared with joint mobilization techniques.

Effect size values, which typically range from 0.00 to 3.00, are calculated by using the means and SDs of a variable from 2 groups. In our scenario above, Dr. Academy could calculate the effect size of the lower extremity stretching protocol by using the postintervention mean of the control group (11.2 degrees ± 1.7 degrees) and the postintervention mean of the experimental group (15.6 degrees ± 2.3 degrees). To calculate effect size, you will use the following equation:

$$d = (m_e - m_c) \div SD$$

d = standardized unit
m_e = mean of experimental group
m_c = mean of control group
SD = higher SD value between the 2 groups

Therefore, the effect size for Dr. Academy's research study is:

$$d = (m_e - m_c) \div SD$$
$$d = (15.6 - 11.2) \div 2.3$$
$$d = 1.91$$

It is important to interpret this value. Although there are no universally accepted definitions for the interpretation of effect size, many researchers use Cohen's definition (Table 4-4). By using these values, we can conclude that the lower extremity stretching protocol had an extremely large effect (d = 1.91) on increasing ankle dorsiflexion range of motion.

Effect size values provide a standardized unit and, therefore, can be compared across different studies when the variables are measured differently. For example, we know that Dr. Academy's study assessed whether a lower extremity stretching protocol increased ankle dorsiflexion range of motion. Now let us say another researcher, Dr. College, also wanted to determine if a lower extremity stretching protocol increased ankle dorsiflexion range of motion but used different stretching techniques than those Dr. Academy incorporated in his protocol. Dr. College included 50 participants in each group, and data analysis revealed the average ankle dorsiflexion range of motion following the lower extremity stretching protocol to be 12.3 degrees ± 3.1 degrees in the experimental group and 10.5 degrees ± 1.4 degrees in the control group. If you compare these findings to Dr. Academy's study (Table 4-5), you see that Dr. Academy's lower extremity stretching protocol appears to be more effective because it produced higher averages of ankle dorsiflexion range of motion. However, since these

Table 4-4. Effect Size Interpretation

EFFECT SIZE VALUE	INTERPRETATION
0.20	Small effect
0.50	Medium effect
0.80	Large effect
1.10	Very large effect
1.40+	Extremely large effect
Adapted from Cohen J. A power primer. *Psychol Bull.* 1992;112(1):155-159.	

Table 4-5. Study Findings From Dr. Academy and Dr. College

Dr. Academy's study	MEAN	SD
Experimental (n=42)	15.6	2.3
Control (n=42)	11.2	1.7
Difference between means	4.4	
Dr. College's study		
Experimental (n=50)	12.3	3.1
Control (n=50)	10.5	1.4
Difference between means	1.8	

2 studies did not have the same methodology or sample size, we are unable to determine which lower extremity stretching protocol is superior. Therefore, to compare these 2 studies, it is necessary to determine the effect size for each study.

To begin, let us calculate the effect size for Dr. College's study:

$$d = (m_e - m_c) \div SD$$
$$d = (12.3 - 10.5) \div 3.4$$
$$d = 0.53$$

Once the values for each study are on a standardized scale, you can compare their effects. Remember, we earlier defined effect size as the magnitude of difference, or the magnitude of a relationship, between 2 variables. Now that you have 2 values on a standardized scale, you can compare the magnitude of the differences between the 2 studies (ie, we can assess the effect size). Referring back to Table 4-4, you can now conclude that Dr. Academy's lower extremity stretching protocol, with an extremely large effect size of 1.91, is more effective at increasing ankle dorsiflexion range of motion than Dr. College's stretching protocol, which had a medium effect size of 0.53.

Types of Error

Along with understanding probability values, CIs, and effect size, it is important to understand how these statistical components can affect a research study. In some instances, the data collected from a research study may lead a researcher to draw inaccurate conclusions about the findings from the investigation as they relate to the population. More specifically, the researcher may commit a type I or type II error.

A **type I error** is caused when a researcher makes an incorrect decision to *reject* the null hypothesis when it is actually true. Remember, the null hypothesis stated that there would be no differences/relationships among groups. By rejecting the null hypothesis (ie, reporting a *false positive*), the researcher is concluding that there is a significant relationship or difference between 2 variables when in fact *there is not*.

A **type II error** is caused when a researcher makes an incorrect decision to *accept* the null hypothesis. By accepting the null hypothesis, the researcher is stating that there is no relationship or difference between 2 variables when in fact *there is*. Committing a type II error could prevent a researcher from discovering important information, and it is also known as a *false negative*. For example, Dr. Academy may commit a type II error if he reports that a lower extremity stretching protocol does not have an effect on improving ankle dorsiflexion, when in fact there is a true difference. A type II error often occurs when there are low participant numbers in a research investigation. Instead of 32 participants per group, let us say Dr. Academy decided to conduct his study on the effects of a lower extremity stretching protocol on a sample group with a low number of participants (eg, 5 participants per group) instead. Data from his study yielded results with a *P* value equal to .023, therefore concluding that there was a significant difference. However, Dr. Academy decided to conduct the same study with a larger number of participants (eg, 100 participants per group), and this time the results yielded a nonsignificant *P* value of .74. Based on this information, we can conclude that Dr. Academy committed a type II error in the first study of only 5 participants per group by indicating that there was a significant difference when in fact there likely was not.

Statistical Power

The results of any study depend on the design's **statistical power**, the ability of a statistical test to detect a significant difference if it truly does exist. Importantly, statistical power helps one to determine the probability of making a correct decision about the findings from a research study. It is particularly crucial in helping to ensure that a researcher does not commit a type II error (ie, accepting that there is no difference between groups when there is).

To help ensure that the appropriate number of participants are included in a research study (not too many and not too few) and to avoid committing a type I or type II error, researchers often calculate statistical power by conducting a power analysis. A **power analysis** is a technique that takes into consideration several components (eg, alpha level, effect size, and sample size). This technique allows a researcher to estimate the value of one of the components, provided that he or she has information for the other 3. For example, if the researcher knows the alpha level, effect size, and the desired power level, he or she will be able to determine the number of subjects needed for the sample size. For a power analysis, the desired power level is typically set at a minimum of 80%.

For example, you are interested in conducting a study to assess the effects of a lower extremity stretching protocol on ankle dorsiflexion range of motion following a lateral ankle sprain. Before you begin your research study, you would like to determine how many participants you will need to be able to estimate that any observed differences are real and not caused by chance. After doing a literature search to determine what research has previously been performed on the topic, you come across a similar study conducted by Dr. College and decide to use the data from the study to help calculate a power analysis. As we previously calculated, the effect size of Dr. College's study is 0.53. Since you already know the effect size, you can use a power table (Figure 4-7) to help you determine the statistical power. By using this table, you can see that, for an effect size of 0.53 and a power set at 80%, you will need at least 50 participants in each group to be able to estimate observed differences if they exist.

By estimating the number of participants required, a researcher will be able to control the probability of committing a type II error. A power analysis is conducted by utilizing tables, simple formulae, or computer software to tabulate the appropriate sample size. G*Power 3.1 (Heinrich-Heine-Universität Düsseldorf, Düsseldorf, Germany) is an example of a type of computer software that will compute a power analysis.

Summary

Comprehending and applying the foundational terms within research and statistics are essential for you to examine information for your clinical practice. Interpretation of the basics, such as CIs, effect sizes, and *P* values, will give you the ability to apply the findings and make adjustments depending on what may be clinically meaningful.

Key Points

- Data are classified as nominal, ordinal, interval, or ratio. Each type of scale provides different information and is defined by how it is collected.
- Research designs include independent variable(s), dependent variable(s), hypothesis, null hypothesis, and possibly a research hypothesis.
- Descriptive statistics cannot be used to draw conclusions about the hypothesis; this type of information can only provide a description of the data.
- Inferential statistics often involve the use of statistical tests to analyze the data and deduce how the findings could potentially represent what may occur in a given patient population.
- If 1 of the 3 assumptions for parametric statistical tests is not met, then nonparametric statistical tests should be utilized.

Bibliography

Cohen J. A power primer. *Psychol Bull.* 1992;112(1):155-159.

Faul F, Erdfelder E, Lang AG, Buchner A. G*Power 3: a flexible statistical power analysis program for the social, behavioral, and biomedical sciences. *Behav Res Methods.* 2007;39(2):175-191.

Greenfield ML, Kuhn JE, Wojtys EM. A statistics primer. Confidence intervals. *AM J Sports Med.* 1998;26(1):145-149.

Greenfield ML, Kuhn JE, Wojtys EM. A statistics primer. P values: probability and clinical significance. *AM J Sports Med.* 1996;24(6):863-865.

Norton BJ, Strube MJ. Understanding statistical power. *J Orthop Sports Phys Ther.* 2001;31(6):307-315.

Oldham J. Statistical tests (part 2): parametric tests. *Nurs Stand.* 1993;7(44):28-30.

Oldham J. Statistical tests (part 3): non-parametric tests. *Nurs Stand.* 1993;7(45):28-30.

Portney LG, Watkins MP. *Foundations of Clinical Research: Applications to Practice.* 3rd ed. Upper Saddle River: Prentice Hall Health; 2009.

d (Effect Size)

n (Number of Participants Needed)	.10	.20	.30	.40	.50	.60	.70	.80	1.00
50	12	26	44	63	80	91	97	99	*
52	13	26	45	65	81	92	97	99	
54	13	27	46	66	83	93	98	99	
56	13	28	47	68	84	93	98	99	
58	13	28	49	69	85	94	98	*	
60	13	29	50	70	86	95	98		
64	14	30	52	73	88	96	99		
68	14	31	54	75	90	97	99		
72	15	33	56	77	91	97	99		
76	15	34	58	79	92	98	*		
80	15	35	60	81	93	98			
84	16	36	61	82	94	99			
88	16	37	63	84	95	99			
92	17	38	65	85	95	99			
96	17	40	66	87	96	99			
100	17	41	68	88	97	*			
120	19	46	75	93	99				
140	21	51	80	95	99				
160	23	56	85	97	*				
180	24	60	88	98					
200	26	64	91	99					
250	30	72	96	*					
300	34	79	98						
350	37	84	99						
400	41	88	*						
450	44	91							
500	47	93							
600	53	97							
700	59	98							
800	64	99							
900	68	*							
1000	72								

Power Level

Figure 4-7. Power table. $P=.05$. (Adapted from Cohen J. *Statistical Power Analysis for the Behavioral Sciences.* 2nd ed. Hillsdale, NJ: Erlbaum; 1988.)

5

Introduction to Critical Appraisal

Now that you have searched the literature to find useful information to help you answer your clinical question and have a good understanding of the foundational concepts involved in research and statistics, it is time to proceed to the next step of the evidence-based practice process: critical appraisal. With the increasing volume of scientific publications each year (ie, more than 200,000 new publications per year), having the skills to critically appraise the information you find is becoming exceedingly important. As a busy clinician, these skills will allow you to reduce the amount of time necessary to find information that will help you make a strong clinical decision. Unfortunately, although most publications undergo a peer review process, publication does not necessarily ensure the quality of a study. In fact, poor-quality intervention studies tend to overestimate the actual benefits received from the intervention by an estimated 30%. Similarly, results gained from diagnostic tests have also been found to exaggerate the accuracy of the test being evaluated. Therefore, critically appraising the evidence may be the most vital step for you to make informed clinical decisions.

Critical appraisal is the process of carefully and systematically examining research to judge its trustworthiness as well as its value and relevance in a particular context. More specifically, the purpose of critical appraisal is to determine whether evidence from a viable source can be translated and applied to help you answer your clinical question. Traditionally, critical appraisal focuses on whether research findings can be applied within your clinical practice. For the purposes of this unit, we will focus on the critical appraisal process as it relates to research literature. However, clinician expertise is also considered a viable source, and information you receive from a fellow clinician should also be appraised and considered when making an informed clinical decision. For example, depending on your topic or target patient population, research literature may not be available to help you answer your clinical question. In this instance, discussion with other athletic trainers or other health care providers who may be familiar with the topic of interest or have provided care for a patient with a similar case presentation will be extremely beneficial in helping you make a clinical decision.

Van Lunen BL, Hankemeier DA, Welch CE.
Evidence-Guided Practice: A Framework for Clinical Decision Making in Athletic Training (pp 59-62).

Throughout the critical appraisal process, there are several questions you should consider to help you determine whether the information will be useful for your patient case or clinical practice setting. Essentially, you should be able to answer 3 general questions for each study that is reviewed:

1. Are the results of the study valid?
2. Are the results of the study reliable?
3. Are the findings of the study clinically relevant and applicable to your clinical question?

Appraising the Validity of a Study

As you are critically appraising a research study to help you answer your clinical question, it is crucial to determine whether the results of the study are valid. More specifically, you will need to determine whether the findings produce answers to what the researcher was initially examining. Ideally, the primary purpose of conducting research is to use systematic approaches to find answers to clinical questions. Although researchers' intentions are to find such answers, there are several factors that can influence the findings of the study and, therefore, affect the validity. These factors are also referred to as threats to validity and must be considered as you are appraising a research study. Conversely, the researcher may have tried to control for these factors during the study, which would therefore increase the strength of the internal validity (how well the study was conducted), but may also decrease the external validity (application to the population). Thus, determining the validity of a research study requires you to appraise the strengths and threats that could influence how valid the findings are. The fewer threats to internal and external validity there are in a study, the more likely the results of that investigation are valid and applicable to the population of interest.

Appraising the Reliability of a Study

Along with assessing the validity of a study, the reliability must be considered. More specifically, it is important to determine whether the findings can be reproduced if the same study was conducted again. If the methodologies of a study were not reproducible, it would be difficult to determine the accuracy of those results as well as how applicable they would be to clinical practice. In addition to the reliability of the results, it is also necessary to appraise the reliability of the tools and equipment used to collect the data for a study. For example, if a researcher collected data to determine dorsiflexion range of motion using a goniometer but that goniometer was not considered a reliable tool (ie, it could not produce the same range of motion value when used on a single patient multiple times), the data from that study will not be useful to you in clinical practice because the likelihood of reproducing similar findings would be unlikely. Therefore, if a protocol used in a study is not reliable, the information from that study is not valuable to you as a clinician because you will not be able to reproduce that information during your patient care.

Appraising the Clinical Applicability of a Study

As is human nature, no single research study is perfect. Being able to identify flaws, limitations, and threats to validity will not necessarily eliminate the study from consideration but will aid you in making a thorough clinical decision. However, it is often easier to identify aspects of a research study that were poorly conducted vs highlighting the parts that were performed correctly.

Table 5-1.
Critical Appraisal Guiding Questions

1. Why was the study performed? What is the guiding clinical question?
2. What study design was utilized? Is it appropriate to answer the clinical question?
3. How was the sample size decided?
4. Were the measurements used valid? Were the measurements reliable?
5. How were the data analyzed?
6. Were there any problems during the study?
7. Was previous research performed in this area? If so, how do these results compare?
8. How does this research influence clinical practice?
9. Can the results from this study be applied to my patient case or population?

Therefore, as you begin to formulate a critical appraisal process that works best for you, it is important to find a balance between identifying the positive aspects of a study as well as the negatives ones. In doing so, you will be able to dissect which information is clinically relevant to your particular clinical question or patient case.

As has been discussed in previous chapters, there are several different ways in which research can be conducted, and as a result, critical appraisal must take into account the characteristics of each type of research study design. Each type of design has its own advantages as well as disadvantages, and it is important for you to be able to recognize both. Therefore, to begin the critical appraisal process, it is necessary to determine whether the type of study design utilized to answer the clinical question is appropriate and well implemented. Simultaneously, it is important to appraise specific aspects of the research study. Table 5-1 provides you with a list of guiding questions to help you navigate through the critical appraisal process. As you progress through this unit, each chapter will provide you with essential information that will help you determine the answers to these guiding questions as you strive to make informed clinical decisions.

The remaining chapters in this unit will highlight various concepts that will be important to comprehend as you strive to critically appraise literature to make informed clinical decisions. Along with providing a foundation of the concepts involved in critical appraisal, this unit includes useful tools that can be used to assist you with the critical appraisal process. It is important to note that critical appraisal seems like a complex and daunting process at first. Similar to many skills you will learn in athletic training, with time and practice, your skills for critically appraising the literature will become a natural part of your daily clinical decision making.

Key Points

- With practice and time, critical appraisal will become a natural part of your daily clinical decision making.
- To begin the critical appraisal process, it is important to determine whether the type of study design utilized is appropriate for the type of clinical question asked.

- Clinician expertise is also a viable source of evidence and should also be appraised and considered when making clinical decisions.

Bibliography

Fineout-Overholt E, Melnyk BM, Schultz A. Transforming health care from the inside out: advancing evidence-based practice in the 21st century. *J Prof Nurs.* 2005;21(6):335-344.

Fisher CG, Wood KB. Introduction to and techniques of evidence-based medicine. *Spine (Phila Pa 1976).* 2007;32(19 suppl):S66-S72.

Forrest JL, Miller SA. Evidence-based decision making in action: part 2—evaluating and applying the clinical evidence. *J Contemp Dent Pract.* 2003;4(1):42-52.

Lijmer JG, Mol BW, Heisterkamp S, et al. Empirical evidence of design-related bias in studies of diagnostic tests. *JAMA.* 1998;282(11):1061-1066.

Moher D, Cook DJ, Jadad AR, et al. Assessing the quality of reports of randomised trials: implications for the conduct of meta-analyses. *Health Technol Assess.* 1998;3(12):i-iv,1-98.

Steves R, Hootman JM. Evidence-based medicine: what is it and how does it apply to athletic training? *J Athl Train.* 2004;39(1):83-87.

Welch CE, Yakuboff MK, Madden MJ. Critically appraised papers and topics part 1: use in clinical practice. *Athl Ther Today.* 2008;13(5):10-12.

6

Selection and Assignment of Participants

As you examine the available evidence, you will need to make decisions about the applicability of the information to the type of patient you are treating. The participants within many research articles are chosen to match criteria that the investigators are interested in; therefore, you need to understand how the selection of the participants relates to what you are able to apply to your patient. This chapter will provide guidance on how participants are chosen and selected, how the participants are assigned to groups, and what it means to blind the participants and possibly the examiners.

Choosing Participants

Prior to conducting a research study, the investigator needs to specify the criteria used to select participants. Typically, this is defined through inclusionary and exclusionary criteria. **Inclusion criteria** are the characteristics and/or traits that are desired for each participant. These could relate to particular demographic characteristics (eg, marital status, sex, age), clinical findings (eg, range of motion, injury status, disability level), or patient-oriented outcomes (eg, health-related quality of life measures, fear of reinjury, patient-reported function). Using inclusionary criteria typically helps to narrow down the sample population and focus on just the participants of interest. For example, a researcher studying the effects of a soft tissue mobilization technique on edema reduction may choose to only include athletic collegiate patients with ankle injuries. When selecting inclusionary criteria, it is important to remember that the more restrictive the criteria, the less likely the results of the study can be generalized to a larger population. If we use the previous example, it would be more restrictive if we chose to use collegiate male basketball patients with a grade III inversion ankle sprain that demonstrated greater than 10 mm of swelling when compared bilaterally. In this case, it would take much longer to get participants that met the criteria, and it would limit how well the results could be related to a different population. For example, information gained from these collegiate male basketball patients may not translate to high school female

Van Lunen BL, Hankemeier DA, Welch CE.
Evidence-Guided Practice: A Framework for Clinical Decision Making in Athletic Training (pp 63-68).

soccer patients. To allow for the findings to be related to a more general population, it is best to limit the inclusion criteria to only a few items of interest. Limiting the inclusion criteria also helps eliminate extraneous factors that could affect the internal validity of the study. Internal validity will be further discussed in the next chapter.

Exclusion criteria are the characteristics that would eliminate an individual from being selected as a participant. Most exclusionary criteria are chosen because they are believed to be considered confounding (ie, complicating) variables to what is being investigated, and these variables may affect the results. If studying the effects of joint mobilizations on patellar mobility, a researcher may choose to eliminate individuals with a recent history of knee injury and those who have a Beighton and Horan Joint Mobility Index score of 4 or greater (indicating significant hypermobility). Both of these characteristics could affect on the mobility of the patella, thus influencing the results of the study in a manner that was not intended. The use of inclusionary and exclusionary criteria help researchers better define the sample of interest.

Methods of Participant Selection

When designing a research study, the researcher wants to try to eliminate as many extraneous variables as possible. To do this, many researchers conduct studies using a **random sampling** or **random selection** of participants. When random selection of participants occurs, every potential participant has the same chance of being selected for inclusion in the study or for a particular treatment. For example, researchers are interested in determining how often athletic trainers (ATs) implement clinical prediction rules in their clinical practice. Instead of asking every AT, they decide to conduct a study assessing a random sample of ATs. The most valid technique of random sampling typically occurs through the use of a computer program or a random numbers table. Using a computer program, the Board of Certification office randomly selects 25% of ATs to participate. Since all ATs are on file with the Board of Certification, every AT has the chance of being chosen to participate. The use of a random sampling technique is thought to be the best way to provide an accurate representation of the population. There are times when random selection can be tedious due to the fact that every individual must be assigned a corresponding number. When this occurs, some researchers will choose to use a **systematic sampling** of participants. Often, potential participants are listed alphabetically or by some other organizational variable. With systematic sampling, the total number of the population available is divided by the number of participants needed to determine what systematic sampling procedure should be used. For example, if there is a population of 300 high school student athletes and the researcher intends to study 50 of those individuals, they could choose to systematically sample those 50 players. To systematically sample this population of 300, it is determined that every sixth student athlete (300/50) on the alphabetical roster will be selected. A random point on the list is determined as the starting point, and then every sixth name is randomly selected to participate. This process allows the researcher to identify the 50 random participants without assigning each a unique number. Many statisticians believe that systematic sampling is just as robust as random sampling.

Another type of sampling is called **stratified random sampling**. Although not as robust as random or systematic sampling approaches, this form of sampling is often used when there is a particular condition of interest to the researcher. In stratified random sampling, researchers stratify the total sample by the condition or variable of interest. If a researcher was interested in studying 100 freshman student athletes (65 males and 35 females) regarding the effect of a new peer tutoring program on academic retention, stratified random sampling would be warranted. Instead of sampling the entire population, the researcher wants to assess a group of 30 total students. They could randomly choose 15 male students and 15 female students to have equal representation from males and females. Since there are more male student athletes than females in the population, a true random sample could produce a group that consists of mostly one sex, which would not be truly representative of the population. To get a better representation of the population, the researcher could conduct **proportional stratified random sampling** by selecting a proportion of male and female students equal to the proportion of the population. For the previous example, the researcher would select 65% of the 30 total students from the males (n = 20) and 35% of the total from the females (n = 10).

In many cases, it is difficult to get access to the entire population of interest. For example, if a researcher is interested in surveying athletic training preceptors, there is no formal list of these individuals. **Cluster sampling** allows the researcher to randomly select a cluster of individuals who meet the inclusionary criteria. To start, the researcher could randomly select 15 states and then randomly select 3 Commission on Accreditation of Athletic Training Education accredited professional athletic training programs from each state (n = 45 programs). From those 45 programs, the researcher then randomly selects 4 preceptors from each athletic training program. This would give you a total participant pool of 180 preceptors in a much more convenient manner. Unfortunately, each step in cluster sampling allows for more sampling error to occur, so choosing a large enough sample at the onset is important.

The final type of sampling is **convenience sampling**. With convenience sampling, all participants are recruited and selected based on convenience and accessibility. With convenience sampling, it is easy to recruit participants, but the ability to generalize the findings to those outside the population is significantly decreased. Often, convenience sampling is used in initial or pilot studies to test study methodology before conducting the study on a larger scale. When conducting a research study, careful consideration regarding the population should be taken into account to obtain the most representative sample. Table 6-1 recaps each of the sampling procedures while also identifying pros and cons for each method.

Participant Assignment to Groups

Once individuals are selected to participate in a research study, they are often allocated into a particular group. **Allocation** refers to how a participant is placed into a group for the duration of the study. Participants can be allocated to receive a particular treatment or to be in a **control group** that receives no treatment. As with sampling, computer randomization is considered the most robust form of allocation. Similar to the randomization sampling procedures, randomization is also used to assign or allocate a participant to a particular intervention. With random assignment, each participant has an equal chance of being allocated to a specific group. For example, if a researcher was conducting a study on the effects of 3 stretching regimens (dynamic stretching, proprioceptive neuromuscular facilitation, or a control group) on hamstring flexibility, each participant would have an equal chance of being selected for any 1 of the 3 treatment groups. While random assignment does not mean that all 3 groups are equal, it does eliminate the possibility that one group would be skewed heavily in one direction.

Control groups are often used in clinical research as a comparison to the intervention of interest. In the example above, 2 stretching protocols are being compared with individuals in a control group. Control groups often receive no intervention, a placebo intervention, or a standard treatment that all individuals would receive. It is also important that the individuals in the control group are similar to those in the intervention groups, which can occur through random assignment. In many athletic training clinical studies, specifically those using patients as research participants, control groups are difficult to use because using the current standard of care as a control does not allow conclusions to be drawn about the actual effectiveness of the intervention. For example, most clinicians initially treat ankle sprains with cryotherapy and compression, which would be considered the standard treatment or control. If the researcher was assessing the effect of cryokinetics or immobilization on ankle swelling, it would be difficult to separate the effect of the standard/control treatment from that of the treatment groups because they have some similar

Table 6-1. Sampling Procedures

SAMPLING METHOD	DESCRIPTION	PROS	CONS
Random sampling	Every person in the population of interest has an equal chance of being chosen	Allows a true representation of the sample of interest	Every person in the population must be given a matching number
Systematic random sampling	Every person in the population of interest is listed by a variable (name, birth date, etc) and then every n^{th} is chosen	Allows simplification of the randomization process without assigning a specific numeric value to each participant	Can be biased depending on how the sample population is listed
Stratified random sampling	When the population of interest includes strati, people from each strati are selected	Allows for equal representation between strati	There is less variety included in the sample
Proportional stratified sampling	Select participants that represent a proportion of the sample of interest	Allows for proportional representation of the sample of interest	The sample is not completely random and does not have variety
Cluster sampling	Breakdown of the larger population of interest to smaller clusters that meet the inclusionary criteria	Allows sampling of a larger population to occur	Larger number of errors can occur when there are several levels to the cluster sample
Convenience sampling	Choosing participants that are easily accessible and meet the inclusionary criteria	Allows an easy selection of participants	Least robust form of sampling

components. Withholding treatment (ie, providing no treatment) in the control group is often impossible because it would involve denying care to the patient. When selecting participants for a study or assigning them into a group, there is no set way to allocate these individuals into groups. The decision on which method should be chosen needs to be based on the research question, the population being studied, and the variables of interest.

Blinding

In experimental studies, there is a potential for bias of the researchers and participants. **Bias** indicates that an individual may be favorable toward one end of a spectrum. For example, if a researcher was trying to determine whether ice massage or cold-water submersion was more effective at reducing pain following an acute ankle sprain, a participant's subjective pain rating may be affected by which treatment they prefer, therefore creating a participant bias. To eliminate bias in studies, many researchers initiate a **blinding** process. Typically, there are 3 groups that can be blinded: the participant, the researcher, or the clinician providing the treatment. If the research participant is blinded, they do not know which treatment they are receiving (eg, experimental treatment or the control). To assist with blinding, participants may receive a placebo or sham treatment so they do not know whether they are receiving the actual treatment. Blinding of participants is easier to achieve in research studies that investigate pharmacological interventions than those receiving an exercise regimen or a specific taping technique because a placebo can be given with a pharmacological intervention. It is extremely difficult to blind an individual to a specific taping technique because the participant will be aware if they are not receiving the taping treatment. When participants cannot be blinded, the research team or clinician taking the measurements may be blinded to which group the participant is allocated. In some instances, there may be a third group, the clinicians taking the measures, who are blinded to the individuals in the treatment groups. These individuals are often different from the research team. There are times when blinding of the researcher is not as vital as that of blinding the clinician because the clinician is the one taking the measurement. If you were assessing the effects of 2 stretching protocols on hamstring flexibility, you may want the researcher to supervise the stretching protocol while a clinician who is blinded to which treatment was administered measures the flexibility. Keeping the role of the researcher and the clinician separate can help to control for bias.

When participants cannot be blinded but the researcher or clinician is blinded, it is considered a **single-blind study** because only one aspect of the study is blinded. To reduce as much bias as possible, it is best for the research team and participant to be unaware of the treatment groups until after the data are collected. This is considered to be a **double-blind study** because neither party is privy to the individuals in the groups or the treatments being administered. If the researchers, participants, and clinicians are unaware of the allocation to groups, it is considered a **triple-blind** study. As with sampling and selection of participants, how the study is blinded depends on several variables. It is important to eliminate as much bias as possible while still being able to effectively perform the research as designed.

Summary

Being able to apply information from various research studies to the patient for whom you are providing care is extremely important. Much of the available research is limited for the athletic population due to the fact that many athletic training facilities monitor injuries and treatments within an isolated environment and it is not used for research purposes. Careful consideration must be taken when selecting participants and assigning them to groups within a research study. It is the goal of the researcher to provide information to clinicians that is applicable in real-life scenarios, but that is often difficult; therefore, you must often examine research outside of the specific patient you are treating to find out information which will affect your plan of care.

Key Points

- Prior to conducting a research study, the investigator needs to specify or define the inclusionary or exclusionary criteria that will be used to select participants.
- When random selection of participants occurs, every potential participant has the same chance of being selected for inclusion in the study or for a particular treatment.
- Participants can be allocated to receive a particular treatment or to be in a control group that received no treatment. As with sampling, computer randomization is considered to be the most robust form of allocation.
- To eliminate bias in studies, many researchers initiate a blinding process that can include the participant, the researcher, or the clinician providing the treatment.

Bibliography

Acharya A, Prakash A, Saxena P, Nigam A. Sampling: why and how of it? *Indian J Med Spec.* 2013;4(2):330-333.

Biernacki P, Waldrof D. Snowball sampling: problems and techniques of chain referral sampling. *Sociol Methods Res.* 1981;10(2):141-163.

Day SJ, Altman DG. Statistics notes: blinding in clinical trials and other studies. *BMJ.* 2000;321(7259):504.

Jadad AR, Moore RA, Carroll D, et al. Assessing the quality of reports of randomized clinical trials: is blinding necessary? *Control Clin Trials.* 1996;17(1):1-12.

Schulz KF, Grimes DA. Blinding in randomised trials: hiding who got what. *Lancet.* 2002;359(9307):696-700.

The Standards of Reporting Trials Group. A proposal for structured reporting of randomized controlled trials. *JAMA.* 1994;272(24):1926-1931.

7

Concepts of Validity

Validity is often discussed in terms of research design and data collection. **Validity** determines if a test or instrument measures what it is intended to measure. Validity can be discussed in several different avenues, such as the structure and design of a research study, the validity of the intervention being assessed, or the validity of the measurements collected in a given study. In each of these 3 cases, validity has a different meaning and is assessed in different ways. This chapter will focus on how you can evaluate the internal, external, and statistical validity of a given study design or measurement. It is important to understand these components of validity assessment because they are often used in the appraisal of research literature.

Threats to Validity

When referring to the experimental design of a study, the internal and external validity of the research design must be assessed. Many research studies are designed to determine a cause and effect relationship or **internal validity** of the study. In other words, the researcher is trying to determine if a given treatment (eg, joint mobilizations) improves the desired outcome (eg, increased range of motion). While it is important to determine that relationship, there are often extraneous factors or threats that can contribute to the change in range of motion outside of the treatment, in this case joint mobilizations. A study design with high validity has attempted to rule out all plausible threats to internal validity. **External validity** aims to explain how results from a particular study can be applied to populations outside of the study. Threats to external validity occur when incorrect conclusions are made beyond the subjects being studied. The threats to internal and external validity are explained throughout this chapter.

Van Lunen BL, Hankemeier DA, Welch CE.
Evidence-Guided Practice: A Framework for Clinical Decision Making in Athletic Training (pp 69-77).

Internal Validity Threats

Internal validity threats can include treatments, procedures, or experiences of the participants that threaten the researcher's ability to draw accurate conclusions from the research. Threats could include aspects related to the participants (ie, maturation, mortality, selection), procedures involved in the experiment (ie, instrumentation, testing procedures), or errors relating to the treatment administered (ie, diffusion, compensatory rivalry).

When research involves human participants, each individual has a different background, making variability between the participants a potential threat to internal validity. Internal validity threats related to the participants include: history, maturation, mortality, selection, and regression.

History refers to the unanticipated concurrent events (eg, natural disaster, change in job) that can occur outside of an experiment, which may potentially change the outcome of the study beyond the experiment. If you are studying the effects of a stretching program over a period of 6 weeks, there is potential for outside events to cause changes within the participants. If participants are allowed to participate in outside stretching activities (ie, yoga classes) this may affect the results of the study, especially if all of the participants are not experiencing the same activities outside of the study. It is important that you try to control the history threat by specifically stating what participants are allowed or not allowed to do outside of the study and also by making sure that you control as many external factors for all participants as possible. For studies that occur over a short period of time, the history threat is not as severe as in those studies that occur over weeks or months. With longer-duration studies, there is more opportunity for uncontrolled outside events to affect the outcomes of the research. While the duration of the study can affect this, it does not mean that you should not conduct studies over an extended period of time, but instead design a study that takes outside influences into account. For example, if you were assessing the long-term effects of a particular anterior cruciate ligament (ACL) reconstruction technique on return to play, you would have to track the participants over several months. During that time, some participants may move, thus making long-term follow-up more difficult.

Maturation refers to the changes (eg, physical, psychological, spiritual, emotional) that occur naturally to a participant over time independent of external events. With each passing day, participants are maturing and changing. While there is nothing that can be done to stop the maturation process of a participant, it is something that needs to be considered. Since each individual matures and changes differently, it may cause changes or differences from one testing period to the next. If you are interested in examining the effects of an 8-week strength training program on high school students, you would want to select participants that are similar in age because adolescents are maturing and changing at a rapid pace. The strength differences from week 1 to week 8 may not all be attributed to the training program, but also to the physiologic changes within the body. If there is a longer time between data collection periods, there will be more of a chance for maturation to adversely affect the outcome. To counteract this threat, many studies complete multiple baseline assessments to ensure that the participant has stabilized on the outcome of interest prior to starting the intervention. For example, if you wanted to assess the effects of a plyometric training program on dynamic balance, you may choose to conduct multiple assessments of dynamic balance until the fluctuations in the participant's balance stabilized. Once multiple trials resulted in the same level of dynamic balance, you could be more confident that changes that occur in dynamic balance could actually be attributed to the intervention and not changes in the participants themselves.

Mortality, also referred to as attrition, indicates the number of participants who drop out of a research study before it is completed. People may drop out of a study prior to completing it because of the time commitment, loss of interest, injuries, dislike of the treatment, or any other reason. A researcher should only analyze the data of those people who completed the study. It is also important for there to be a description of the number of people who did not complete the study and the reason for their attrition. Providing this information allows the reader of the research to

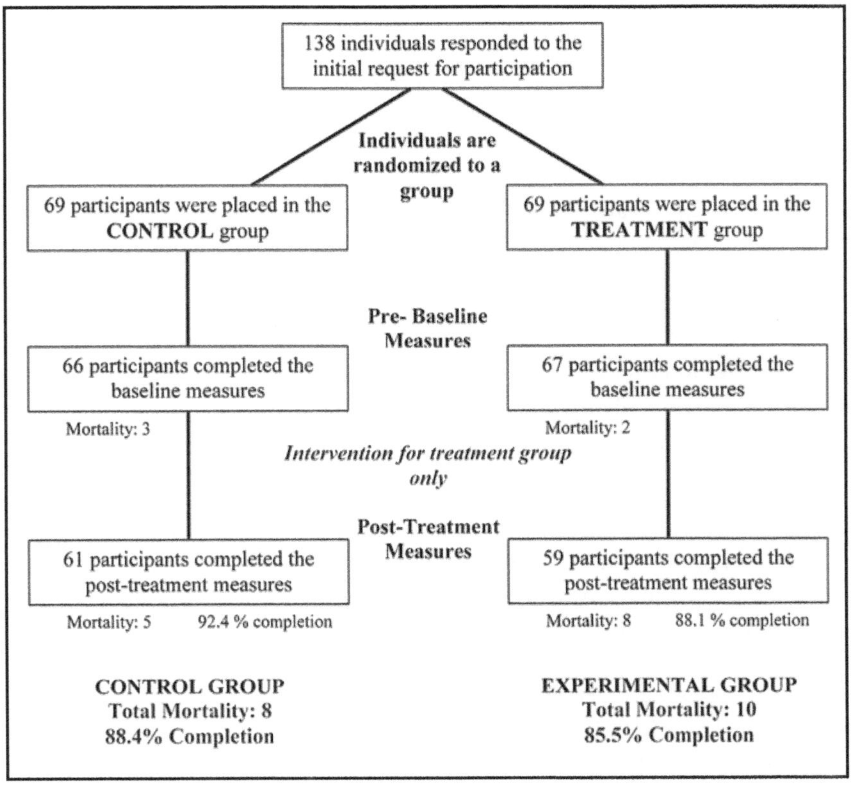

Figure 7-1. Participant mortality.

understand where and why the mortality occurred. Figure 7-1 provides an example of how mortality could be tracked in a study. In the figure, you see that 69 individuals were randomly assigned to control and treatment groups, but some individuals dropped out prior to the prebaseline measures. Even more individuals dropped out prior the posttreatment measures. To determine the total mortality of each group, individuals who did not complete the study should be added together for each group. Tracking the participants who withdraw from a study is important because it may be that the individuals who drop out are the ones who are of most interest. For example, if there are total of 20 participants in a study with 10 in a control group and 10 in the treatment group, it would be important to understand that 4 participants dropping out from the treatment group could be problematic. It could indicate that there is a problem with the treatment, thus causing more attrition. If participants dropped out of both groups equally, it may not be as much of a concern. Completely controlling for individuals who will not finish the study is often impossible, but measures should be taken to ensure as much compliance as possible. When recruiting participants for a study, it is important to thoroughly explain all of the procedures and to discuss the potential time commitment necessary to complete the study. Doing this, along with eliminating any factors that could cause physical or emotional harm, will help decrease the amount of mortality associated with study. It is also important to select a larger number than what you believe is necessary to account for the mortality that will occur.

Selection or selection bias is another internal validity threat; the previous chapter on sampling and participant selection discussed the criticality of this step in the research process. If you do not use random sampling to select individuals for your study, you risk selection bias. Using a convenience sample may be easier for you as the researcher, but it may also include biases that could change the results of the study. If you were interested in studying the effects of body fat composition on the incidence of heat illness in collegiate football athletes, you would want to examine a variety of body fat percentage groupings. If you chose to only study individuals with more than 30% body fat, you would not be able to determine if the incidence of heat illness was directly related to body fat percentage since you did not assess those individuals with a low body fat percentage. The use of more inclusive sampling measures that better represent the population of interest will help to counteract the selection threat.

The final internal validity threat related to the participant is referred to as **regression**. Regression, or regression toward the mean, occurs when unreliable testing procedures are used or when there are extreme group scores. If the measures are not reliable, there is a tendency for error to occur, thus causing the scores to go toward the mean. Additionally, if you have a group of scores that are extremely high and another group of scores that are extremely low on the first assessment, there is a tendency for the scores to stay the same or go toward the mean, respectively. For example, if an examination was given on the first day of class, there would be individuals who scored really well and those who scored poorly. A week later, another examination was given, and those with poor scores tended to do better than on the previous test, while those who did well the previous time stayed about the same. Since one group increased their scores and the other stayed the same, it is seen as the scores improving toward the mean. This can be easily avoided if there is random selection of participants instead of choosing participants that are on one extreme end of the spectrum. Random selection helps to ensure that the participants are evenly distributed, whereas convenience sampling may lead to individuals who are more alike and, thus, regress more toward the mean. The regression threat can be easily counteracted by using reliable testing procedures and random selection of participants.

Using **matched pairs** is another strategy to counteract the selection bias and regression threats. When using a matched pair, individuals are matched together based on a common variable, such as isotonic strength. If you are interested in determining the effects of a plyometric training program on vertical jump height, you could equally distribute your strongest and weakest individuals in the experimental and control groups. You would take the 2 strongest individuals and place 1 in the experimental group and 1 in the control group. Then, you would do the same with the second strongest pair and continue down the list until all people are equally distributed. While this eliminates the option to use the random assignment approach for sampling, it does help to ensure that the control and experimental groups are similar at the start of the intervention. It is also possible that if you choose strength as your matching variable, you may be inadvertently discriminating against another variable (eg, sex, sport position) that you did not intend. Using matched pairs is not always recommended, but it is an option that can be used to better equalize groups.

In addition to internal validity threats that are associated with the participants, there are also internal validity threats that are directly related to the experimental procedures used in conducting the research. When conducting research, there is always a potential for error to occur during data collection. **Testing** is a threat to internal validity that occurs when participants become familiar with the testing procedures. Learning effects can change pre- and post-test scores, so it is important to try to counteract the learning effect of the testing procedures if possible. When assessing body fat composition with hydrostatic weighing, participants are not typically comfortable with the testing procedures as it calls for one to expel all of their air and then submerge themselves under water. If the participant does not feel comfortable with the testing, their initial pretest may not be truly reflective of their body composition. As participants become more comfortable with the assessment through repeated administrations, they tend to improve based solely on the fact that they have learned how to do the assessment better. In instances where there is a large learning effect for the testing procedures, it is recommended that you do some familiarization sessions with the participant to minimize this threat. Another method of counteracting the testing threat is to randomly change the order of testing among participants so that the same test or measurement is not performed first every time. This helps to decrease the effect the first test has on subsequent tests. In addition to a learning effect, a tester or researcher can also influence the performance of a participant. If the tester is extremely encouraging for only some participants, there is a potential for their encouragement to affect the outcomes of the study. A researcher can help counteract this threat by asking the tester to use standardized testing scripts and procedures for each participant.

As discussed with the regression threat, the reliability of measures is extremely important. The use of reliable testing procedures and **instrumentation** helps to reduce this threat. You should make sure that you use instruments and equipment that are regularly calibrated and have been assessed for reliability. You do not want to assume that the scale you are using is accurate at determining an individual's weight, so you would want to calibrate the scale prior to collecting data. Depending on the measure you are taking and the instruments being used, you may need to calibrate your equipment prior to collecting data on each person, but some cases may only require calibration at the commencement of data collection. In addition to instrumentation faults, the testers using the instrumentation can also be a threat to validity. Determining the reliability of the testers is extremely important. Over the course of repeated measurements, the testers will often improve if they were not completely comfortable with the measure initially. This is typically counteracted by having several practice and training sessions with all involved testers. The training helps standardize the testing procedures, and use of instrumentation in practice sessions allow the testers to become more confident and reliable in their measures. Reliability of testers will be discussed in much greater detail in the upcoming chapter.

The final type of internal validity threats are related to the interventions that are administered. **Diffusion** or imitation of treatments refers to when participants of the control group and experimental group are in communication with each other. There are times when blinding cannot occur, so every participant knows the treatment they are receiving. If participants in the experimental group share their treatment experiences with members of the control group, there is diffusion of information between the groups that may not be wanted. If you are treating individuals who have a grade 3 ankle sprain with the experimental treatment (cryokinetics) and a control treatment (cryotherapy and modality), the participants in the control group may discuss their treatment with those in the experimental group. Upon finding out that the participants in the experimental group were completing more exercises and performing active rehabilitation, the participants in the control group may decide to start doing their own exercise program. This would affect the outcome of your study because they are no longer receiving the intended treatment. To counteract the diffusion of treatments threat, it is important to limit communication between participants. This can be achieved by asking participants to keep information to themselves or by physically separating the 2 groups. To separate the groups, you could conduct the study at multiple facilities. Everyone in the control group participates at one facility, and the experimental group is based at a different facility.

Compensatory equalization of treatments is a threat that occurs when a clinician or tester knows that the participant may not be getting the best treatment, so they work extra hard to help a member of the control group compensate for the lack of treatment they are receiving. If you want to study the effects of Kinesio tape (Kinesio) and massage on edema reduction, you could have the experimental group receive Kinesio tape and massage while the control group receives massage only. If the clinician working with members of the control group knows that they are not receiving the full experimental treatment, they may do extra work with the massage treatment to help make up for not receiving the Kinesio taping treatment. To counteract this threat, it is important to blind the clinicians to the different types of treatments being administered if possible. Once again, multiple clinics are often used to minimize this threat, as it eliminates interaction between testers.

The final 2 threats to internal validity are compensatory rivalry and resentful demoralization of respondents. **Compensatory rivalry** occurs when a participant who receives a less desirable treatment or is part of the control group tries to compensate by working harder to make up for the lack of treatment. This is similar to compensatory equalization, but in this case, it is the patient who is putting in extra effort, and they often do not know the other treatment that is being administered. **Resentful demoralization** is the opposite phenomenon and occurs with a participant in the control group who feels devalued and demoralized. Because the participant does not feel as if they are a valuable asset to the research, they may give a lower performance, thus inflating the results of the experimental group. Counteracting this threat is often difficult if you are not able to physically separate the members of the control and experimental group. Blinding and random sampling can help, but they cannot always eliminate this threat.

There are many threats to internal validity, but with stringent sampling procedures and research design methods, you can counteract many of the threats. It is nearly impossible to control for every threat to internal validity; therefore, it is important to identify and control the areas that would be most detrimental to the study. In doing so, you may expose a smaller, less harmful threat. It is important to weigh everything based on the purpose of your study and research questions.

External Validity Threats

External validity explains the ability of a study to be generalized to populations outside of the controlled study. **External validity threats** occur when researchers draw incorrect conclusions or inferences to populations or settings other than what was originally studied. There is a fine line between controlling for all of the external validity threats and designing a study that can be applied in a clinical setting. You can have a study that is extremely well designed in terms of controlling all of the threats to external validity, but you may find that results obtained in the study would never occur in the clinical setting because there is no way to control for everything in the real world. There are 3 main threats to external validity: interaction of treatment and selection, interaction of treatment and setting, and interaction of treatment and history.

Interaction of treatment and selection refers to the selection of participants and the inferences you can make based on the treatment. If the experiment has a narrow range of participants with homogenous characteristics, the researcher cannot generalize the findings to individuals who do not have the same characteristics as the study participants. For example, if a study investigated the effects of intermittent compression on edema at the knee in adolescent patients, it would not be appropriate to infer that intermittent compression is suitable to reduce edema at the knee in a more heterogeneous population (eg, elderly patients, college students, or working adults). Due to the maturation differences in these populations, you would not be able to safely conclude that the effects found on adolescents would be similar to elderly patients.

Interaction of treatment and setting describes the ability of the researcher to generalize the results of the study to a setting that is different from the one where the experiment was conducted. For example, if patients were able to improve strength and range of motion in a supervised rehabilitation setting, it would be important to investigate whether the same results could be obtained via an at-home rehabilitation program. Again, it would be inappropriate to assume that the same results could be obtained in both settings. It would be best for the researcher to implement the same study in the other setting to see if similar results occur.

Another threat to external validity is the **interaction of treatment and history**. Results from an experiment can only be generalized to the current experiment and should not be applied to past or future situations. If you want to apply the results of a previous study, it is important to make sure that the results have been replicated in additional studies and that this research confirms the findings of the previous study. Using treatments from studies several years old could be detrimental because knowledge and protocols change over time, so it is important to use the most current information. For example, several years ago, it was common practice and supported in research literature that casting a patient following ACL reconstruction would result in a better outcome. This threat specifically demonstrates the need for continual research. Research now shows that casting following ACL reconstruction is not supported and could actually be detrimental to the long-term outcomes of the patient.

As in internal validity, there are many external validity threats that need to be controlled. The interaction that treatments have with other treatments and with participants' histories should be considered. Similar to internal validity threats, you need to weigh all of the potential interactions and design a study that will minimize the potential threats as much as possible. When the internal and external validity threats have been controlled for as much as possible, it is then important to address the statistical validity.

Statistical Validity

Statistical conclusion validity addresses whether there is a relationship between the dependent and independent variables. If a researcher draws inaccurate conclusions about the data because of improper statistical analysis or power, then the study has low statistical validity. Many of the statistical threats are described in depth in future chapters, so they are only briefly be discussed here. **Statistical power** addresses the ability to accurately document that there is a defined relationship between the independent and dependent variable. If a study has low statistical power, it typically means that the sample size for the study was not adequate. Other threats to statistical validity include error rate and violated assumptions of statistical tests. The **error rate** becomes a threat when the number of repeated statistical tests increases, leading to incorrect conclusions. There are several types of statistical tests (eg, independent *t*-test, analysis of variance) that can be used to analyze data. It is up to the researcher to ensure that he or she has an appropriate understanding of the differences in these tests so the appropriate statistical analysis can be applied. If the researcher uses the correct statistical analysis for the data type and the measures that were taken, the error rate threat is usually controlled. Implementing the appropriate statistical analysis will also help to control against the **violated assumptions of statistical tests**. Each statistical test has a variety of assumptions that must be met for that statistical test to be accurately applied, so if an incorrect test is used, these assumptions may not be met. Another threat to statistical validity is due to **reliability and variance**. Conclusions drawn from statistical analysis can be vulnerable to variations in the data that may be caused by lack of a formal collection protocol, unreliable measurements, or subjects that differ greatly. For example, if the researcher does not standardize the data collection procedures across patients and does not measure each person in the same manner, there may be variability in the data that are collected.

Validity of Measurements

Controlling the threats to internal and external validity is extremely important to ensure any survey instruments, questionnaires, or outcome measures are also valid. When addressing the **validity of a measurement**, you are concerned about whether a particular instrument or assessment measures what it is intended to measure. For example, a radiograph is a valid measurement of bone integrity, but it is not as valid at assessing soft tissue; thus, it is not intended to measure these structures. There are 4 types of measurement validity: face validity, content validity, criterion-related validity, and construct validity.

Face validity is the least rigorous form of validity because it is often determined by expert opinion or the subjective assessment of a few individuals. Face validity indicates that the instrument or measurement appears to assess what it is supposed to. If creating an assessment to evaluate a patient's satisfaction with their treatment plan, there may be several questions that address concepts of satisfaction. With face validity, this assessment would appear to meet the spirit of the intended assessment, but there are no statistical tests or measurements that are conducted to demonstrate that the instrument measures patient satisfaction. Due to the weakness of this form of validity, some statistical experts would argue that face validity is not a true type of validity.

Content validity refers to the adequacy with which the particular measurement assesses all plausible constructs (ie, a theory to explain a relationship between attitudes and behaviors) it is intended to measure. Content validity is of particular importance in surveys, questionnaires, and interviews because it is important to make sure that all facets of the experience are captured. If an athletic training education program wanted to assess how graduating students rated their experience as an athletic training student, it would be important for questions to be asked about all aspects of the experience, which may include clinical placements, interaction with clinical preceptors, major courses, and internships. If the program's assessment only included questions about the didactic coursework but did not address any of the clinical education requirements, it would not have very strong content validity. Face and content validity are often thought of as interchangeable, but content validity is more rigorous. Content validity is typically assessed by a panel of experts who evaluate the instrument to determine if all intended components are addressed. The panel of experts is usually composed of individuals who have experience with the particular type of assessment or those who have a direct understanding of the subject matter. In the example used above about assessing the experience of graduating students, the panel might consist of the following: alumni of the program, faculty of the athletic training program, department administrators, program director/faculty of a different athletic training program, among others. By including individuals who are familiar and unfamiliar with the program, it would help to ensure that a well-rounded instrument is created. When using a panel of experts, the assessment and revision of an instrument can result in several drafts until all parties determine that there is an adequate representation of all components in the final version of the instrument.

If you are interested in assessing the ability of one test to predict the outcome of another external test, you are using a measure of **criterion-related validity**. This type of validity uses a gold standard reference criterion that is already established to be valid. The **gold standard** is used as the criterion to predict the outcome of your intended test. When choosing a criterion or gold standard, it must be reliable, free of bias, and relevant to what you are intending to measure. For example, if you were interested in determining if a new test was accurate at diagnosing a fracture, you would choose radiography as your gold standard or reference criterion. Criterion-related validity is separated into 2 areas: concurrent validity and predictive validity.

When comparing the results of one test (eg, Lachman's test) against the gold standard (ie, magnetic resonance imaging) simultaneously, you are assessing **concurrent validity**. Typically, to assess concurrent validity, measures of both tests are taken at the same time. Diagnostic or screening tests are often assessed with concurrent validity. For example, if you were interested in assessing body fat percentage, you may consider using the gold standard of hydrostatic weighing. Unfortunately, not all athletic trainers have access to this measurement technique, so you decide to utilize the Cooper Clinic guidelines for skinfold assessment of body fat percentage. If this method had not already been validated, you would need to go through the validation process. To validate a new measurement, it would be best to assess multiple individuals using both techniques to determine whether the skinfold technique was an accurate method of assessing body fat percentage. If you are trying to validate an assessment where there is no gold standard with which to compare it, there is a challenge in establishing the validity. In these cases, other forms of testing must be utilized to establish validity of the instrument or measurement.

Predictive validity is used when you are trying to establish a predictor of a future criterion score. To assess predictive validity, you would need to give your assessment (eg, college entrance examination) in one session and then wait until the criterion score is obtained (eg, final college grade point average). You are trying to determine the relationship between the 2 variables to see if the score on the entrance examination can predict a student's college success as determined by their grade point average. Predictive validity is used to predict risk of injury, to determine a prognosis, or to determine outcomes. Due to the time between measures that occurs in predictive validity that does not occur in concurrent validity, there are limitations in follow-up and tracking subjects through completion of both measures.

The ability of an instrument or assessment to measure a more abstract concept is referred to as **construct validity**. When assessing the concept of function, it is a multifaceted construct that could be assessed in several ways; function is not an absolute or directly observable construct;

therefore, it is difficult to determine if you are actually measuring the variable of interest. When you think about a person's function, measurements of pain, range of motion, strength, balance, and other factors could all play a part. A survey instrument could have 25 items that address each of the different functional tasks with a portion related to each strength, pain, balance, etc. There are specific statistical analyses that can be used to determine the validity of these separate components (ie, range of motion, strength, pain) on the construct of function. A factor analysis will determine which components best fit within the construct of function, thus helping to validate each construct within the instrument.

Summary

As you apply the concepts of validity, it is important to remember that the threats are numerous and must be considered when evaluating information or when designing a study. Not all threats to validity are equal; therefore, you must prioritize them and weigh the outcome if you are not addressing a particular threat. Research studies are far from perfect; however, consideration of aspects of validity may assist you in making a clinical decision that benefits your patient in the short or long term.

Keys Points

- When research involves human participants, each individual has a different background, thus making variability between the participants a potential threat to internal validity.
- It is also important to select a larger number than what you believe is necessary to account for the mortality that will occur.
- Face and content validity are often thought of as interchangeable, but content validity is more rigorous.
- Content validity is typically assessed by a panel of experts who evaluate the instrument to determine if all intended components are addressed. The panel of experts usually comprises individuals who have experience with the particular type of assessment or those who have a direct understanding of the subject matter.

Bibliography

Behi R, Nolan M. Causality and control: threats to internal validity. *Br J Nurs.* 1996;10(5):374-377.
Downing SM. Validity: on the meaningful interpretation of assessment data. *Med Educ.* 2003;37(9):830-837.
Ferguson L. External validity, generalizability, and knowledge utilization. *J Nurs Scholarsh.* 2004;36(1):16-22.
Greenfield ML, Kuhn JE, Wojtys EM. A statistics primer. *Am J Sports Med.* 1996;24(3):393-395.
Sim J, Arnell P. Measurement validity in physical therapy research. *Phys Ther.* 1993;73(2):102-110.
Turlik M. Evaluating the internal validity of a randomized controlled trial. *FAOJ.* 2009;2(3):5.

8

Measures of Reliability

Reliability refers to the consistency of a specific measurement or data point. For example, when you are appraising research, it can be thought of as a means of determining if a measure is consistent or error free. You can assess reliability in terms of raters, instruments, or testing procedures. If we do not have reliability, then we cannot be sure that data we collect are consistent. In this chapter, we discuss the different types of reliability and introduce the most common statistical operations utilized to assess each type of reliability.

Rater Reliability

Intrarater reliability (ie, within or inside) refers to the consistency of data recorded by one individual across multiple trials. If you were going to assess range of motion at the humeroulnar joint, you would want to make sure that the rater measuring the range of motion was reliable. To do this, you would ask the rater to measure the available range of motion at the humeroulnar joint over several trials (more than 2) on multiple people. Table 8-1 provides 3 trials of 1 rater for 4 subjects. From a quick view, it is apparent that rater A is consistent in the measurements for each of the subjects.

Interrater reliability (ie, between or among) refers to the consistency of data recorded by multiple individuals who measure the same group of subjects. If you were going to use multiple athletic trainers to assess balance by using the Balance Error Scoring System (BESS) during a preparticipation examination, you would want to make sure that all of the raters scoring the BESS were reliable (ie, they score the same errors during the test). To assess the interrater reliability, you would have at least 2 people score the BESS on multiple individuals. Having each rater watch the BESS trial simultaneously allows for the measurement error to be further reduced because each rater is viewing the same thing, allowing for a representation of the true difference in scores. It is important that before you try to establish interrater reliability, you first determine the individual reliability (ie, intrarater reliability) for each rater. In Table 8-2, you can see that rater B has

Van Lunen BL, Hankemeier DA, Welch CE.
Evidence-Guided Practice: A Framework for Clinical Decision Making in Athletic Training (pp 79–86).

Table 8-1.
Intrarater Reliability of Humeroulnar Flexion Range of Motion

	SUBJECT 1			SUBJECT 2			SUBJECT 3			SUBJECT 4		
Trial	T1	T2	T3	T1	T2	T3	T1	T2	T3	T1	T2	T3
Rater A	145	142	142	138	138	137	140	141	142	132	132	132

Table 8-2.
Interrater Reliability of the Balance Error Scoring System

	BESS SCORE SUBJECT 1 (TOTAL NO. OF ERRORS)	BESS SCORE SUBJECT 2 (TOTAL NO. OF ERRORS)	BESS SCORE SUBJECT 3 (TOTAL NO. OF ERRORS)
Rater A	12	20	18
Rater B	14	23	19

Abbreviation: BESS, Balance Error Scoring System.

consistently higher scores than rater A each time, but the discrepancies between the raters are not drastically different. To determine if the raters have good reliability, an intraclass correlation coefficient (ICC) should be used.

Statistical Application for Rater Reliability

An ICC is most commonly used to determine if the reliability of one rater or a group of raters is consistent. The ICC is a reliability coefficient statistical measure that is sensitive to changes between raters and/or between trials. There are 3 common ICC models that are used to assess reliability data (Table 8-3). This table explains how raters are selected and how data are assessed for each ICC model. Additionally, the table provides the mathematical formula for calculating the ICC value for each model. When discussing the ICC models, it is important to understand that the values in the parentheses indicate the model and form, respectively. An ICC (2,1) indicates that it is model 2 and form 1. The **model** (first number) differs in accordance to how the raters are chosen within a study and how they are assigned to the subjects. The **form** (second number) is determined if you are using an average of measures (referred to as k) or a single measure (referred to as 1).

The practice of using an ICC (1,1) or (1,k) model is rarely performed in reliability studies because each subject is being assessed by a different rater. It would be extremely difficult to assess the reliability if all subjects were being assessed by a different rater. Intraclass correlation coefficient models (2,1) and (2,k) are chosen when the subjects and raters are considered to be randomly selected from the larger population, thus allowing the results to be generalized outside the study. For example, if you wanted to assess the ability of athletic training students to accurately assess dorsiflexion range of motion, you would randomly select students from all over the country. The students are selected from the larger population, so an ICC model 2 would be best because those students are a representative sample of all athletic training students. Intraclass correlation

Table 8-3.
Intraclass Correlation Coefficient Models

MODEL	FORMULA	DESCRIPTION
ICC (1,1)	$\frac{BMS - WMS}{BMS + (k - 1)\ WMS}$	• Used when each subject is assessed by a different set of randomly selected raters • Uses a single measure, not an average of measures
ICC (1,k)	$\frac{BMS - WMS}{BMS}$	• Used when each subject is assessed by different set of randomly selected raters • Uses the average of the raters' measurements
ICC (2,1)	$\frac{BMS - EMS}{BMS + (k - 1)\ EMS + k\ (TMS - EMS)/n}$	• Used to make generalizations across raters • All subjects are tested by the same raters who represent a random sample of all possible raters • Uses a single measure, not an average of measures
ICC (2,k)	$\frac{BMS - EMS}{BMS + (TMS - EMS)/n}$	• Used to make generalizations across raters • Uses the same assumptions about the raters but uses an average of measures
ICC (3,1)	$\frac{BMS - EMS}{BMS + (k - 1)EMS}$	• Used when you do not want to make generalizations across raters • Uses a single measure, not an average of measures
ICC (3,k)	$\frac{BMS - EMS}{BMS}$	• Used when you do not want to make generalizations across raters • Uses the same assumptions about the raters but uses an average of measures

Abbreviations: BMS, between mean square; EMS, error mean square; ICC, intraclass correlation coefficient; k, number of trials; n, number of subjects; TMS, trial mean square; WMS, within mean square.

coefficient models (3,1) and (3,k) should be used to assess intrarater reliability because only a single rater is used. Since intrarater reliability is only concerned with the reliability of one person, model 3 should be used because it accounts for making generalizations across raters. For interrater

Table 8-4.
Interclass Correlation Coefficient Value Interpretation

SOURCE	LEVEL OF RELIABILITY	ICC VALUE
Shrout[1]	Substantial reliability	.81 to 1.00
	Moderate reliability	.61 to .80
	Fair reliability	.41 to 60
	Slight reliability	.11 to .40
	No reliability	.00 to .10
Portney & Watkins[2]	Good reliability	.75 to 1.00
	Poor to moderate reliability	≤.75
Abbreviation: ICC, interclass correlation coefficient.		

reliability, ICC model 2 or 3 can be used depending on whether generalization across raters is not needed (model 3) or if the raters are representative of the larger population (model 2).

An ICC value commonly ranges from 0.00 to 1.00, with higher values representing stronger reliability. There is a potential for the ICC value to be negative when certain calculations are performed. There are several guidelines for interpretation of reliability values. Two commonly used interpretation scales are shown in Table 8-4. Regardless of the guidelines used, a researcher or clinician must be able to justify their interpretation of the reliability coefficients. If you were measuring the reliability of a blood test to determine if someone has high cholesterol, you would want to ensure that test has high reliability, so more stringent reliability values[1] would be warranted. If we use the BESS example in which rater B was consistently higher than rater A, the ICC value of their reliability with each other is .786. If we look at the table, we can see that this value indicates moderate[1] or good[2] reliability.

Instrument Reliability

Test-retest reliability is a form of reliability that assesses the stability of an instrument. To assess test-retest reliability, a group of individuals is assessed in the same manner on 2 different occasions. All testing conditions should remain as close to the same as possible. Typically, test-retest reliability is used for survey instruments, psychological measures, and instances in which raters are not involved. Since you are trying to assess the reliability of an instrument, it is important to keep the time in between administrations of the instrument in mind. If you want to assess the consistency of a health-related quality of life questionnaire that is 100 questions long, you would not want to give the assessment on back-to-back days because answer fatigue may set in. The participant may not want to truthfully answer the questions a second time since they just did it the day before, or they may remember the answers they chose the day before. However, you do not want to allow too much time to pass during administrations because that could allow actual health changes to occur, which would also affect the results. The length of time depends on what instrument you are trying to assess, so make sure that you consider all variables when selecting your testing periods. Test-retest reliability is often used when analyzing the reliability of knowledge assessments. If you wanted to assess the test-retest reliability of a 50-question multiple choice examination, you would ask participants to take the examination and then ask them to repeat the

Table 8-5.
Percent Agreement

		Rater 1	
		Within Normal Limits	*Not Within Normal Limits*
RATER 2	*Within Normal Limits*	60[a]	15
	Not Within Normal Limits	10	15[a]

[a]Indicates exact agreement.

examination 1 week later. You would then compare the participants' responses on both administrations of the examination. To ensure that you get the most reliable information, it would be best to ask participants to refrain from looking up information they did not know the first time, so the responses the second time do not change due to an increase in knowledge they obtained after the first administration of the examination.

Test-retest reliability can also be used on assessments that evaluate an individual's ability or level of preparedness. You would ask the individual to rate him- or herself and then repeat the assessment a week later. With any type of test-retest reliability, you are aiming to see similar results from one administration to the next, indicating that the instrument has good reliability. Clinically, neurocognitive tests after a concussion (eg, ImPACT test) require high test-retest reliability because the test is administered on multiple occasions, and you want to make sure changes that are seen are due to the patient changing, not because the test is unreliable.

Internal consistency is another form of reliability used to assess the characteristics of a group of items. Internal consistency is often used to evaluate scale items of surveys or assessments. To have good internal consistency, you want to have good homogeneity of all the items in the scale. If you have an assessment of 15 scale items measuring concepts (eg, physical function, psychological function, and cognitive function), you would expect that the 5 questions assessing cognitive function should be moderately correlated with each other. Likewise, you would expect the physical function items (n = 5) and the psychological items (n = 5) to be correlated within each category.

Statistical Application for Instrument Reliability

To assess test-retest reliability, ICCs are the preferred method since they account for correlation and agreement. When using an ICC for test-retest reliability for an instrument, you should think of it similarly to that of using a single rater, so ICC (3,1) is often used. Percent agreement is one of the simplest forms of reliability assessment. **Percent agreement** is determined by taking the sum of observed agreements divided by the number of paired scores obtained. For this example, 2 raters assessing subjective hamstring flexibility placed individuals in 1 of 2 categories: within normal limits or not within normal limits. The 2 raters each assessed 100 individuals and placed them into 1 of the 2 categories using a 2-by-2 contingency table (Table 8-5). To determine the percent agreement, you add the number of exact agreements by both raters and divide it by the number of possible agreements. The annotated values in the table show exact agreement between both raters for number of possible agreements. The number of exact agreements is 75 out of a possible 100 agreements, indicating a 75% agreement. This value is high, but there is a possibility that some of these agreements happened by chance. Although percent agreement can be used to demonstrate instrument reliability, it can also be used to show the basic agreement of other measures as well (eg, correct diagnoses).

Table 8-6.
Kappa Example

	ANTERIOR PELVIC TILT (NO. OF INDIVIDUALS)	POSTERIOR PELVIC TILT (NO. OF INDIVIDUALS)
Rater A	28	22
Rater B	35	15

Table 8-7.
Weighted Kappa

	ANTERIOR PELVIC TILT (NO. OF INDIVIDUALS)	NEUTRAL PELVIS (NO. OF INDIVIDUALS)	POSTERIOR PELVIC TILT (NO. OF INDIVIDUALS)
Rater A	15	25	10
Rater B	20	23	7

To measure internal consistency of instrument scales, **Cronbach's alpha** (α) is used. Cronbach's alpha values range from 0.0 to 1, with values around 0.90 considered to be highly reliable. When assessing scale items of surveys or assessments, it is often recommended that strong internal consistency be found with values between 0.7 and 0.9.[3,4] If values are found to be too high, it may indicate that items within the scale are redundant and could be replaced, while values that are too low indicate that they are measuring different ideas that are not intended.

Statistical Application for Nominal Reliability Data

The statistical applications discussed previously are used specifically for ratio and interval data. Because nominal data are categorical in nature, they do not have a numeric value, so the kappa statistic is most often used. Unlike percent agreement, a **kappa statistic** is used with categorical data to assess the proportion of observed agreements as well as the agreements expected by chance. A 2-by-2 contingency table is often used when analyzing data with the kappa statistic because each rater places data into a predetermined category. The kappa is a measure of true agreement and is written as a formula, (k = observed agreement - chance agreement/1 - chance agreement). Kappa ratings can range from –1 to 1, although most values fall between 0 and 1. A rating of 0 would indicate that agreement is no better than what is expected by chance, which means that the raters would have guessed at every rating. Kappa statistics are often used when there are only 2 categories to rate. For example, if you were going to ask 2 raters to assess pelvic tilt on 50 patients, you may ask each rater to classify each patient with anterior or posterior pelvic tilt (Table 8-6). From the data in the table, you can see that the raters looked at the patients very differently. Based on these data, you may find that you cannot classify each person into one of these categories because some individuals have a neutral pelvis (Table 8-7). In this case, you would need to add another category; thus, you need to use a weighted kappa statistic. **Weighted kappa statistics** account for the number of categories and penalize the disagreement in terms of seriousness.

Table 8-8.
Weighted Kappa With One Category Unfilled

	ANTERIOR PELVIC TILT (NO. OF INDIVIDUALS)	NEUTRAL PELVIS (NO. OF INDIVIDUALS)	POSTERIOR PELVIC TILT (NO. OF INDIVIDUALS)
Rater A	15	25	10
Rater B	23	27	0

Table 8-9.
Kappa Coefficient Values

LEVEL OF AGREEMENT	KAPPA VALUE
Almost perfect agreement	.81 to 1.00
Substantial agreement	.61 to .80
Moderate agreement	.41 to 60
Fair agreement	.21 to .40
Slight agreement	.01 to .20
Poor agreement	≤0

Adapted from Landis JR, Koch GG. The measurement of observer agreement for categorical data. *Biometrics.* 1977;33(1):159-174.

For example, if you rate someone as having anterior pelvic tilt, but the other rater classifies the same subject as having a neutral pelvis, there is a disagreement between raters, but that disagreement is not as severe as if one rater classified as a pelvic tilt as anterior and the other rater classified it as posterior. Using a weighted kappa statistic allows for more categories to be utilized, and it takes into account the amount of disagreement. To effectively use a kappa statistic, the data obtained from the measurements of each rater must be present in each category. If one rater did not rate anyone with a posterior pelvic tilt but the other rater had subjects in each of the 3 categories, a kappa statistic cannot be used (Table 8-8). When this situation occurs, percent agreement must be used to determine the agreement between the 2 raters. Like ICC values, there are several interpretation guidelines for the kappa coefficient. Table 8-9 shows one of the recommended guidelines to use for the kappa coefficient.

Summary

For a clinical test to be used within clinical practice, you will need to determine aspects of reliability that could affect the outcome. Reliability focuses on the reproducibility of a test or examiner and is an essential attribute to consider. Reliability can be assessed in a variety of ways depending upon the type of data with which you are dealing. In the end, you want your instrument or tester to be as reliable and consistent as possible.

Key Points

- Without reliability, we cannot be sure that the data we collect are consistent. Regardless of the guidelines used, a researcher or clinician must be able to justify their interpretation of the reliability.
- Reliability can refer to rater reliability or instrument reliability.
- Intraclass correlation coefficients consist of determining a model (how raters are chosen and assigned) and a form (using an average of measures or a single measure).
- Kappa statistics are used with nominal data to assess the proportion of observed agreements as well as the agreements expected by chance.

References

1. Shrout PE. Measurement reliability and agreement in psychiatry. *Stat Methods Med Res.* 1998;7(3):301-317.
2. Portney LG, Watkins MP. *Foundations of Clinical Research: Applications to Practice.* 3rd ed. Upper Saddle River, NJ: Pearson Prentice Hall; 2009.
3. Boyle GJ. Does item homogeneity indicate internal consistency or item redundancy in psychometric scales? *Personality Individ Differences.* 1991;12:291-294.
4. Cronbach LJ. Coefficient alpha and the internal structure of tests. *Psychometrika.* 1951;16:297-334.

Bibliography

Boyle GJ. Does item homogeneity indicate internal consistency or item redundancy in psychometric scales? *Personality Individ Differences.* 1991;12:291-294.

Cohen J. Weighted kappa: nominal scale agreement with provision for scaled disagreement or partial credit. *Psychol Bull.* 1968;70(4):213-220.

McGinn T, Wyer PC, Newman TB, et al. Tips for learners of evidence-based medicine: 3. Measures of observer variability (kappa statistic). *CMAJ.* 2004;171(11):1369-1373.

Shrout PE, Fleiss JL. Intraclass correlations: uses in assessing rater reliability. *Psychol Bull.* 1979;86:420-428.

Sim J, Wright CC. The kappa statistic in reliability studies: use, interpretation and sample size requirements. *Phys Ther.* 2005;85(3):257-268.

Viera AJ, Garrett JM. Understanding interobserver agreement: the kappa statistic. *Fam Med.* 2005;37(5):360-363.

Weir JP. Quantifying test-retest reliability using the intraclass correlation coefficient and the SEM. *J Strength Cond Res.* 2005;19(1):231-240.

9

Diagnostic Accuracy

The use of valid diagnostic tests in your clinical practice is vital to making grounded decisions for the assessment of your patients. Athletic training competencies no longer encompass detailed lists of clinical diagnostic tests (eg, tissue tests, special tests) that must be included within didactic curricula. The competencies merely state that athletic training students must be able to assess and interpret findings from a physical examination that is based on the patient's clinical presentation. To determine which clinical diagnostic tests are most relevant for a condition, the test must be examined for various concepts.

When a patient presents to you with an injury, it is up to you to conduct a thorough examination to decide how to direct the treatment plan. Many available clinical diagnostic tests have been identified as being able to correctly identify a condition (eg, rotator cuff tear, foot metatarsal fracture); however, if you examine the tests a bit more in depth, you may see that much of the information is not as helpful as previously thought. For example, the pivot shift test is purported to be clinically useful in confirming anterior cruciate ligament (ACL) tears; however, this test is often not conclusive due to muscle guarding or the absence of the shift within certain patients who actually have an ACL tear.

The validity of a clinical diagnostic test is measured through mathematical equations that compare the clinical diagnostic test to a reference standard. This is often demonstrated within a 2-by-2 contingency table (Figure 9-1), which will be explained within this section. The contingency table incorporates all of the individuals who were examined with the clinical diagnostic test and compares the findings (positive or negative) with the reference or gold standard findings (positive or negative). A **reference standard** represents the most accurate tool (eg, radiograph to confirm a fracture, arthroscopy to confirm a ligament injury) available for assessing a current condition or determining an outcome. Reference standards are often expensive, difficult to access, labor intensive, or invasive; therefore, you will often seek other clinical alternatives to determine an outcome. The reference standard is something that clearly determines that the condition exists. In orthopedic examinations, the reference standard is usually visual inspection during a surgical intervention, but you will often see other reference standards, such as radiographs, magnetic

Van Lunen BL, Hankemeier DA, & Welch CE.
Evidence-Guided Practice: A Framework for Clinical Decision Making in Athletic Training (pp 87-99).

(A)		Reference Standard	
		Reference Standard Positive	Reference Standard Negative
Clinical Diagnostic Test Result	Clinical Diagnostic Test Positive	a **True Positive**	b False Positive
	Clinical Diagnostic Test Negative	c False Negative	d **True Negative**

(B)		Reference Standard		
		Arthroscopic Examination Positive	Arthroscopic Examination Negative	
Tibiofemoral Test	Tibiofemoral Test Positive	a **True Positive (8)**	b False Positive (2)	Total = 10
	Tibiofemoral Test Negative	c False Negative (7)	d **True Negative (23)**	Total = 30
		Total =15	Total = 25	Overall Total = 40

Figure 9-1. (A) Reference standard and clinical diagnostic test comparison. (B) Application of the tibiofemoral test within a 2-by-2 contingency table.

resonance images, and bone densitometry. As a health care provider, you will tend to err on the side of caution when managing an injury; therefore, if a good clinical diagnostic test or set of tests is not available, you would seek confirmation from more expensive tests to determine the outcome.

To explain the components of a contingency table, we will use a fictitious clinical diagnostic test, the tibiofemoral stress test, which will be used for diagnosing an ACL injury. You would perform the tibiofemoral stress test on every individual during the year if you suspected ACL involvement. Let us say that you had 40 individuals sustain a potential ACL knee injury over the course of the year and you had 10 with a positive finding on the tibiofemoral stress test. You would then record your findings for the clinical diagnostic test as being positive for 10 individuals and negative for 30 individuals. Then, when the patient underwent arthroscopic examination, you would record a positive or negative reference standard finding. The 10 individuals whom you found to have had a positive clinical diagnostic test may not necessarily be part of the group that will have a positive reference standard test. Let us say that the arthroscopic examination confirmed that there were 15 positive findings and 25 negative findings for ACL injury. Now it is time to put all of this information into the contingency table so that you can see it all come together.

The 2-by-2 contingency table (see Figure 9-1) includes verbiage related to the comparisons between the clinical diagnostic test and reference standard. The **true positives** include those individuals for whom the clinical diagnostic test was positive and the reference standard was positive, indicating that there was agreement. To apply this to our example, we need to input the values (see Figure 9-1) for each patient; if patient 1 had a positive clinical diagnostic test (ie, tibiofemoral stress test) and had a positive reference standard test (ie, arthroscopic examination), then they would be counted within box a of the contingency table. For the purposes of our example, we determined that there were 8 true positives for the sample. The **true negatives** include those individuals for whom the clinical diagnostic test was negative and the reference standard was negative, also

		Reference Standard		
		Arthroscopic Examination Positive	Arthroscopic Examination Negative	
Powden Test	Powden Test Positive	a **True Positive (100)**	b False Positive (50)	Total = 150
	Powden Test Negative	c False Negative (30)	**d** **True Negative (80)**	Total = 110
		Total = 130	Total = 130	Overall Total = 260

Figure 9-2. Contingency table for the Powden test to detect meniscal injury.

indicating agreement. Again, we would enter our information from our findings and put patients in box d if both tests were negative for the patient. Together, the true positives and the true negatives form the foundation of the testing, and the **percent accuracy** of the clinical diagnostic test can be derived by combining these values and dividing the sum by the total number of tests performed. You will need to multiply the outcome by 100 to get a percentage value.

$$\text{Percent Accuracy} = \frac{\text{True Positives} + \text{True Negatives}}{\text{Total No. of Patients}}$$

The disagreement between the clinical diagnostic test and reference standard is represented by the **false negative** (negative clinical diagnostic finding but positive reference standard finding) and **false positive** (positive clinical diagnostic finding but negative reference standard finding) results. If we applied this information to our example using the tibiofemoral stress test, then our contingency table (see Figure 9-1) would contain:

- 8 true positives (both tests agreed that the ACL was torn; box a)
- 23 true negatives (both tests agreed that the ACL was not torn; box d)
- 7 false negatives (reference standard indicated injury to the ACL but diagnostic test did not; box c)
- 2 false positives (reference standard indicated no injury to the ACL but clinical diagnostic test did; box b)

The percent accuracy of the clinical diagnostic test seems to be fairly high:

$$\text{Percent Accuracy} = \frac{\text{True Positives} + \text{True Negatives}}{\text{Total No. of Patients}} = \frac{8+23}{40} = 77.5\%$$

However, in the case of this example, it is easy to see that the clinical diagnostic test was not in agreement for some of the individuals with an actual ACL injury (7 individuals). A valid clinical diagnostic test consistently produces true positives, true negatives, or both.

This is further explained through another example. Figure 9-2 provides information on all individuals who underwent a fictitious clinical diagnostic test, the Powden test, for meniscal injury. The reference standard used to confirm meniscal injury was arthroscopic examination. Each cell of the contingency table can be interpreted as follows:

- Box a represents the individuals who had a positive Powden test and a positive meniscal tear confirmed by arthroscopic examination (true positives).

- Box b represents the individuals who had a positive Powden test but for whom no meniscal tear was found during arthroscopic examination (false positives).
- Box c represents the individuals who had a negative Powden test but for whom a meniscal tear was confirmed by arthroscopic examination (false negatives).
- Box d represents the individuals who had a negative Powden test and for whom no meniscal tear was found during arthroscopic examination (true negatives).

Based upon the information provided within Figure 9-2, it appears that the Powden Test has similar results as findings upon arthroscopic examination for 180 (true positives + true negatives) of the individuals; however, there is disagreement for the remaining 80 patients (percent accuracy: 180/260 = 69%).

$$\text{Percent Accuracy} = \frac{\text{True Positives} + \text{True Negatives}}{\text{Total No. of Patients}} = \frac{100+80}{260} = 69.0\%$$

To examine the information from the contingency table findings in more depth, additional mathematical equations are applied to understand what everything truly means. Just obtaining the accuracy of a clinical diagnostic test should not be satisfactory because you want to know how your other findings (false positives and false negatives) affect the meaning of the findings. Sensitivity and specificity calculations are often conducted to further explain these findings. **Sensitivity** refers to the capability of the diagnostic test to correctly classify individuals with the condition of interest (true positives). Sensitivity can be calculated by taking all the individuals with the condition who test positive on the clinical test (box a from the table in Figures 9-1 and 9-2) and dividing that value by all the patients who are confirmed as having the condition with the reference test (boxes a + c from the table). You will need to multiply the outcome by 100 to get a percentage value.

$$\text{Sensitivity} = \frac{\text{True Positives}}{(\text{True Positives} + \text{False Negatives})} \text{ OR } \frac{\text{Box a}}{(\text{Boxes a} + \text{c})}$$

Utilizing the Powden contingency table, you would use box a (100) and divide it by boxes a + c (130) for a sensitivity value of .77, or 77%. A sensitivity of 77% indicates that the Powden test is able to detect meniscal injury 77% of the time.

$$\text{Sensitivity} = \frac{\text{Box a}}{(\text{Boxes a} + \text{c})} \text{ OR } \frac{100}{(100+30)} = 77\%$$

Specificity refers to the capability of the diagnostic test to correctly classify individuals who do not have the condition. Specificity can be calculated by taking all of the patients who had a negative diagnostic test (box d from the table) and dividing that value by all the patients who are confirmed as not having the condition with the reference test (boxes d + b from the table). You will need to multiply the outcome by 100 to get a percentage value.

$$\text{Specificity} = \frac{\text{True Negatives}}{(\text{True Negatives} + \text{False Positives})} \text{ OR } \frac{\text{Box d}}{(\text{Boxes d} + \text{b})}$$

Utilizing the Powden contingency table, you would use box d (80) and divide it by boxes d + b (130) for a specificity value of .62, or 62%. A specificity value of 62% indicates that the Powden test correctly classifies an individual as not having a meniscal injury 62% of the time.

$$\text{Specificity} = \frac{\text{Box d}}{(\text{Boxes d} + \text{b})} \text{ OR } \frac{80}{(80+50)} = 62\%$$

You seek to find a clinical diagnostic test with high sensitivity and specificity, but this is often difficult, as there are factors that affect the outcome values. As you recall, the percent accuracy of the Powden test for classifying whether an individual had a meniscal injury was 69%. Accuracy is heavily influenced by the prevalence of the condition, so you still do not know much about the

(A)

Study 1: Harrison et al, 2009 *(referred patients with meniscal tears)*		Reference Standard		
		Arthroscopic Examination Positive	Arthroscopic Examination Negative	
Thessaly Test	Thessaly Test Positive	a **True Positive (65)**	b False Positive (1)	Total = 66
	Thessaly Test Negative	c False Negative (7)	d **True Negative (43)**	Total = 50
		Total = 72	Total = 44	Overall Total = 116

(B)

Study 2: Mirzatolooei et al, 2010 *(Patients with ACL tear as the primary condition)*		Reference Standard		
		Arthroscopic Examination Positive	Arthroscopic Examination Negative	
Thessaly Test	Thessaly Test Positive	a **True Positive (31)**	b False Positive (24)	Total = 55
	Thessaly Test Negative	c False Negative (8)	d **True Negative (17)**	Total = 25
		Total = 39	Total = 41	Overall Total = 80

Figure 9-3. Contingency tables for the Thessaly test to detect meniscal injury in studies (A) 1 and (B) 2.

usefulness of the test. **Prevalence** refers to the number of cases of a condition existing in a given population at any one time. If a condition happens to be prevalent within the sample that is being examined, then more individuals will already potentially have the condition of interest, making it easier to detect. Prevalence of a condition changes based on the group being studied. For example, the prevalence of eating disorders from a study in 2004 is higher in athletes (28%) than in controls (10%), higher in female athletes (20%) than in male athletes (8%), and more common among those competing in leanness-dependent and weight-dependent sports than in other sports. Therefore, when determining if your patient may test positive with the diagnostic test that you are using, knowing the prevalence of the condition in the population may affect your outcomes.

Let us consider findings from 2 separate studies concerning the use of the Thessaly test for detecting meniscal tears (Figure 9-3).

- Study 1 included patients who were referred by primary care providers to the Department of Orthopedic Surgery for suspected meniscal pathology.
- Study 2 included individuals with magnetic resonance imaging–confirmed ACL injury and unknown involvement of the menisci.

Upon initial review of Figure 9-3, it is evident that study 1 reported higher accuracy, specificity, and sensitivity. This is most likely due to the fact that the individuals were referred primarily because the physicians thought there was some type of meniscal injury. In fact, when conducting the mathematical equations for diagnostic accuracy of the Thessaly test, the values demonstrated a 94% accuracy for study 1 and a 60% accuracy for study 2.

NAME OF TEST	EQUATION	STUDY 1	STUDY 2
Accuracy	a+d/(a+b+c+d)	109/116=94%	48/80=60%
Sensitivity	a/(a+c)	65/72=90%	31/39=79%
Specificity	d/(b+d)	43/44=98%	17/41=41%

In study 2, the focus was on ACL injury, and meniscal involvement may have also been associated with the condition. Therefore, the prevalence in the sample was already lower because the primary injury was to the ACL; therefore, applying the Thessaly test in this situation was more difficult because of the inherent pain and instability from the injury to the ACL.

Other pieces of the puzzle that should be examined include **positive predictive values** (PPVs) and **negative predictive values** (NPVs) that are derived from the contingency table and are related to disease prevalence, which assists you with applying the information within the clinical realm. The PPV is an estimate of a diagnostic test to correctly determine the proportion of patients with the disease from all of the patients with positive test results.

$$\text{PPV} = \frac{\text{True Positives (box a)}}{\text{True Positives and False Positives (boxes a + b)}} \text{ OR } \frac{\text{Patients With Condition Who Test Positive}}{\text{All Patients With Positive Test Results}}$$

The NPV is an estimate of a diagnostic test to correctly determine the proportion of patients without the disease from all of the patients with negative test results.

$$\text{NPV} = \frac{\text{True Negatives (box d)}}{\text{False Negatives and True Negatives (boxes c + d)}} \text{ OR } \frac{\text{Patients Without Condition Who Test Negative}}{\text{All Patients With Negative Test Results}}$$

From our Powden meniscal test example, the PPV and NPV would equate to:

$$\text{PPV} = \frac{\text{box a}}{\text{boxes a + b}} = \frac{100}{100 + 50} = 67\%$$

$$\text{NPV} = \frac{\text{box d}}{\text{boxes c + d}} = \frac{80}{80 + 30} = 73\%$$

The PPV of 67% means that the estimated probability that the patient has the disease in question given a positive test is 67%, while the NPV means that the estimated probability that the patient does not have the disorder given a negative test is 73%. This information provides you with estimates for the predictive value of the diagnostic test; however, these values are affected by the prevalence of the condition. Close scrutiny must be taken when examining the source of the findings. For example, if more individuals who are truly expected to have the condition of interest are in the study, then the diagnostic test may be more apt to identify them as having the condition (high PPV).

Diagnostic tests are utilized to help you make a decision about whether an individual patient may have a certain condition. You usually have an idea as to what condition a patient may have prior to doing any type of physical examination because you have discussed the history of injury thoroughly and obtained feedback from the patient through visual observation. This idea has been identified as **pretest probability**, or the odds/probability that a patient has a condition based on clinical presentation before a diagnostic test is conducted. You will use your clinical experiences, best judgment, and information from the literature to determine what you believe to be the pretest probability that the patient has the condition. Remember, you can make a good estimate if you understand what the prevalence of the condition is within the population that is linked to your patient. For example, you know that females have a higher rate of ACL injury than males, and you also have an idea of what sports are linked with higher rates of ACL injury. Therefore, if a female basketball player presents to you with a clinical presentation of an ACL injury, then the ligamentous integrity test (ie, Lachman's test) you choose to assess the patient will most likely identify a positive test. You can find the prevalence of an injury in a particular study by dividing the total number of subjects who have the condition (boxes a + c) by the total number of subjects in the study. For example, the prevalence within the Powden example would be:

$$\text{Powden Study Prevalence} = (100 + 30)/260 \quad \text{OR} \quad .50 \text{ or } 50\%$$

The calculation of prevalence in the Powden example can be used for the patient's/client's pretest probability of the condition if a known prevalence of the condition in the population is not known.

These pretest probabilities are used in conjunction with the likelihood of an individual to have or not have the condition (likelihood ratios [LRs]) to determine posttest probabilities. Likelihood ratios combine sensitivity and specificity to evaluate the diagnostic accuracy of a test for an individual patient and are termed as positive or negative. A **positive likelihood ratio** (LR+) indicates that a positive test result was obtained in a person with the condition as compared with a person without the condition and is expressed as a ratio. It is a ratio of sensitivity to 1-specificity and is expressed as:

$$LR+ = \frac{\text{Sensitivity}}{1 - \text{Specificity}} \quad \text{OR} \quad \frac{(a/a + c)}{\left[1 - (d/b + d)\right]}$$

This ratio provides you with an estimate as to whether an individual with a disease is more likely to test positive compared with someone without the disease. A good test will have a high LR+ (values greater than 2). However, a **negative likelihood ratio** (LR–) indicates the likelihood that a negative test result was observed in a person with the condition compared with a person without the condition. It is a ratio of 1-Sensitivity to Specificity and is expressed as:

$$LR- = \frac{1 - \text{Sensitivity}}{\text{Specificity}} \quad \text{OR} \quad \frac{\left[1 - (a/a + c)\right]}{(d/b + d)}$$

This ratio provides you with an estimate of how much less likely someone with a disease is to test negative than someone without the disease. A good test will have a very low LR– (value closer to zero). Let us return to our example for the hypothetical Powden test (see Figure 9-2) used to detect meniscal injury and calculate the LR+ and LR–:

$$LR+ = \frac{.77}{1 - .62} \quad \text{OR} \quad \frac{1(00/100 + 30)}{\left[1 - (80/50 + 8\ 0)\right]} = \frac{.77}{.38} = 2.03$$

$$LR- = \frac{1 - .77}{.62} \quad \text{OR} \quad \frac{\left[1 - (100/100 + 30)\right]}{(80/50 + 80)} = \frac{.23}{.62} = .37$$

The LR+ of 2.03 indicates that a positive Powden test obtained in a person with the condition is twice as likely to have the condition of interest compared with a person without the condition. The LR– of .37 indicates that individuals with a negative Powden test have .37 times lesser likelihood of having the condition. Likelihood ratios have values that are greater than or equal to zero, and an LR+ will have values greater than 1, while an LR– will have values less than 1. The following guidelines for interpreting LRs include:

LIKELIHOOD RATIO RANGE	MEANING
LR+ > 10 or LR– < .10	Large and conclusive change from pre- to posttest probability
LR+ = 5 to 10 or LR– = 0.10 to 0.20	Moderate change from pre- to posttest probability
LR+ = 2 to 5 or LR– = .20 to .50	Small but sometimes important change from pre- to posttest probability
LR+ = 1 – 2 or LR– = .50 to 1.0	Negligible change in pretest probability

The closer the LR+ and LR– are to 1, the less accurate the diagnostic test because that is equivalent to flipping a coin to determine the outcome. Likelihood ratios are being reported more within textbooks and other publications because they are independent of disease prevalence, making them applicable across settings and patients.

The LRs can now be used to figure out posttest probability. Because you may already know your pretest probability from the literature or calculated the prevalence within your sample and now you have LRs, you can revise your probability values to be more confident in the diagnosis and improve certainty. This is done by finding the **posttest probability**, which is the revised probability, and this is performed through the use of a nomogram. The **nomogram** (Figure 9-4) can be used to determine whether performing the test will provide enough additional information so that it is worth conducting the test on a patient.

Let us take the information from the Powden meniscal test that we have and apply it to the nomogram:

$$\text{Prevalence}\left(\text{in study}\right) = 50\%$$

$$\text{LR} + = 2.03$$

$$\text{LR} - = .37$$

You would plot the pretest probability using the calculated prevalence from your study (in this case since the population prevalence is not known) on the line on the lefthand side of the nomogram (Figure 9-5). Secondly, plot the LR on the middle line. Lastly, you would then connect the dots by using a straight edge and continuing that line across the posttest probability (right-hand side of the nomogram). For the Powden meniscal test, the posttest probability would be approximately 67% for the LR+ of 2.03 when the pretest probability is 50%; therefore, the LR+ of 2.03 increases the probability that an individual has a meniscal injury to about 67%. The dashed line indicates that an LR– of .37 decreases the probability that an individual has a meniscal injury to approximately 25%.

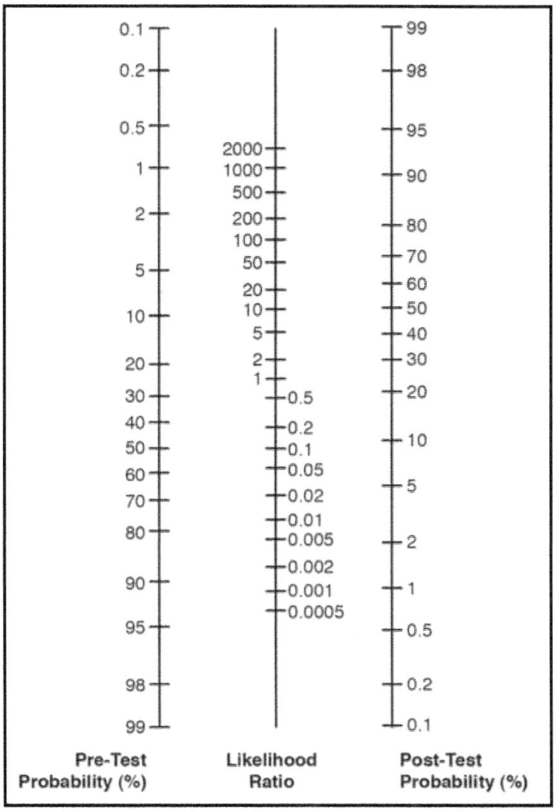

Figure 9-4. Nomogram for plotting pretest probability and likelihood ratios. (Reprinted with permission from Fagan TJ. Letter: Nomogram for Bayes theorem. *N Engl J Med.* 1975;293(5):257. Copyright © 1975 Massachusetts Medical Society.)

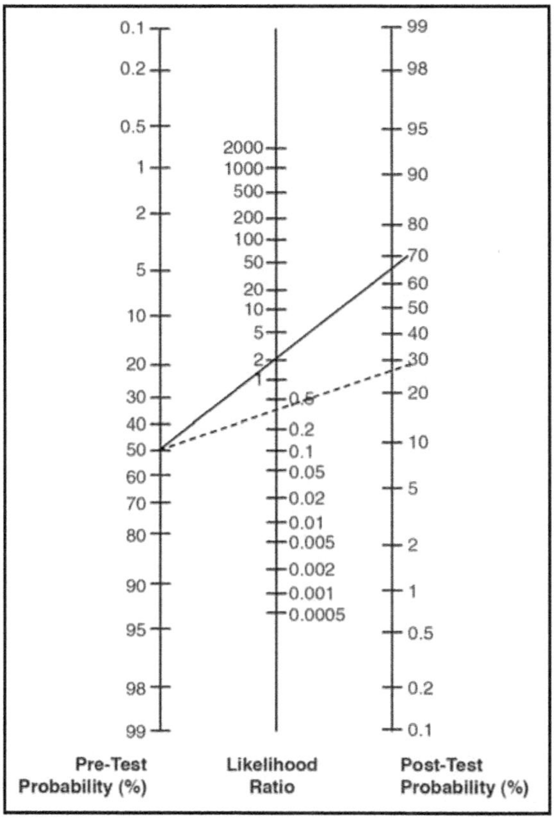

Figure 9-5. Nomogram for Powden meniscal test. Solid line represents positive likelihood ration. Dashed line represents negative likelihood ratio. (Adapted from Fagan TJ. Letter: Nomogram for Bayes theorem. *N Engl J Med.* 1975;293(5):257. Copyright © 1975 Massachusetts Medical Society.)

The shift from pre- to posttest probabilities can all be calculated using the calculations provided by Sackett et al.[1] This involves converting the probabilities to odds and then using these values to calculate the new posttest probability. The formulae include:

TERM	CALCULATION
Pretest odds	$\frac{\text{Pretest probability}}{1 - \text{pretest probability}}$
Posttest odds	Pretest odds x likelihood ratio
Posttest probability	$\frac{\text{Posttest odds}}{\text{Posttest odds} + 1}$

These formulae may be easier for you to use in clinical practice than the nomogram because the calculations are performed with simple math and can be remembered fairly easily. If we apply these formulae to our Powden meniscal example, the calculations would result in this:

TERM	FORMULA	CALCULATIONS	OUTCOME
Pretest odds	$\frac{\text{Pretest probability}}{1 - \text{pretest probability}}$	$\frac{.50}{1 - .50}$	1
Posttest odds	Pretest odds x likelihood ratio	1 x 2.03	2.03
Posttest probability	$\frac{\text{Posttest odds}}{\text{Posttest odds} + 1}$	$\frac{2.03}{2.03 + 1}$	67%

Let us use all the information that you now have and apply it to a research study example for using the Thessaly test to detect meniscal injury.[2] All of the values that we need to complete the calculations are derived from the 2-by-2 contingency table (Figure 9-6). The information gained from calculating the various components of the diagnostic test allows you to make a clinical decision about including the Thessaly test when evaluating potential meniscal injury. However, the results from this particular study may not be as applicable as you would like because the individuals had a primary ACL injury as well. The following are 2 websites that you can use to assist you in calculating the various aspects for diagnostic tests:

- *Australian Prescriber*: http://www.australianprescriber.com/magazine/26/5/111/13
- Diagnostic Test Calculator, version 2010042101: http://araw.mede.uic.edu/cgi-bin/testcalc.pl

Another tool that you can use to assist you with making a clinical decision is the utilization of a **receiver operating characteristic** (ROC) curve, which uses specificity and sensitivity information from continuous data to determine a cutoff score for decision making. The **cutoff score** is a specific score used to determine at which point the value of the test can be used to make a decision for the next course of action (ie, treatment, risk of injury increase). For example, what if you wanted to use a test (fictitious Ankle Injury Assessment Tool [AIAT]) to determine at which point individuals who have ankle instability are at a greater risk of reinjury. For you to do this, you would need to consider the range of scores and at which score there was the most risk of being more susceptible to a reinjury. Let us say that lower scores on the AIAT are indicative of increased ankle instability and you want to determine the cutoff score for the AIAT at which you should implement an intervention. To do this, the sensitivity and specificity for each cutoff score must be calculated

Study 2: Mirzatolooei et al, 2010 *(Patients with ACL tear as the primary condition)*		Reference Standard		
		Arthroscopic Examination Positive	Arthroscopic Examination Negative	
Thessaly Test	Thessaly Test Positive	a **True Positive (31)**	b False Positive (24)	Total = 55
	Thessaly Test Negative	c False Negative (8)	d **True Negative (17)**	Total = 25
		Total = 39	Total = 41	Overall Total = 80

Diagnostic Accuracy	**(a + d)/N**	**(31+17)/80 = 48/80 or 60%**	
Sensitivity	**a/(a + c)**	**31/(31 +8) = 31/39 or 79%**	
Specificity	**d/(b + d)**	**17/(24+17) = 17/41 or 41%**	
Prevalence	**(a + c)/N**	**(31 + 8)/80 = 39/80 or 49%**	
Positive Predictive Value	**a/(a + b)**	**31/(31 + 24) = 31/55 or 56%**	
Negative Predictive Value	**d/(c + d)**	**17/(8 + 17) = 17/25 or 68%**	
LR+	**(a/a+c)/[1-(d/b+d)]**	**(31/31+8)/[1-(17/24+17)] =**	**1.34**
LR-	**[1-(a/a+c)]/(d/b+d)**	**[1-(31/31+8)]/(17/24+17) =**	**.51**
Pretest Probability	**determined from literature or your study for this example = 49%**		
Post-test Probability (LR+)	**USE Sacketts formula or nomogram**	**56%**	
Post-test Probability (LR-)	**USE Sacketts formula or nomogram**	**33%**	

Figure 9-6. Overall summary of the contingency table for the Thessaly test to detect meniscal injury. ACL = anterior cruciate ligament.

so that you can plot the information on the ROC curve. An ROC curve is plotted graphically, with the y-axis representing sensitivity (true-positive rate) and the x-axis representing 1 – specificity (false-positive rate) (Figure 9-7). The information plotted on the ROC curve from the continuous data will assist you in identifying critical points, which will guide your clinical practice, and you will then be able to determine cutoff points (ie, a value for ankle instability from the AIAT), which will be used to determine who should receive an intervention. If the plotted data result in a perfect diagonal line as represented in Figure 9-7, then the test produces the same value of true-positive and false-positive results for any score, and it is the same result you would get from flipping a coin. When the plotted values for a test equate to high sensitivity and high specificity (or a low false-positive score), then most of the graph will be shaded (Figure 9-8). Due to the fact that most tests are imperfect, the cutoff score is the point at which the curve starts to bend away from the y-axis because the false-positive rate increases. This cutoff score will represent the score for which you may want to use to make your clinical decisions about a course of action.

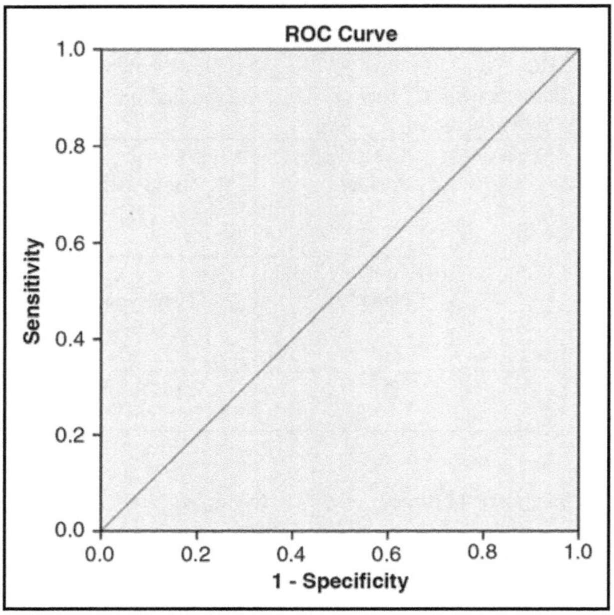

Figure 9-7. A receiver operating characteristic (ROC) curve for a test that is equal to chance. Anything higher than the line indicates the test is better than guessing.

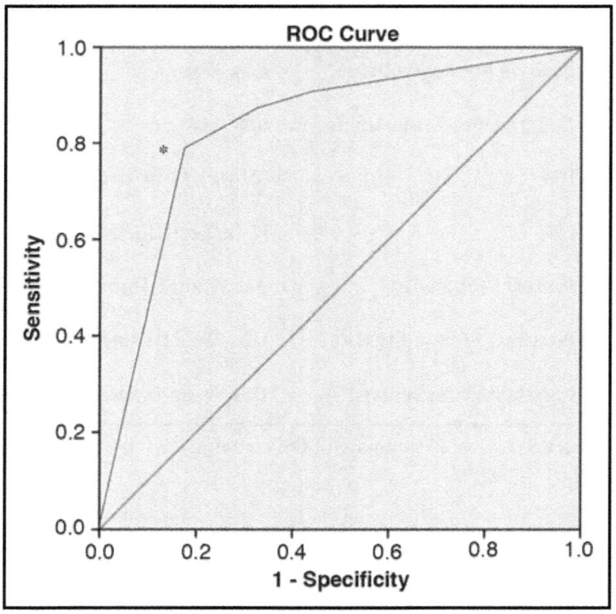

Figure 9-8. A receiver operating characteristic (ROC) curve for a test that has a high sensitivity and low false positive rate (1-Specificity). *Cutoff score.

Summary

You will utilize many diagnostic tests and clinical measures within your clinical practice; therefore, you must be able to determine whether the tests and measures you have chosen can assist you with a clinical decision. It is becoming more common for authors to provide you with values related to sensitivity, specificity, NPVs and PPVs, and LRs when reporting information concerning diagnostic tests. This information is useful for your clinical practice as long as you remember to apply it to the prevalence of the condition for the specific individual for whom you are making a decision.

Key Points

- The validity of a clinical diagnostic test is measured through mathematical equations that compare the clinical diagnostic test to a reference standard.
- Diagnostic tests are utilized to help you make a decision about whether an individual patient has a certain condition.
- You will use your clinical experiences, best judgment, and information from the literature to determine what you believe to be the pretest probability that the patient has the condition. Remember, you can make a good estimate if you understand what the prevalence of the condition is within the population that is linked to your patient.

References

1. Sackett D. *Evidence-Based Medicine: How to Practice and Teach EBM.* 2nd ed. London, UK: Churchill Livingtone; 2000.
2. Mirzatolooei F, Yekta Z, Bayazidchi M, Ershadi S, Afshar A. Validation of the Thessaly test for detecting meniscal tears in anterior cruciate deficient knees. *Knee.* 2010;17:221-223.

Bibiography

Campo M, Shiyko MP, Lichtman SW. Sensitivity and specificity: a review of related statistics and controversies in the context of physical therapist education. *J Phys Ther Educ.* 2010;24(3):69-78.

Carvajal DN, Rowe PC. Sensitivity, specificity, predictive values, and likelihood ratios. *Pediatr Rev.* 2010;31(12):511-513.

Collier J, Huebscher R. Sensitivity, specificity, positive and negative predictive values: diagnosing purple mange. *J Amer Acad Nurse Pract.* 2010;22(4):205-209.

Harrison BK, Abell BE, Gibson TW. The Thessaly test for detection of meniscal tears: validation of a new physical examination technique for primary care medicine. *Clin J Sport Med.* 2009;19(1):9-12.

Lalkhen AG, McCluskey A. Clinical tests: sensitivity and specificity. *Contin Educ Anaesth Crit Care Pain.* 2008;8(6):221-223.

Parikh R, Mathai A, Parikh S, Sekhar GC, Thomas R. Understanding and using sensitivity, specificity and predictive values. *Indian J Ophthalmol.* 2008;56(1):45-50.

Parikh R, Parikh S, Arun E, Thomas R. Likelihood ratios: clinical application in day-to-day practice. *Indian J Ophthalmol.* 2009;57(3):217-221.

Sundgot-Borgen J, Torstveit MK. Prevalence of eating disorders in elite athletes is higher than in the general population. *Clin J Sport Med.* 2004;14(1):25-32.

10

Levels of Evidence and Grades of Recommendation

An evidence-guided approach to clinical practice is based upon input from many available sources. It will be up to you to decide if the sources are worthy of consideration when you are making a clinical decision. Fortunately, a hierarchy of evidence exists to guide decision making and should be used when you need to examine the available evidence. The 2 most commonly utilized scales for examining the evidence are the Oxford Centre for Evidence-Based Medicine (CEBM) scale and the Strength of Recommendation Taxonomy (SORT). The purpose of these scales is to organize the evidence into categories so that you will then be able to determine the strength of the evidence. Each scale will assist you with (1) determining the level of evidence and (2) assigning a grade of recommendation.

A **level of evidence** is defined as the critical evaluation of a research article that rates the quality of evidence based on the research design of the study. A level of evidence is provided through a numeric rating system (eg, 1, 2, 3) and is assigned to an individual study to depict the validity of the study. This rating, however, does not necessarily take clinical applicability into consideration. A **grade of recommendation** is a letter rating system (eg, A, B, C) assigned to a body of evidence by examination of a group of articles relating to the same topic. Along with the validity of the studies, a grade of recommendation also considers other factors, such as cost, ease of implementation, and reproducibility throughout various clinical settings.

These scales allow us to identify the value of the research evidence and determine whether it can be applied to clinical practice. You must realize that there are more than 100 grading scales in use within the medical literature. When one group of articles has a grade of B assigned to it, that may mean something totally different when comparing it to another group of articles that also were given a grade B because the scales used to assess the information were different.

Van Lunen BL, Hankemeier DA, Welch CE.
Evidence-Guided Practice: A Framework for Clinical Decision Making in Athletic Training (pp 101-117).

Oxford Centre for Evidence-Based Medicine Scale

The CEBM levels of evidence were first produced in 1998 and updated in 2009 to make the process of finding appropriate evidence feasible and to demonstrate that the evidence reflected was clearly categorized. The initial scale involved 5 levels of evidence with subcategories within most of the levels. The most current version, the 2011 CEBM levels, has eliminated the subcategories and just focuses on the original 5 levels.

The CEBM scale for determining levels of evidence is formulated around 5 levels that are used to rate the quality of a particular study, with Level 1 corresponding with the highest level of evidence and Level 5 with the lowest. Generally, you begin to examine your clinical question by investigating whether a systematic review exists on the topic, as systematic reviews are usually at the highest level of evidence. If that does not exist, then you may decide to look for individual randomized, clinical trials within the same area and then work your way down the hierarchy to determine what level of evidence is available for the question that you are asking. Level 1 studies generally include evidence from randomized, controlled trials and can be in the form of systematic reviews or meta-analyses. Level 2 evidence involves prospective cohort studies in which baseline measurements are taken before any interventions are implemented. Level 3 evidence consists of case control studies that are retrospective in design due to the fact that outcomes of the groups have been examined after the interventions have already been implemented. Level 4 evidence is composed of case series designs, which do not include a control group; therefore, the internal validity of the study is in question. Level 5 evidence consists of expert opinion and disease-oriented evidence (intermediate, histopathologic, physiologic, or surrogate [alternate]) that may reflect improvement in patient outcomes because they are not supported with facts or are not associated with patient-oriented evidence.

The general hierarchy of the 2009 CEBM Levels of Evidence 1 is depicted in Figure 10-1. Table 10-1 further delineates utilization of the general model but provides an approach for examining different types of research questions related to therapy/prevention/etiology/harm, prognosis, diagnosis, differential diagnosis/system prevalence study, and economic and decision analyses. These levels of evidence were revised in 2011 in light of new concepts and data. The 2011 CEBM Levels of Evidence 2 begins with asking the clinical question, and then you are able to choose the appropriate level based upon what type of clinical question you may have (Table 10-2). The changes were intended to lend to the clinical decision-making process, while also providing clinicians with essential rules of thumb to make the decision in a real environment. This often requires limited available time, so an efficient process is warranted. The 2011 structure also has fewer footnotes, making it easier to use, and it is accompanied by an extensive glossary. Lastly, you are now able to use it even if there are no systematic reviews available for your type of clinical question. Table 10-2 is intended to be used alongside the accompanying "Introductory Document" and "Background Document" that are provided by the CEBM. The "Introductory Document" provides additional insight on considerations that you need to keep in mind when using the CEBM 2011 Levels of Evidence, such as what the 2011 CEMB Levels of Evidence is and is not. The "Background Document" provides an overview of the reasons why the instrument was created, what was revised from the previous version, how the tables utilized for describing the levels have changed, limitations of the document, and future directions.

An example utilizing the PICO clinical question format is:

In acute knee-injured patients (P), is the Thessaly test (I) compared with the McMurray test (C) more accurate in diagnosing a meniscal injury (O)?

Because your clinical question is diagnostic, you would proceed by aligning your question with the second row of Table 10-1, which reads, "Is this diagnostic or monitoring test accurate?" If you locate a systematic review that contained multiple cross-sectional studies that had consistently applied a reference standard (possibly arthroscopic surgery) and had blinding of the testers, then

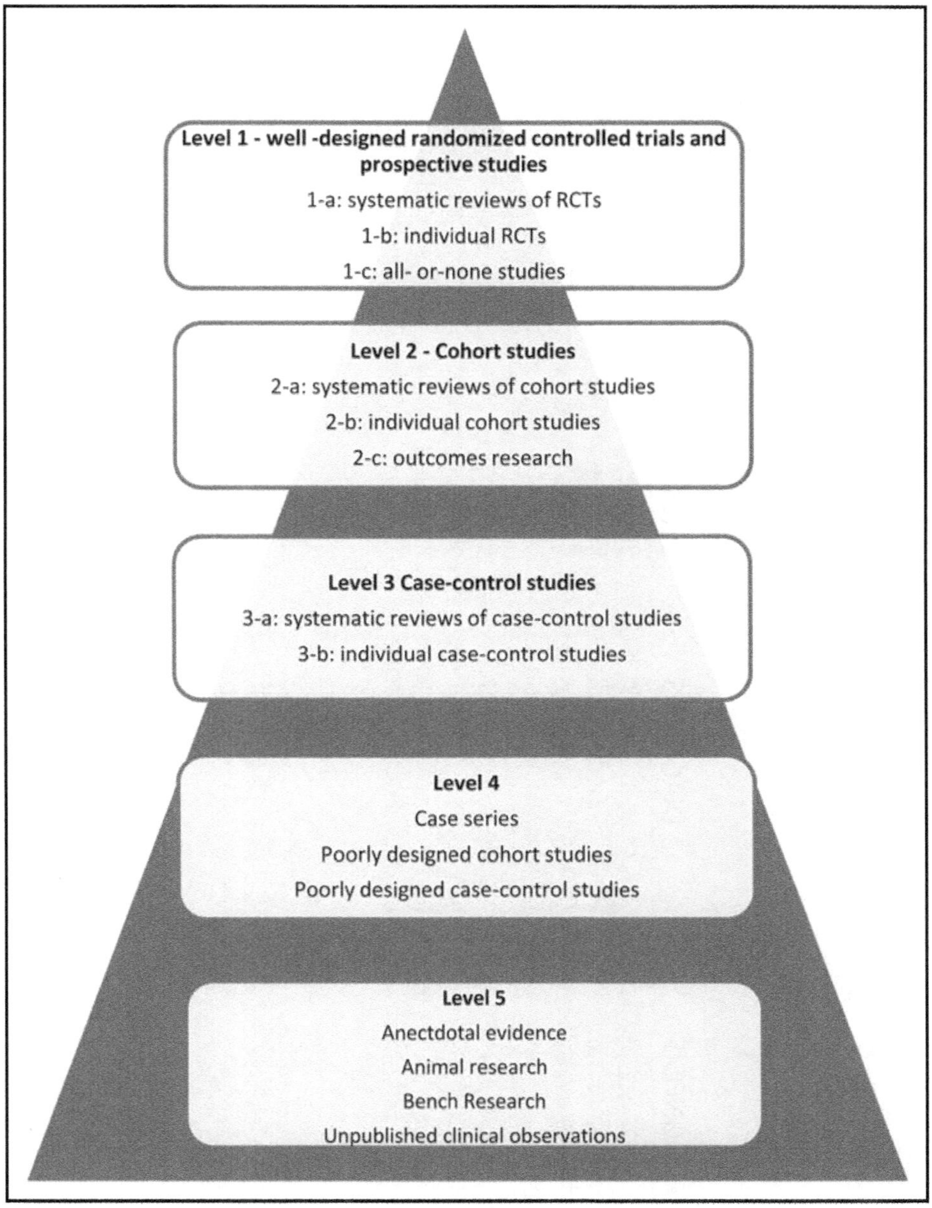

Figure 10-1. Oxford Centre for Evidence-Based Medicine hierarchy, 2009. Abbreviation: RCTs, randomized controlled trials.

you would consider that study to be a Level 1 Diagnostic study. However, if the study you located is merely a single cross-sectional study with a consistent reference standard (possibly arthroscopic surgery) and had blinding of the testers, then you would consider that to be a Level 2 Diagnostic study. The only difference between the 2 studies is that one is a systematic review (several studies that were reviewed and summated) and the other is a single study. The important component of using this table in clinical practice is that you will need to have a solid understanding of the types of research designs and terms before you can assign a level of evidence.

Grades of recommendation are used when a body of information is available on a particular topic. The CEBM grades range from A, highest grade of evidence, to D, the lowest grade (Table 10-3). When evidence receives an A designation, the information can strongly be argued for or

Table 10-1. Oxford Centre for Evidence-Based Medicine Levels of Evidence 2009

LEVEL	THERAPY/ PREVENTION, ETIOLOGY/ HARM	PROGNOSIS	DIAGNOSIS	DIFFERENTIAL DIAGNOSIS/ SYMPTOM PREVALENCE STUDY	ECONOMIC AND DECISION ANALYSES
1a	SR (with homogeneity*) of RCTs	SR (with homogeneity*) of inception cohort studies; CDR† validated in different populations	SR (with homogeneity*) of Level 1 diagnostic studies; CDR† with 1b studies from different clinical centres	SR (with homogeneity*) of prospective cohort studies	SR (with homogeneity*) of Level 1 economic studies
1b	Individual RCT (with narrow confidence interval‡)	Individual inception cohort study with >80% follow-up; CDR† validated in a single population	Validating** cohort study with good††† reference standards; or CDR† tested within one clinical centre	Prospective cohort study with good follow-up****	Analysis based on clinically sensible costs or alternatives; systematic review(s) of the evidence; and including multi-way sensitivity analyses
1c	All or none§	All or none case series	Absolute SpPins and SnNouts††	All or none case series	Absolute better-value or worse-value analyses††††

(continued)

Table 10-1. (continued)
Oxford Centre for Evidence-Based Medicine Levels of Evidence 2009

LEVEL	THERAPY/ PREVENTION, ETIOLOGY/ HARM	PROGNOSIS	DIAGNOSIS	DIFFERENTIAL DIAGNOSIS/ SYMPTOM PREVALENCE STUDY	ECONOMIC AND DECISION ANALYSES
2a	SR (with homogeneity*) of cohort studies	SR (with homogeneity*) of either retrospective cohort studies or untreated control groups in RCTs	SR (with homogeneity*) of Level > 2 diagnostic studies	SR (with homogeneity*) of 2b and better studies	SR (with homogeneity*) of Level > 2 economic studies
2b	Individual cohort study (including low-quality RCT [eg, < 80% follow-up])	Retrospective cohort study or follow-up of untreated control patients in an RCT; Derivation of CDR† or validated on split-sample§§§ only	Exploratory** cohort study with good††† reference standards; CDR† after derivation, or validated only on split-sample§§§ or databases	Retrospective cohort study, or poor follow-up	Analysis based on clinically sensible costs or alternatives; limited review(s) of the evidence, or single studies; and including multi-way sensitivity analyses
2c	"Outcomes" research; ecological studies	"Outcomes" research		Ecological studies	Audit or outcomes research

(continued)

Table 10-1. (continued)

Oxford Centre for Evidence-Based Medicine Levels of Evidence 2009

LEVEL	THERAPY/ PREVENTION, ETIOLOGY/ HARM	PROGNOSIS	DIAGNOSIS	DIFFERENTIAL DIAGNOSIS/ SYMPTOM PREVALENCE STUDY	ECONOMIC AND DECISION ANALYSES
3a	SR (with homogeneity*) of case-control studies		SR (with homogeneity*) of 3b and better studies	SR (with homogeneity*) of 3b and better studies	SR (with homogeneity*) of 3b and better studies
3b	Individual case-control study		Nonconsecutive study; or without consistently applied reference standards	Nonconsecutive cohort study or very limited population	Analysis based on limited alternatives or costs, poor quality estimates of data, but including sensitivity analyses incorporating clinically sensible variations.
4	Case series (and poor-quality cohort and case-control studies§§)	Case series (and poor-quality prognostic cohort studies***)	Case-control study, poor or nonindependent reference standard	Case series or superseded reference standards	Analysis with no sensitivity analysis

(continued)

Table 10-1. (continued)

Oxford Centre for Evidence-Based Medicine Levels of Evidence 2009

LEVEL	THERAPY/ PREVENTION, ETIOLOGY/ HARM	PROGNOSIS	DIAGNOSIS	DIFFERENTIAL DIAGNOSIS/ SYMPTOM PREVALENCE STUDY	ECONOMIC AND DECISION ANALYSES
5	Expert opinion without explicit critical appraisal, or based on physiology, bench research or "first principles"	Expert opinion without explicit critical appraisal, or based on physiology, bench research or "first principles"	Expert opinion without explicit critical appraisal, or based on physiology, bench research or "first principles"	Expert opinion without explicit critical appraisal, or based on physiology, bench research or "first principles"	Expert opinion without explicit critical appraisal, or based on economic theory or "first principles"

For definitions of terms used, see glossary at http://www.cebm.net/?o=1116.

Notes

Users can add a minus-sign "–" to denote the level of that fails to provide a conclusive answer because:

EITHER a single result with a wide Confidence Interval

OR a Systematic Review with troublesome heterogeneity.

Such evidence is inconclusive, and therefore can only generate Grade D recommendations.

* By homogeneity we mean a systematic review that is free of worrisome variations (heterogeneity) in the directions and degrees of results between individual studies. Not all systematic reviews with statistically significant heterogeneity need be worrisome, and not all worrisome heterogeneity need be statistically significant. As noted above, studies displaying worrisome heterogeneity should be tagged with a "–" at the end of their designated level.

† Clinical Decision Rule. (These are algorithms or scoring systems that lead to a prognostic estimation or a diagnostic category.)

(continued)

Table 10-1. (continued)
Oxford Centre for Evidence-Based Medicine Levels of Evidence 2009

‡See previous note for advice on how to understand, rate, and use trials or other studies with wide confidence intervals.

§Met when all patients died before the prescription became available but some now survive on it; or when some patients died before the perscription became available but none now die on it.

§§By poor-quality cohort study, we mean one that failed to clearly define comparison groups and/or failed to measure exposures and outcomes in the same (preferably blinded) objective way in both exposed and nonexposed individuals and/or failed to identify or appropriately control known confounders and/or failed to carry out a sufficiently long and complete follow-up of patients. By poor-quality case-control study, we mean one that failed to clearly define comparison groups and/or failed to measure exposures and outcomes in the same (preferably blinded) objective way in both cases and controls and/or failed to identify or appropriately control known confounders.

§§§Split-sample validation is achieved by collecting all the information in a single tranche, then artificially dividing this into "derivation" and "validation" samples.

††An "Absolute SpPin" is a diagnostic finding whose specificity is so high that a positive result rules in the diagnosis. An "Absolute SnNout" is a diagnostic finding whose sensitivity is so high that a negative result rules out the diagnosis.

‡‡Good, better, bad, and worse refer to the comparisons between treatments in terms of their clinical risks and benefits.

†††Good reference standards are independent of the test and applied blindly or objectively to applied to all patients. Poor reference standards are haphazardly applied but are still independent of the test. Use of a nonindependent reference standard (where the test is included in the reference, or where the testing affects the reference) implies a level 4 study.

††††Better-value treatments are clearly as good but cheaper or are better at the same or reduced cost. Worse-value treatments are as good and more expensive or are worse and equally or more expensive.

** Validating studies test the quality of a specific diagnostic test based on prior evidence. An exploratory study collects information and trawls the data (eg, using a regression analysis) to find which factors are significant.

*** By poor-quality prognostic cohort study, we mean one in which sampling was biased in favor of patients who already had the target outcome, or the measurement of outcomes was accomplished in <80% of study patients, or outcomes were determined in an unblinded, nonobjective way, or there was no correction for confounding factors.

**** Good follow-up in a differential diagnosis study is >80%, with adequate time for alternative diagnoses to emerge (eg, 1 to 6 months acute, 1 to 5 years chronic).

Adapted from OCEBM Levels of Evidence Working Group. Levels of Evidence [March 2009]. Oxford Centre for Evidence-Based Medicine. http://www.cebm.net/oxford-centre-evidence-based-medicine-levels-evidence-march-2009/.

Table 10-2.
Oxford Centre for Evidence-Based Medicine Levels of Evidence 2011

Question	STEP 1 LEVEL 1*	STEP 2 LEVEL 2*	STEP 3 LEVEL 3*	STEP 4 LEVEL 4*	STEP 5 LEVEL 5*
How common is the problem?	Local and current random sample surveys (or censuses)	Systematic review of surveys that allow matching to local circumstances**	Local nonrandom sample**	Case series**	n/a
Is this diagnostic or monitoring test accurate? (Diagnosis)	Systematic review of cross-sectional studies with consistently applied reference standard and blinding	Individual cross-sectional studies with consistently applied reference standard and blinding	Nonconsecutive studies or studies without consistently applied reference standards**	Case-control studies or poor or nonindependent reference standard**	Mechanism-based reasoning
What will happen if we do not add a therapy? (Prognosis)	Systematic review of inception cohort studies	Inception cohort studies	Cohort study or control arm of randomized trial*	Case series, case-control, or historically controlled studies**	N/A
Does this intervention help? (Treatment benefits)	Systematic review of randomized trials or n-of-1 trials	Randomized trial or observational study with dramatic effect	Nonrandomized controlled cohort/follow-up study**		Mechanism-based reasoning

(continued)

Table 10-2. (continued)
Oxford Centre for Evidence-Based Medicine Levels of Evidence 2011

Question	STEP 1 LEVEL 1*	STEP 2 LEVEL 2*	STEP 3 LEVEL 3*	STEP 4 LEVEL 4*	STEP 5 LEVEL 5*
What are the COMMON harms? (Treatment harms)	Systematic review of randomized trials, systematic review of nested case-control studies, n-of-1 trial with the patient you are raising the question about, or observational study with dramatic effect	Individual randomized trial or (exceptionally) observational study with dramatic effect	Nonrandomized controlled cohort/follow-up study (post-marketing surveillance) provided there are sufficient numbers to rule out a common harm. (For long-term harms, the duration of follow-up must be sufficient.) **	Case series, case-control, or historically controlled studies**	Mechanism-based reasoning
What are the RARE harms? (Treatment harms)	Systematic review of randomized trials or n-of-1 trials	Randomized trial or (exceptionally) observational study with dramatic effect			
Is this (early detection) test worthwhile? (Screening)	Systematic review of randomized trials	Randomized trial	Nonrandomized controlled cohort/follow-up study**	Case series, case-control, or historically controlled studies**	Mechanism-based reasoning

*Level may be graded down on the basis of study quality, imprecision, indirectness (study PICO does not match questions PICO), because of inconsistency between studies, or because the absolute effect size is very small; level may be graded up if there is a large or very large effect size.

**As always, a systematic review is generally better than an individual study.

Reprinted from OCEBM Levels of Evidence Working Group. The Oxford 2011 Levels of Evidence. Oxford Centre for Evidence-Based Medicine. http://www.cebm.net/index.aspx?o=5653.

Table 10-3. CEBM Grading Scale for Bodies of Evidence

GRADES OF RECOMMENDATION	
A	Consistent Level 1 studies
B	Consistent Level 2 OR 3 studies or extrapolations from Level 1 studies
C	Level 4 studies OR extrapolations from Level 2 or 3 studies
D	Level 5 evidence or troublingly inconsistent or inconclusive studies of any level
Extrapolations are where data are used in a situation that has potentially clinically important differences than the original study situation.	

Reprinted from OCEBM Levels of Evidence Working Group. The Oxford 2011 Levels of Evidence. Oxford Centre for Evidence-Based Medicine. http://www.cebm.net/index.aspx?o=5653.

against a particular intervention as it is usually consistent and comes from high-quality Level 1 evidence. A grade B recommendation denotes research evidence from the CEBM Levels 2 or 3 OR extrapolations from Level 1 studies, which include inconsistent results that show promise. A grade C is associated with Level 4 evidence OR extrapolations from Level 2 or 3 studies in which there were inconsistent results, while a grade D (also depicted as I for insufficient) concludes that the available research is inadequate to make a sound clinical recommendation.

Application of this hierarchy is used within many instances, but you would be able to recognize it fairly easily within a critically appraised topic. The authors of a critically appraised topic provide you with the information regarding the level of evidence with which each individual study is associated (usually from the CEBM Levels of Evidence 1), followed by a grade of recommendation for the grouping of articles. For example, a critically appraised topic on "the effectiveness of injury-prevention programs in reducing the incidence of anterior cruciate ligament sprains in adolescent athletes" indicates that 4 articles were included, which received level of evidence scores of 1B (n = 2) and 2B (n = 2). Upon further examination of the content, the authors provide a grade of recommendation of B, which provides the reader with a summary of the 4 articles.

The CEBM is one of the most common hierarchies used to classify studies and is widely known across disciplines. The scale has the ability to differentiate between studies based upon the specific criteria used to categorize each study. This advantage can also be viewed as a disadvantage due to the fact that it requires more time to accurately categorize the study. Additionally, the information within an individual article may dictate which level the study falls into because the authors did not provide enough information concerning the design to properly categorize the study. The levels are not intended to provide you with a definitive answer about the quality of evidence, as there are many other factors (ie, design specifics, patient sample, clinical relevance, importance of another treatment) that may influence your clinical decision making.

Strength of Recommendation Taxonomy

The SORT (Table 10-4) was developed in 2004 by the editors of the United States family medicine and primary care journals to utilize a unified taxonomy (classification). They intended to have a taxonomy that should (1) be uniform in most family medicine journals and electronic databases; (2) allow authors to evaluate the strength of recommendation of a body of evidence; (3)

allow authors to rate the level of evidence for an individual study; (4) be comprehensive and allow authors to evaluate studies of screening, diagnosis, therapy, prevention, and prognosis; (5) be easy to use and not too time consuming for authors, reviewers, and editors who may be content experts but not experts in critical appraisal or clinical epidemiology; and (6) be straightforward enough that primary care physicians can readily integrate the recommendations into daily practice.

To understand how the SORT is utilized, you will need to be familiar with the differences between disease-oriented outcomes and patient-oriented outcomes. **Disease-oriented outcomes** include intermediate, histopathologic, physiologic, or surrogate (alternate) results that may or may not reflect improvement in patient outcomes. These may include such outcomes as blood sugar levels, blood pressure, respiratory flow rate, or coronary plaque thickness. **Patient-oriented outcomes** are things that matter to the patient and help them live longer or better lives. These types of outcomes may include reduced morbidity, reduced mortality, symptom improvement, improved quality of life, or lower cost.

Similar to the CEBM, the SORT is used to examine the quality of individual studies through a numeric rating system (ie, 1, 2, 3; Figure 10-2) and to determine the strength of recommendation based on a body of evidence through the use of a lettering system (ie, A, B, C; Figure 10-3). A Level 1 study has the highest amount of quality and contains patient-oriented evidence, while a Level 2 study decreases in quality but still has the patient-oriented evidence component. A Level 3 study is classified as other evidence, as it does not contain aspects related to what matters to the patient but does provide information that may be useful in clinical decision making, such as blood pressure values following implementation of a structured dietary plan for a patient with an eating disorder.

The strength of recommendation based on a body of evidence, grades A, B, and C, is utilized if there are enough articles on a particular topic area. The intent for this scale is to have a way to clearly group studies in a simple and useful way across various journals so that the readers could apply the information gained more readily. These grades follow a similar concept to the Level system in that the highest 2 grades (A and B) are associated with patient-oriented evidence, while the lowest grade (C) is not. The algorithm in Figure 10-3 provides additional information as to the distinction between components of grades A and B.

The proposed advantages of the SORT include the straightforward and comprehensive scale that can easily be applied by physicians and researchers and the ability to explicitly address the importance and role of patient- versus disease-oriented evidence. Although the taxonomy may not be as detailed in its assessment of study designs compared with other scales, it provides a clear recommendation that is strong (A), moderate (B), or weak (C) in support of a particular intervention. Disadvantages of the SORT include that its applicability is limited by the information that the authors provided in the article because if the authors did not provide enough detail, often due to word limit restrictions, then the article may not receive the appropriate grade. Additionally, this taxonomy can be viewed as being too general and not able to really distinguish between studies due to the lack of specifics needed to categorize information.

Comparing the Oxford Centre for Evidence-Based Medicine Scale and the Strength of Recommendation Taxonomy

The ability for taxonomies to be compared is useful, as it allows you to be able to put things in perspective when determining whether a study or group of studies may be similar in strength. A suggested comparison between the CEBM and SORT has been proposed by the authors of the SORT for readers and authors to use them more effectively. The SORT Level 1 corresponds with Level 1 of the CEBM, Level 2 corresponds with Levels 2 to 3 and sometimes with Levels 2 to 4 of the

Table 10-4.
Components of the Strength of Recommendation Taxonomy

I. *Utilize this table to determine whether a study measuring patient-oriented outcomes is of good or limited quality and whether the results are consistent or inconsistent between studies.*

STUDY QUALITY	DIAGNOSIS	TREATMENT/ PREVENTION/ SCREENING	PROGNOSIS
Level 1 Good-quality patient-oriented evidence	• Validated clinical decision rule • SR/meta-analysis of high-quality studies • High-quality diagnostic cohort study*	• SR/meta-analysis of RCTs with consistent findings • High-quality individual RCT† • All-or-none study‡	• SR/meta-analysis of good-quality cohort studies • Prospective cohort study with good follow-up
Level 2 Limited-quality patient-oriented evidence	• Unvalidated clinical decision rule • SR/meta-analysis of lower-quality studies or studies with inconsistent findings • Lower-quality diagnostic cohort study or diagnostic case-control study‡	• SR/meta-analysis of lower-quality clinical trials or of studies with inconsistent findings • Lower-quality clinical trial† • Cohort study • Case-control study	• SR/meta-analysis of lower-quality cohort studies or with inconsistent results • Retrospective cohort study or prospective cohort study with poor follow-up • Case-control study • Case series
Level 3 Other evidence	Consensus guidelines, extrapolations from bench research, usual practice, opinion, disease-oriented evidence (intermediate or physiologic outcomes only), or case series for studies of diagnosis, treatment, prevention, or screening		

II. *Determine the consistency across the studies.*

Consistent = Most studies found similar or at least coherent conclusions (coherence means that differences are explainable) OR if high-quality and up-to-date systematic reviews or meta-analyses exist, they support the recommendation.

Inconsistent = Considerable variation among study findings and lack of coherence OR if high-quality and up-to-date systematic reviews or meta-analyses exist, they do not find consistent evidence in favor of the recommendation.

III. *Determine the strength of recommendation for the body of evidence found.*

(continued)

Table 10-4. (continued)
Components of the Strength of Recommendation Taxonomy

STRENGTH OF RECOMMENDATION	DEFINITION
A	Recommendation based on consistent and good-quality patient-oriented evidence§
B	Recommendation based on inconsistent or limited-quality patient-oriented evidence§
C	Recommendation based on consensus, usual practice, opinion, disease-oriented evidence,§ or case series for studies of diagnosis, treatment, prevention, or screening

Abbreviations: RCT, randomized, controlled trial; SR, systematic review.
*High-quality diagnostic cohort study: cohort design, adequate size, adequate spectrum of patients, blinding, and a consistent, well-defined reference standard.
†High-quality RCT: allocation concealed, blinding if possible, intention-to-treat analysis, adequate statistical power, adequate follow-up (>80%).
‡In an all-or-none study, the treatment causes a dramatic change in outcomes, such as antibiotics for meningitis or surgery for appendicitis, which precludes study in a controlled trial.
§Patient-oriented evidence measures outcomes that matter to patients, such as morbidity, mortality, symptom improvement, cost reduction, and quality of life.
Reprinted with permission from Ebell MH, Siwek J, Weiss BD, et al. Strength of Recommendation Taxonomy (SORT): a patient-centered approach to grading evidence in the medical literature. *J Am Board Fam Med.* 2004;17(1):59-67.

CEBM, and Level 3 of the SORT corresponds with Levels 4 to 5 of the CEBM. The body of evidence for grading is also comparable between the 2 taxonomies, and the comparisons are located within Table 10-5. The commonality of rating individual studies and then grouping bodies of evidence for each scale is something that is easy to remember. The biggest difference between the 2 scales is that the SORT concentrates on the value of patient-oriented evidence as one of the key factors within the hierarchy. In the end, you must be able to understand how to apply the evidence to your clinical practice, and you must decide how your patient population, setting, and individual patient goals align with the evidence.

Summary

Determining the level of evidence for a particular article will assist you with understanding the quality, while a grade is given to a body of evidence. Utilization of a common hierarchy for evidence within athletic training will make it easier for you to compare evidence, thereby bringing consistency to interpretation within your clinical practice.

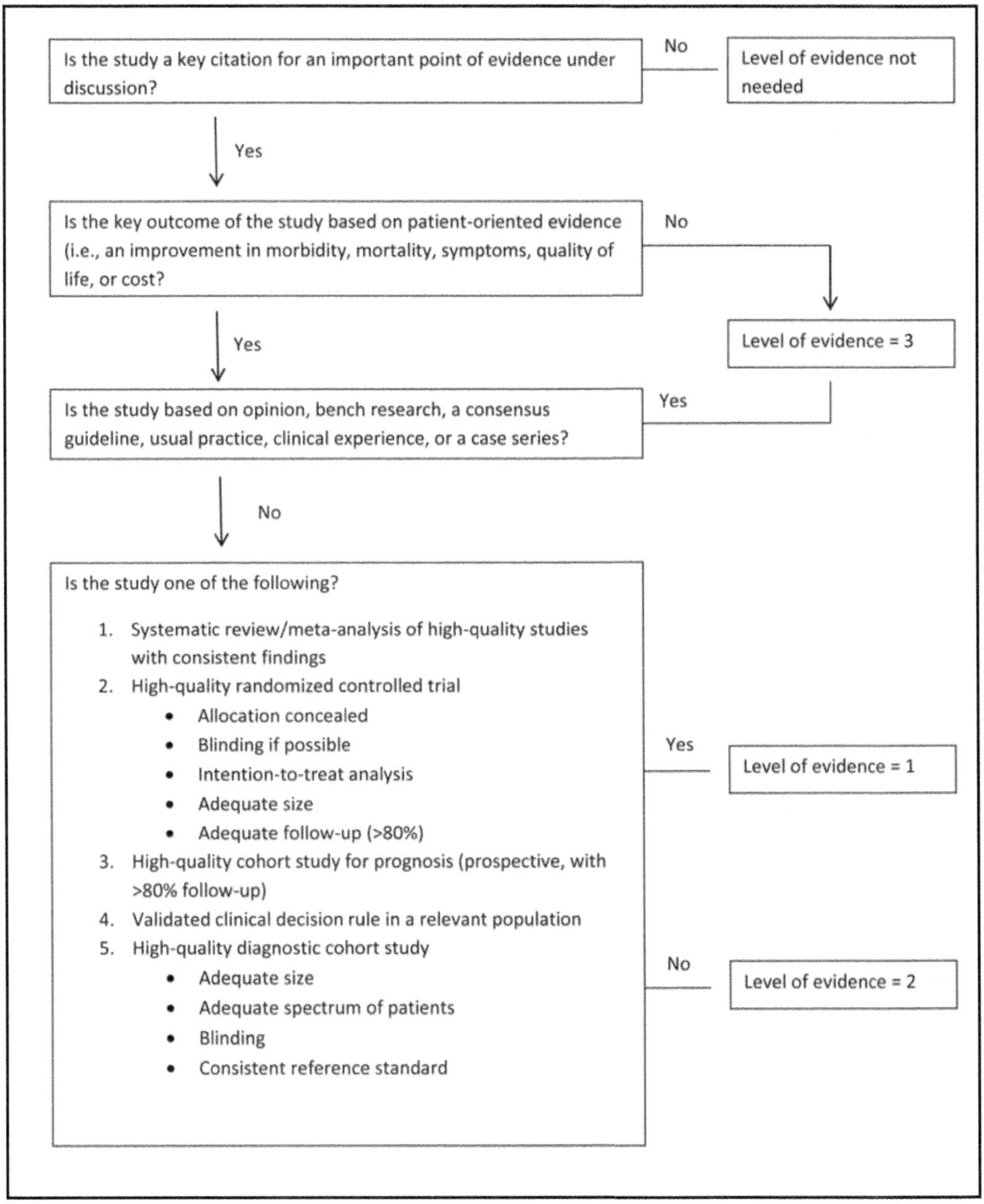

Figure 10-2. Algorithm for determining the level of evidence for an individual study. (Reprinted with permission from Ebell MH, Siwek J, Weiss BD, et al. Strength of Recommendation Taxonomy [SORT]: a patient-centered approach to grading evidence in the medical literature. *J Am Board Fam Med.* 2004;17[1]:59-67. © 2004 American Board of Family Medicine, Inc.)

Key Points

- A hierarchy of evidence exists to guide decision making in an evidence-guided approach to clinical practice and should be used when examining the available evidence.
- Organized scales of evidence should assist you in determining the level of evidence and a grade of recommendation.

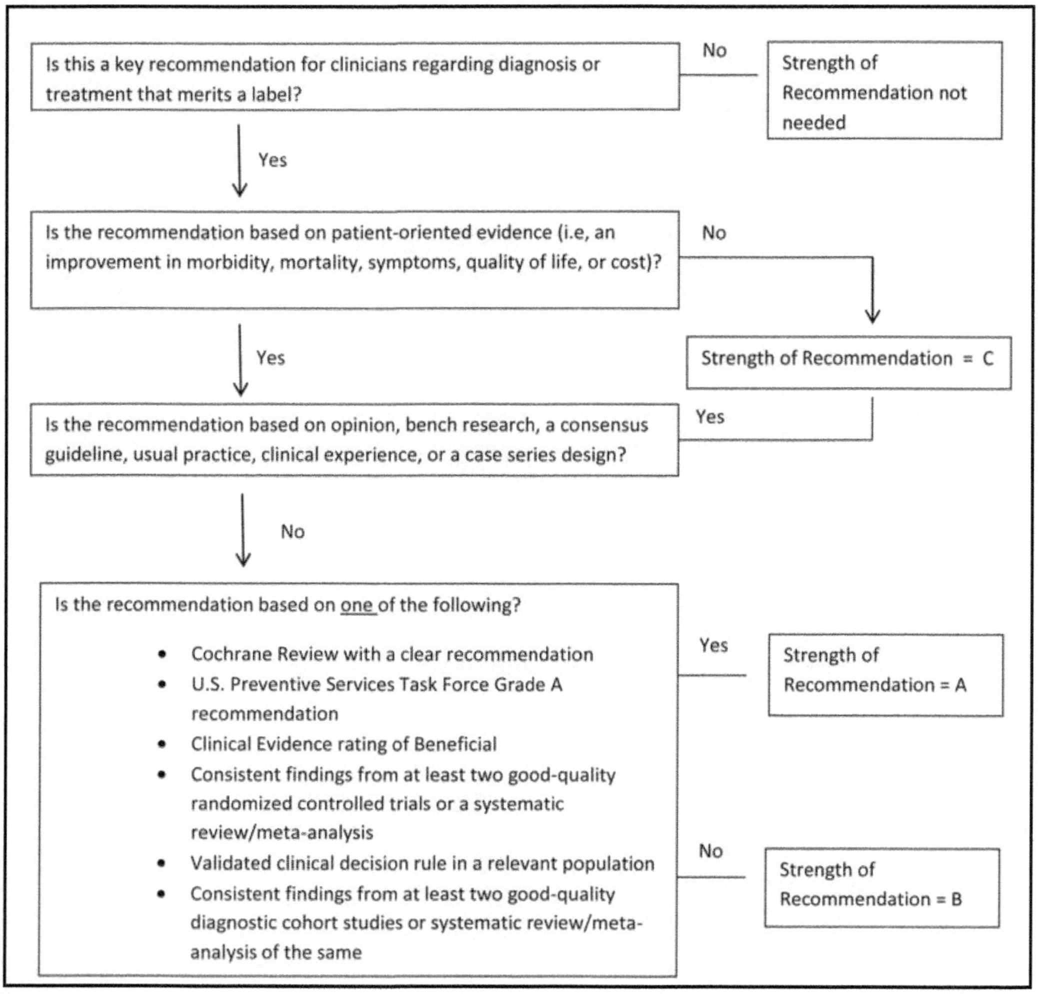

Figure 10-3. Algorithm for determining the strength of a recommendation based on a body of evidence (applies to clinical recommendations regarding diagnosis, treatment, prevention, or screening). (Reprinted with permission from Ebell MH, Siwek J, Weiss BD, et al. Strength of Recommendation Taxonomy [SORT]: a patient-centered approach to grading evidence in the medical literature. *J Am Board Fam Med.* 2004;17[1]:59-67. © 2004 American Board of Family Medicine, Inc.)

Bibliography

Ebell MH, Siwek J, Weiss BD, et al. Simplifying the language of evidence to improve patient care: strength of recommendation taxonomy (SORT): a patient-centered approach to grading evidence in the medical literature. *Am Fam Physician.* 2004;69(3):549-557.

Ebell MH, Siwek J, Weiss BD, et al. Strength of recommendation taxonomy (SORT): a patient-centered approach to grading evidence in the medical literature. *J Am Board Fam Pract.* 2004;17(1):59-67.

Ebell MH, Siwek J, Weiss BD, et al. Strength of recommendation taxonomy (SORT): a patient-centered approach to grading evidence in the medical literature. *J Fam Pract.* 2004;53(2):111-120.

Howick J, Chalmers I, Glasziou P, et al. Explanation of the 2011 Oxford Centre for Evidence-Based Medicine (OCEBM) Levels of Evidence (Background Document). *Oxford Centre for Evidence-Based Medicine.* http://www.cebm.net/index.aspx?o=5653. Accessed October 13, 2013.

Howick J, Chalmers I, Glasziou P, et al. The 2011 Oxford CEBM Levels of Evidence (Introductory Document). *Oxford Centre for Evidence-Based Medicine.* http://www.cebm.net/index.aspx?o=5653. Accessed October 13, 2013.

OCEBM Levels of Evidence Working Group. The Oxford Levels of Evidence 2. *Oxford Centre for Evidence-Based Medicine.* http://www.cebm.net/index.aspx?o=5653 Accessed October 13, 2013.

Table 10-5.
Comparisons Between the Strength of Recommendation Taxonomy and Centre for Evidence-Based Medicine Grades of Recommendation

STRENGTH OF RECOMMENDATION TAXONOMY	CENTRE FOR EVIDENCE-BASED MEDICINE
Grade A: Recommendation based on consistent and good-quality patient-oriented evidence	Grade A: Consistent Level 1 studies
Grade B: Recommendation based on inconsistent or limited-quality patient-oriented evidence	Grade B: Consistent Level 2 or 3 studies or extrapolations from Level 1 studies Grade C: Level 4 studies or extrapolations from Level 2 or 3 studies
Grade C: Recommendation based on consensus, usual practice, disease-oriented evidence, case series for studies of treatment or screening, and/or opinion	Grade D: Level 5 evidence or troublingly inconsistent or inconclusive studies of any Level

Paszkewicz J, Webb T, Waters B, Welch McCarty C, Van Lunen B. The effectiveness of injury-prevention programs in reducing the incidence of anterior cruciate ligament sprains in adolescent athletes. *J Sport Rehabil.* 2012;21(4):371-377.

Phillips B, Ball C, Sackett D, et al. *Oxford Centre for Evidence-based Medicine Levels of Evidence.* http://www.cebm.net/oxford-centre-evidence-based-medicine-levels-evidence-march-2009/. Published November 1998. Updated March 2009. Accessed September 13, 2013.

Weiss BD. SORT: strength of recommendation taxonomy. *Fam Med.* 2004;36(2):141-143.

11

Scales and Checklists for Critical Appraisal

The amount of available evidence that athletic trainers can utilize to assist them with clinical decision making has increased significantly in the past several years. Therefore, it is important that there are systematic ways for you to assess the value of this evidence. Appraisal scales and checklists are instruments used by researchers, clinicians, and reviewers to examine research quality or to guide construction of viable research studies. **Appraisal scales** produce numeric scores based on the incorporation of specific criteria, while checklists serve more as a guide when establishing study parameters. Both can be used to establish study procedures. Some of these instruments are used by readers and reviewers to appraise the quality of evidence, while others are used as guidelines for authors to enhance the quality of their article. Appraising evidence, for use in clinical practice, is an important component that needs to be performed before you can make a decision about the usefulness and applicability of the information. Critical appraisal is essential; however, the score given to an article must be interpreted with caution because the item will not be given a score if the authors did not decide to report the information.

The decision concerning which appraisal or checklist tool to utilize for a given task revolves around identification of what type of study you wish to evaluate or produce. Appraisal scales and checklists are designed for use with specific study designs, so matching your design to the appropriate appraisal or checklist instrument is paramount. This chapter will introduce some of the available appraisal scales and checklists available for use within health care–related research and has been organized by study design to more easily facilitate your implementation within clinical practice.

Van Lunen BL, Hankemeier DA, Welch CE.
Evidence-Guided Practice: A Framework for Clinical Decision Making in Athletic Training (pp 119-149).

Appraisal Scales and Checklists for Randomized, Controlled Trials

The **Physiotherapy Evidence Database (PEDro) scale** was developed by physiotherapists to initially rate methodological quality of randomized, controlled trials (RCTs) on the PEDro scale (www.pedro.fhs.usyd.edu.au). The PEDro scale is an 11-item scale in which each item receives a yes or no score. Satisfied items (except for item 1, which pertains to external validity) contribute 1 point to the total PEDro score (range, 0 to 10 points; Table 11-1). The PEDro score allocates up to 3 points for the level of masking or blinding achieved (eg, masking of subject, therapist, and assessor), 2 points for randomization procedures (random allocation, concealment of allocation), 3 points for the reporting of appropriate data (baseline characteristics, between-group comparisons, and point and range estimates of efficacy), and 1 point each for analysis of data (intention-to-treat analysis) and adequacy of follow-up (Table 11-2). In addition to the scoring, it affords the opportunity for you to record where the information was found within the manuscript.

The advantages of using the PEDro for scoring RCTs are that it has acceptable reliability, is fairly easy to use and interpret because each criteria is well defined, and includes similar items to those used for the abbreviated 3-item Jadad scale. The disadvantages of using the PEDro scale for scoring are that it has 3 separate blinding criteria, which makes it difficult to attain high quality if blinding was not utilized; it has an increased number of criteria, therefore making it more difficult to depict high quality ratings; it was originally designed for RCTs, so it cannot be accurately applied to other study designs; and the score given to an article may often be misleading because the authors may have performed one of the items but merely did not report it.

You will commonly see the PEDro utilized within critically appraised topic manuscripts if RCTs are utilized because it allows the author to compare and contrast the methods of each study. There are no ranges for poor, acceptable, or outstanding scores in relation to the PEDro; however, a higher score may mean that the authors of the research manuscript addressed many of the 10 scoring items within the paper. These scores help you to judge the quality and usefulness of RCTs to inform your clinical decision making because, generally, the higher the score, the higher the quality of the study.

The **Jadad scale** was originally developed as an appraisal tool that focused on appraisal of pain research. Similar to the PEDro scale, the Jadad Scale assesses the quality of RCTs. More specifically, this scale determines the effects of rater blinding and randomization in addition to patient **withdrawals** and dropouts.

The Jadad scale is based on 3 main criteria (randomization, blinding, and withdrawals/dropouts) and can assign a maximum score of 5. The Jadad scale scoring procedure is described in Figure 11-1. **Randomization** is defined as the allocation of subjects in which each subject is allowed the same chance of receiving the intervention and the investigators cannot predict which treatment is next. A study is regarded as **double-blind** if neither the person administering the assessment nor the subject can identify the intervention being assessed. If you are unable to find a statement including the words double-blind, a study is still said to have met this criterion if the use of placebos is mentioned. Subjects who were included in the study but did not complete the entire observation period (full length of the study) or were excluded from analysis are considered to be withdrawals or dropouts. The reason for these instances and the number of withdrawals/dropouts needs to be explained for each group in the report. Additionally, if there were no withdrawals or dropouts from the study, you should be able to find a statement within the article. A "no" is awarded for this criterion if the authors fail to discuss withdrawals and dropouts (or the absence of) in the study.

The advantages of using the Jadad scale for appraising an article are related to the fact that it can be completed within 10 minutes once the article has been read. Although it was initially developed to assess pain research, the criterion are generalized; therefore, you can utilize it to assess

Table 11-1. The PEDro Appraisal Scale

1*	Eligibility criteria were specified (*not part of total score)	☐No	☐Yes	Where:
2	Subjects were randomly allocated to groups (in crossover study, subjects were randomly allocated in order in which treatments were received)	☐No	☐Yes	Where:
3	Allocation was concealed	☐No	☐Yes	Where:
4	The groups were similar at baseline regarding the most important prognostic indicators	☐No	☐Yes	Where:
5	There was blinding of all subjects	☐No	☐Yes	Where:
6	There was blinding of all therapists who administered the therapy	☐No	☐Yes	Where:
7	There was blinding of all assessors who measured at least one key outcome	☐No	☐Yes	Where:
8	Measurements of at least one key outcome were obtained from more than 85% of the subjects initially allocated to groups	☐No	☐Yes	Where:
9	All subjects for whom outcomes measurements were available received the treatments or control condition as allocated, or where this was not the case, data for at least one key outcome were analyzed by "intention to treat"	☐No	☐Yes	Where:
10	The results of between-group statistical comparisons are reported for at least one key outcome	☐No	☐Yes	Where:
11	The study provides both point measurements and measurements of variability for at least one key outcome	☐No	☐Yes	Where:
Total score (max = 10)				

Reprinted with permission from The George Institute for Global Health. www.pedro.org.au/english/downloads/pedro-scale. Updated January 12, 2015. Accessed April 10, 2013.

research from other health care issues. The disadvantages to utilizing it are that (1) it is difficult to execute a true double-blind methodology in athletic training–related research; (2) the criteria used for this appraisal scale are also incorporated in other scales (ie, PEDro scale), which assess more criteria as well; (3) it does not include items to assess the effects of treatments and interventions that are typically important in athletic training research; and (4) it does not assess the reported results of the study. Due to these disadvantages, you will not see the Jadad scale utilized often within the literature you will be reading.

Table 11-2. Notes on Administration of the PEDro Scale

CRITERION	EXPLANATION
All criteria	Points are only awarded when a criterion is clearly satisfied. If on a literal reading of the trial report it is possible that a criterion was not satisfied, a point should not be awarded for that criterion.
Criterion 1*	This criterion is satisfied if the report describes the source of subjects and a list of criteria used to determine who was eligible to participate in the study. *Not given a point within the possible 10-point final score.
Criterion 2	A study is considered to have used random allocation if the report states that allocation was random. The precise method of randomization need not be specified. Procedures such as coin-tossing and dice-rolling should be considered random. Quasi-randomization allocation procedures such as allocation by hospital record number or birth date, or alternation, do not satisfy this criterion.
Criterion 3	*Concealed allocation* means that the person who determined if a subject was eligible for inclusion in the trial was unaware, when this decision was made, of which group the subject would be allocated to. A point is awarded for this criteria, even if it is not stated that allocation was concealed, when the report states that allocation was by sealed opaque envelopes or that allocation involved contacting the holder of the allocation schedule who was "off-site."
Criterion 4	At a minimum, in studies of therapeutic interventions, the report must describe at least one measure of the severity of the condition being treated and at least one (different) key outcome measure at baseline. The rater must be satisfied that the groups' outcomes would not be expected to differ, on the basis of baseline differences in prognostic variables alone, by a clinically significant amount. This criterion is satisfied even if only baseline data of study completers are presented.
Criteria 4, 7 to 11	*Key outcomes* are those outcomes which provide the primary measure of the effectiveness (or lack of effectiveness) of the therapy. In most studies, more than one variable is used as an outcome measure.
Criteria 5 to 7	*Blinding* means the person in question (subject, therapist or assessor) did not know which group the subject had been allocated to. In addition, subjects and therapists are only considered to be "blind" if it could be expected that they would have been unable to distinguish between the treatments applied to different groups. In trials in which key outcomes are self-reported (eg, visual analogue scale, pain diary), the assessor is considered to be blind if the subject was blind.

(continued)

Table 11-2. (continued)
Notes on Administration of the PEDro Scale

CRITERION	EXPLANATION
Criterion 8	This criterion is only satisfied if the report explicitly states *both* the number of subjects initially allocated to groups *and* the number of subjects from whom key outcome measures were obtained. In trials in which outcomes are measured at several points in time, a key outcome must have been measured in more than 85% of subjects at one of those points in time.
Criterion 9	An *intention to treat* analysis means that, where subjects did not receive treatment (or the control condition) as allocated, and where measures of outcomes were available, the analysis was performed as if subjects received the treatment (or control condition) they were allocated to. This criterion is satisfied, even if there is no mention of analysis by intention to treat, if the report explicitly states that all subjects received treatment or control conditions as allocated.
Criterion 10	A *between-group* statistical comparison involves statistical comparison of one group with another. Depending on the design of the study, this may involve comparison of two or more treatments, or comparison of treatment with a control condition. The analysis may be a simple comparison of outcomes measured after the treatment was administered, or a comparison of the change in one group with the change in another (when a factorial analysis of variance has been used to analyze the data, the latter is often reported as a group × time interaction). The comparison may be in the form hypothesis testing (which provides a "p" value, describing the probability that the groups differed only by chance) or in the form of an estimate (for example, the mean or median difference, or a difference in proportions, or number needed to treat, or a relative risk or hazard ratio) and its confidence interval.
Criterion 11	A *point measure* is a measure of the size of the treatment effect. The treatment effect may be described as a difference in group outcomes, or as the outcome in (each of) all groups. *Measures of variability* include standard deviations, standard errors, confidence intervals, interquartile ranges (or other quantile ranges), and ranges. Point measures and/or measures of variability may be provided graphically (for example, SDs may be given as error bars in a figure) as long as it is clear what is being graphed (for example, as long as it is clear whether error bars represent SDs or SEs). Where outcomes are categorical, this criterion is considered to have been met if the number of subjects in each category is given for each group.

Reprinted with permission from The George Institute for Global Health. http://www.pedro.org.au/english/downloads/pedro-scale/. Updated January 12, 2015. Accessed April 10, 2013.

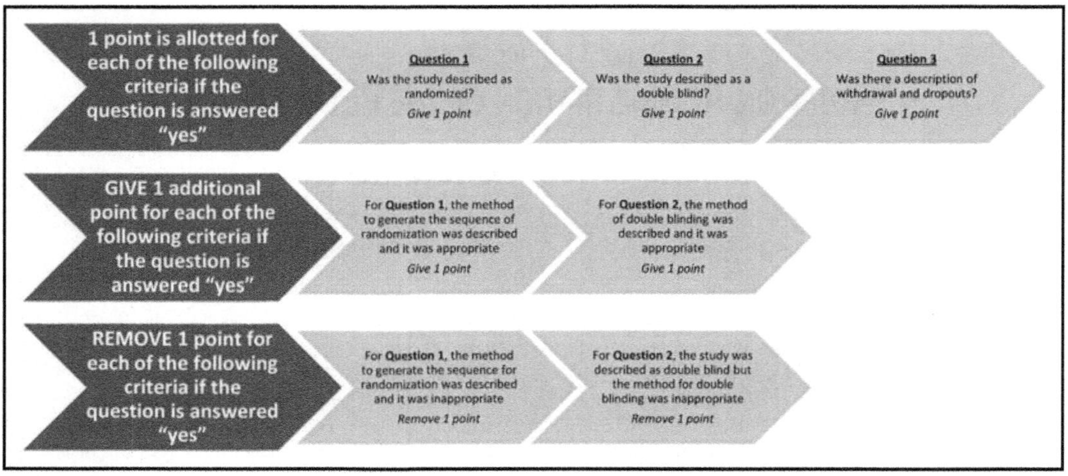

Figure 11-1. Jadad scale and score calculation (highest score = 5 points). (Adapted from Jadad AR, Moore RA, Carroll D, et al. Assessing the quality of reports of randomized clinical trials: is blinding necessary? *Controlled Clin Trials*. 1996;17:1-12.)

The **Consolidated Standards of Reporting Trials (CONSORT) statement** was developed to provide guidelines and offer a standard way of reporting RCTs. This 25-item checklist (Table 11-3) includes a minimum set of recommendations for authors as they prepare RCTs for publication. The checklist items pertain to the content of the (1) title, (2) abstract, (3) introduction, (4) methods, (5) results, (6) discussion, and (7) other information. In addition to the 25-item checklist, a flow diagram (Figure 11-2) was developed for reporting subject progress throughout the study. The flow diagram is intended to depict the movement of participants through the enrollment, intervention allocation, follow-up, and analysis of an RCT. Utilization of the CONSORT statement can help authors ensure that all features of the RCT are included in the publication. Additionally, the CONSORT statement is a good instrument for journal reviewers and readers to use when appraising an RCT because it allows them to make sure all the necessary components are there.

It is strongly recommended that the CONSORT Statement be used in conjunction with the CONSORT Explanation and Elaboration document. These documents are intended to enhance the use, understanding, and dissemination of the CONSORT Statement. The meaning and rationale for each checklist item is presented in the document, which is referenced in several sources and can be located at www.consort-statement.org.

The **Quality of Reports of Meta-Analyses of Randomized Controlled Trials (QUORUM)** was originally created by a group of 30 individuals (including clinical epidemiologists, clinicians, statisticians, editors, and researchers) to establish specific guidelines for reviewing and reporting meta-analyses that pertain to RCTs. The QUORUM comprises a checklist of standards, broken into various sections, that identifies the preferred way to present the title, abstract, introduction, methods, results, and discussion sections of a meta-analysis (Table 11-4).

The first section of the QUORUM checklist focuses on the title, abstract, and introduction of the meta-analysis. More specifically, this section assesses the following:

1. Whether the title clearly identifies the article as a meta-analysis of RCTs.
2. Whether the abstract clearly identifies the objectives, data sources, review methods, results, and conclusions.
3. Whether the introduction details the clinical problem and rationale for the review.

The next portion of the QUORUM examines the methods section of the meta-analysis. Within this section, the article is being assessed for its description of the search process, selection process, validity assessment, data abstraction, study characteristics, and quantitative data synthesis. The final 2 sections of the QUORUM involve the results and discussion. The results section assesses

Table 11-3.
CONSORT 2010 Checklist of Information to Include When Reporting a Randomized Trial*

SECTION/TOPIC	ITEM NO	CHECKLIST ITEM	REPORTED ON PAGE NO
Title and abstract	1a	Identification as a randomised trial in the title	
	1b	Structured summary of trial design, methods, results, and conclusions (for specific guidance see CONSORT for abstracts)	
Introduction			
Background and objectives	2a	Scientific background and explanation of rationale	
	2b	Specific objectives or hypotheses	
Methods			
Trial design	3a	Description of trial design (such as parallel, factorial) including allocation ratio	
	3b	Important changes to methods after trial commencement (such as eligibility criteria), with reasons	
Participants	4a	Eligibility criteria for participants	
	4b	Settings and locations where the data were collected	
Interventions	5	The interventions for each group with sufficient details to allow replication, including how and when they were actually administered	

(continued)

Table 11-3. (continued)
CONSORT 2010 Checklist of Information to Include When Reporting a Randomized Trial*

SECTION/TOPIC	ITEM NO	CHECKLIST ITEM	REPORTED ON PAGE NO
Outcomes	6a	Completely defined prespecified primary and secondary outcome measures, including how and when they were assessed	
	6b	Any changes to trial outcomes after the trial commenced, with reasons	
Sample size	7a	How sample size was determined	
	7b	When applicable, explanation of any interim analyses and stopping guidelines	
Randomization:			
Sequence generation	8a	Method used to generate the random allocation sequence	
	8b	Type of randomization; details of any restriction (such as blocking and block size)	
Allocation concealment mechanism	9	Mechanism used to implement the random allocation sequence (such as sequentially numbered containers), describing any steps taken to conceal the sequence until interventions were assigned	
Implementation	10	Who generated the random allocation sequence, who enrolled participants, and who assigned participants to interventions	
Blinding	11a	If done, who was blinded after assignment to interventions (eg, participants, care providers, those assessing outcomes) and how	
	11b	If relevant, description of the similarity of interventions	
Statistical methods	12a	Statistical methods used to compare groups for primary and secondary outcomes	
	12b	Methods for additional analyses, such as subgroup analyses and adjusted analyses	

(continued)

Table 11-3. (continued)

CONSORT 2010 Checklist of Information to Include When Reporting a Randomized Trial*

SECTION/TOPIC	ITEM NO	CHECKLIST ITEM	REPORTED ON PAGE NO
Results			
Participant flow (a diagram is strongly recommended)	13a	For each group, the numbers of participants who were randomly assigned, received intended treatment, and were analyzed for the primary outcome	
	13b	For each group, losses and exclusions after randomization, together with reasons	
Recruitment	14a	Dates defining the periods of recruitment and follow-up	
	14b	Why the trial ended or was stopped	
Baseline data	15	A table showing baseline demographic and clinical characteristics for each group	
Numbers analyzed	16	For each group, number of participants (denominator) included in each analysis and whether the analysis was by original assigned groups	
Outcomes and estimation	17a	For each primary and secondary outcome, results for each group, and the estimated effect size and its precision (such as 95% confidence interval)	
	17b	For binary outcomes, presentation of both absolute and relative effect sizes is recommended	
Ancillary analyses	18	Results of any other analyses performed, including subgroup analyses and adjusted analyses, distinguishing prespecified from exploratory	
Harms	19	All important harms or unintended effects in each group (for specific guidance see CONSORT for harms)	
Discussion			
Limitations	20	Trial limitations, addressing sources of potential bias, imprecision, and, if relevant, multiplicity of analyses	

(continued)

Table 11-3. (continued)

CONSORT 2010 Checklist of Information to Include When Reporting a Randomized Trial*

SECTION/TOPIC	ITEM NO	CHECKLIST ITEM	REPORTED ON PAGE NO
Generalizability	21	Generalizability (external validity, applicability) of the trial findings	
Interpretation	22	Interpretation consistent with results, balancing benefits and harms, and considering other relevant evidence	
Other information			
Registration	23	Registration number and name of trial registry	
Protocol	24	Where the full trial protocol can be accessed, if available	
Funding	25	Sources of funding and other support (such as supply of drugs), role of funders	

*We strongly recommend reading this statement in conjunction with the CONSORT 2010 Explanation and Elaboration for important clarifications on all the items. If relevant, we also recommend reading CONSORT extensions for cluster randomized trials, noninferiority and equivalence trials, nonpharmacological treatments, herbal interventions, and pragmatic trials. Additional extensions are forthcoming: for those and for up-to-date references relevant to this checklist, see www.consort-statement.org.

Reprinted from CONSORT 2010. CONSORT Transparent Reporting of Trials website. www.consort-statement.org/consort-statement/. Accessed April 10, 2013.

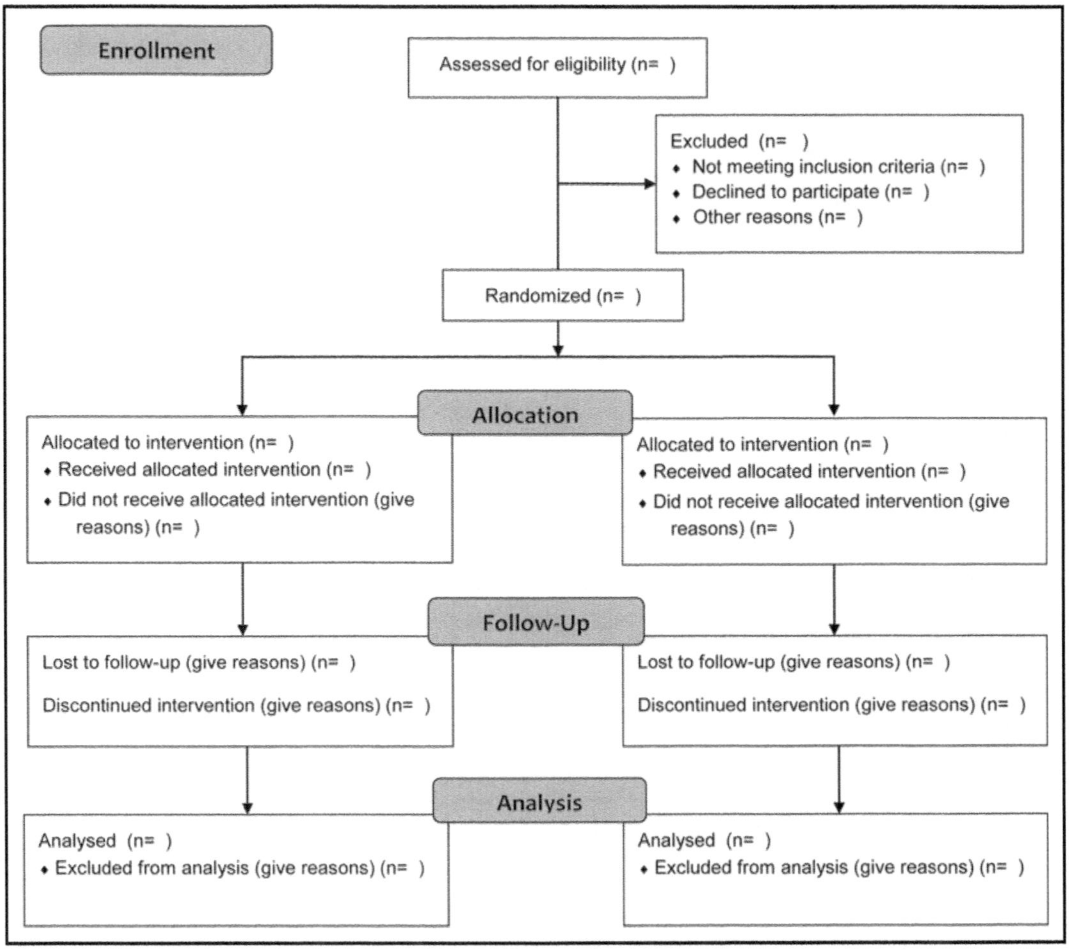

Figure 11-2. Consolidated Standards of Reporting Trials 2010 flow diagram. (Reprinted from Schulz KF, Altman DG, Moher D, for the CONSORT Group. CONSORT 2010 Statement: updated guidelines for reporting parallel group randomised trials. *J Clin Epi.* 2010; 63[8]:834-840.)

whether the article includes details of the trial flow (eg, number of RCTs identified, included, and excluded), individual study characteristics, and quantitative data synthesis. The discussion section focuses on whether the following were discussed:

1. Key findings
2. Clinical inferences (based on internal and external validity)
3. Interpretation of the results
4. Description of potential biases
5. Suggestions for future research

The developers of the QUORUM also produced a flow diagram for authors to use to detail the RCT selection process within a meta-analysis. The chart (Figure 11-3) was created in an effort to provide a standardized process for reporting article selection to allow for easier comprehension for the readers. At each level of the process, authors are asked to also provide the number of RCTs excluded and the reasons for excluding them. The QUORUM statement was an initial attempt to standardize the examination of meta-analyses, and as it has been utilized over time, updates have led to its evolution into a different instrument.

Table 11-4.
QUORUM Checklist

HEADING	SUBHEADING	DESCRIPTOR	REPORTED? (Y/N)	PAGE NUMBER
Title		Identify the report as a meta-analysis (or systematic review) of RCTs		
Abstract		Use a structured format		
	Objectives	The clinical question explicitly		
	Data sources	The databases (ie, list) and other information sources		
	Review methods	The selection (ie, population, intervention, outcome, and study design); methods for validity assessment, data abstraction, and study characteristics; and quantitative data synthesis in sufficient detail to permit replication		
	Results	Characteristics of the RCTs included and excluded, qualitative and quantitative findings (ie, point estimates and confidence intervals), and subgroup analyses		
	Conclusion	The main results		
Introduction		The explicit clinical problem, biological rationale for the intervention, and rationale for review		
Methods	Searching	The information sources, in detail (eg, databases, registers, personal files, expert informants, agencies, hand-searching), and any restrictions (years considered, publication status, language of publication)		
	Validity assessment	The criteria and process used (eg, masked conditions, quality assessment, and their findings)		

(continued)

Table 11-4. (continued)

QUORUM Checklist

HEADING	SUBHEADING	DESCRIPTOR	REPORTED? (Y/N)	PAGE NUMBER
	Data abstraction	The process or processes used (eg, completed independently, in duplicate)		
	Study characteristics	The type of design, participants' characteristics, details of intervention, outcome definitions, etc, and how clinical heterogeneity was assessed		
	Quantitative data synthesis	The principal measures of effect (eg, relative risk), method of combining results (statistical testing and confidence intervals), handling of missing data; how statistical heterogeneity was assessed; a rationale for any a-priori sensitivity and subgroup analyses; and any assessment of publication bias		
Results	Trial flow	Provide a meta-analysis profile summarizing trial flow		
	Study characteristics	Present descriptive data for each trial (eg, age, sample size, intervention, dose, duration, follow-up period)		
	Quantitative data synthesis	Report agreement on the selection and validity assessment; present simple summary results (for each treatment group in each trial, for each primary outcome); present data needed to calculate effect sizes and confidence intervals in intention-to-treat analyses (eg, 2-by-2 tables of counts, means and standard deviations, proportions)		
Discussion		Summarize key findings, discuss clinical inferences based on internal and external validity, interpret the results in light of the totality of available evidence, describe potential biases in the review process (eg, publication bias), and suggest a future research agenda		

Abbreviation: RCT, randomized, controlled trial.

Adapted from Moher D, Cook DJ, Eastwood S, Olkin I, Rennie D, Stroup DF. Improving the quality of reports of meta-analyses of randomized controlled trials: the QUOROM statement. *Lancet*. 1999;354(9193):1896-1900..

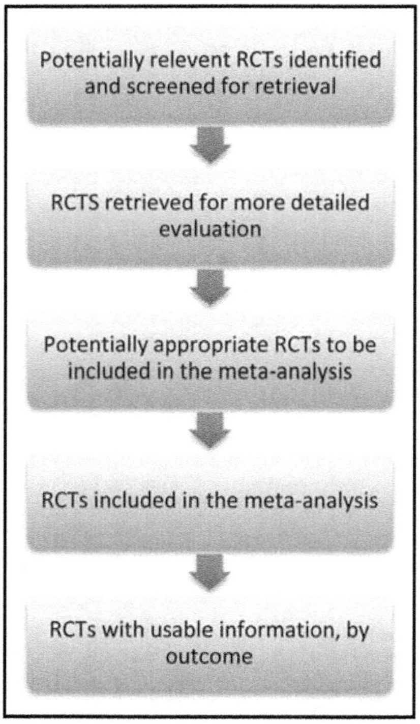

Figure 11-3. Flow diagram for the Quality of Reports of Meta-Analyses and Randomized, Controlled Trials (RCTs). (Adapted from Moher D, Cook DJ, Eastwood S, Olkin I, Rennie D, Stroup DF. Improving the quality of reports of meta-analyses of randomized controlled trials: the QUOROM statement. *Lancet.* 1999;354[9193]:1896-1900.)

Preferred Reporting Items for Systematic Reviews and Meta-Analyses (PRISMA) is an update and expansion of the QUORUM Statement. It was created to ensure that authors had a transparent and complete reporting mechanism for systematic reviews and meta-analyses through a 27-item checklist and a 4-phase diagram. The PRISMA is not intended to be a quality assessment tool, and it should not be used in that manner. The checklist and flow diagram should be accompanied by the PRISMA Explanation and Elaboration document, which is used to enhance the use, understanding, and dissemination of the PRISMA Statement. The Explanation and Elaboration document provides each checklist item, followed by a published example of good reporting for that item, and it is further supported by an explanation of the issue and the rationale for including the item. The checklist items (Table 11-5) pertain to the content of the systematic review and meta-analyses and include items related to the title, abstract, methods, results, discussion, and funding. The following is a breakdown of the topics included within each of the sections:

1. Title
2. Abstract: Structured summary
3. Introduction: Rationale, objectives
4. Methods: Protocol and registration, eligibility criteria, information sources, search, study selection, data collection process, risk of bias in individual studies, summary measures, synthesis of results, risk of bias across studies, additional analyses
5. Results: Study selection, study characteristics, risk of bias within studies, results of individual studies, synthesis of results, risk of bias across studies, additional analysis
6. Discussion: Summary of evidence, limitations, conclusions
7. Funding

The flow diagram depicts the flow of information through the different phases of a systematic review and maps out the number of records identified, included and excluded, and the reasons for exclusions (Figure 11-4). You should utilize the PRISMA when considering the information within

Table 11-5. PRISMA 2009 Checklist

SECTION/TOPIC	#	CHECKLIST ITEM	REPORTED ON PAGE #
Title			
Title	1	Identify the report as a systematic review, meta-analysis, or both.	
Abstract			
Structured summary	2	Provide a structured summary including, as applicable: background; objectives; data sources; study eligibility criteria, participants, and interventions; study appraisal and synthesis methods; results; limitations; conclusions and implications of key findings; systematic review registration number.	
Introduction			
Rationale	3	Describe the rationale for the review in the context of what is already known.	
Objectives	4	Provide an explicit statement of questions being addressed with reference to participants, interventions, comparisons, outcomes, and study design (PICOS).	
Methods			
Protocol and registration	5	Indicate if a review protocol exists, if and where it can be accessed (eg, web address), and, if available, provide registration information including registration number.	
Eligibility criteria	6	Specify study characteristics (eg, PICOS, length of follow-up) and report characteristics (eg, years considered, language, publication status) used as criteria for eligibility, giving rationale.	
Information sources	7	Describe all information sources (eg, databases with dates of coverage, contact with study authors to identify additional studies) in the search and date last searched.	

(continued)

Table 11-5. (continued)

PRISMA 2009 Checklist

SECTION/TOPIC	#	CHECKLIST ITEM	REPORTED ON PAGE #
Search	8	Present full electronic search strategy for at least one database, including any limits used, such that it could be repeated.	
Study selection	9	State the process for selecting studies (ie, screening, eligibility, included in systematic review, and, if applicable, included in the meta-analysis).	
Data collection process	10	Describe method of data extraction from reports (eg, piloted forms, independently, in duplicate) and any processes for obtaining and confirming data from investigators.	
Data items	11	List and define all variables for which data were sought (eg, PICOS, funding sources) and any assumptions and simplifications made.	
Risk of bias in individual studies	12	Describe methods used for assessing risk of bias of individual studies (including specification of whether this was done at the study or outcome level), and how this information is to be used in any data synthesis.	
Summary measures	13	State the principal summary measures (eg, risk ratio, difference in means).	
Synthesis of results	14	Describe the methods of handling data and combining results of studies, if done, including measures of consistency (eg, I2) for each meta-analysis.	
Risk of bias across studies	15	Specify any assessment of risk of bias that may affect the cumulative evidence (eg, publication bias, selective reporting within studies).	
Additional analyses	16	Describe methods of additional analyses (eg, sensitivity or subgroup analyses, meta-regression), if done, indicating which were pre-specified.	

(continued)

Table 11-5. (continued)

PRISMA 2009 Checklist

SECTION/TOPIC	#	CHECKLIST ITEM	REPORTED ON PAGE #
Results			
Study selection	17	Give numbers of studies screened, assessed for eligibility, and included in the review, with reasons for exclusions at each stage, ideally with a flow diagram.	
Study characteristics	18	For each study, present characteristics for which data were extracted (eg, study size, PICOS, follow-up period) and provide the citations.	
Risk of bias within studies	19	Present data on risk of bias of each study and, if available, any outcome level assessment (see item 12).	
Results of individual studies	20	For all outcomes considered (benefits or harms), present, for each study: (a) simple summary data for each intervention group (b) effect estimates and confidence intervals, ideally with a forest plot.	
Synthesis of results	21	Present the main results of the review. If meta-analyses are done, include for each, confidence intervals and measures of consistency.	
Risk of bias across studies	22	Present results of any assessment of risk of bias across studies (see Item 15).	
Additional analysis	23	Give results of additional analyses, if done (eg, sensitivity or subgroup analyses, meta-regression [see Item 16]).	

(continued)

Table 11-5. (continued)
PRISMA 2009 Checklist

SECTION/TOPIC	#	CHECKLIST ITEM	REPORTED ON PAGE #
Discussion			
Summary of evidence	24	Summarize the main findings including the strength of evidence for each main outcome; consider their relevance to key groups (eg, health care providers, users, and policy makers).	
Limitations	25	Discuss limitations at study and outcome level (eg, risk of bias), and at review-level (eg, incomplete retrieval of identified research, reporting bias).	
Conclusions	26	Provide a general interpretation of the results in the context of other evidence and implications for future research.	
Funding			
Funding	27	Describe sources of funding for the systematic review and other support (eg, supply of data); role of funders for the systematic review.	

Reprinted from Moher D, Liberati A, Tetzlaff J, Altman DG, The PRISMA Group. Preferred reporting items for systematic reviews and meta-analyses: the PRISMA statement. *PLoS Med*. 2009;6(6):e1000097. For more information, visit www.prisma-statement.org.

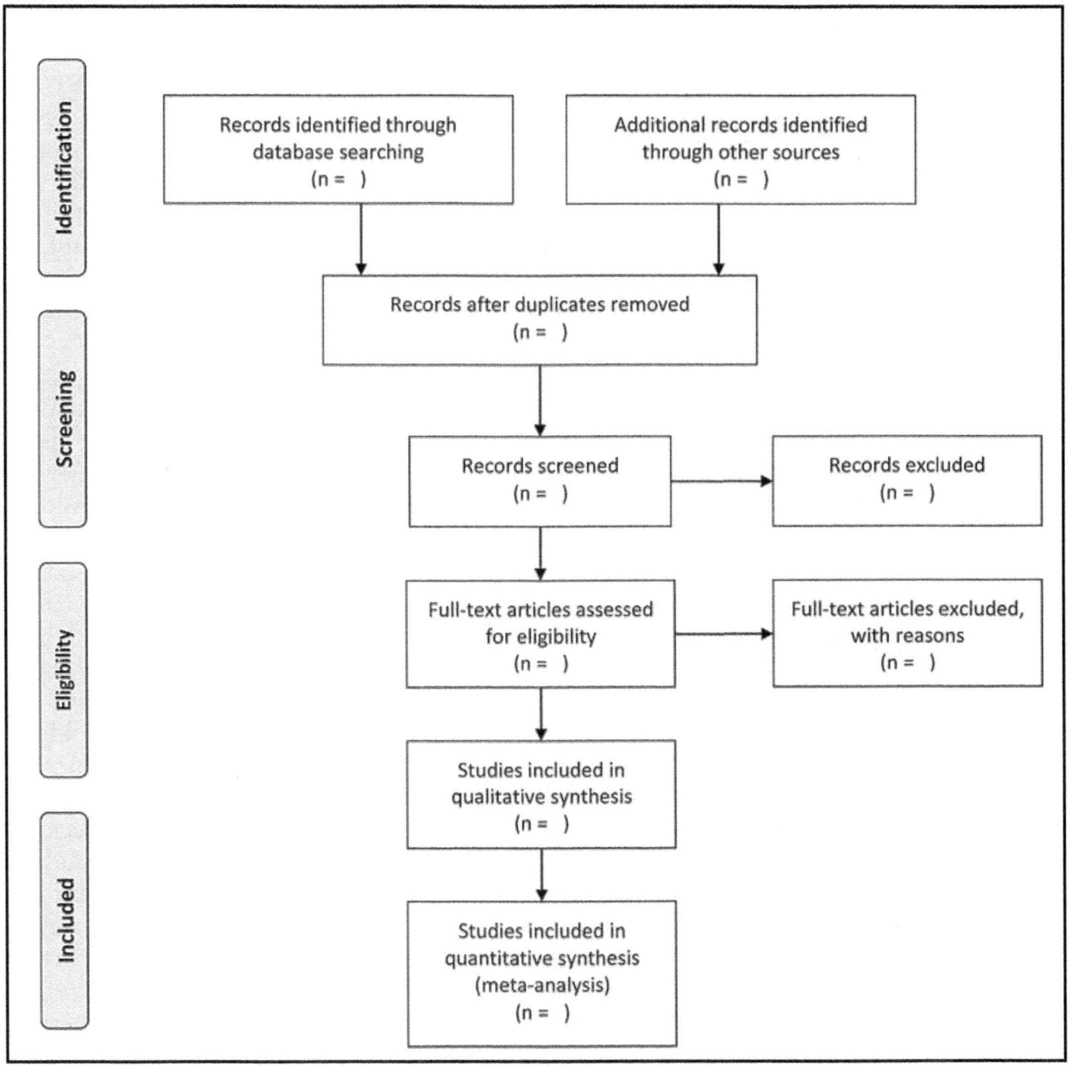

Figure 11-4. Preferred Reporting Items for Systematic Reviews and Meta-Analyses 2009 flow diagram. (Reprinted from Moher D, Liberati A, Tetzlaff J, Altman DG, The PRISMA Group. Preferred reporting items for systematic reviews and meta-analyses: the PRISMA statement. *PLoS Med.* 2009;6[6]:e1000097. http://www.prisma-statement.org.)

a systematic review or meta-analysis for use in your clinical practice, as it will assist you with determining whether all of the key items have been addressed. Because PRISMA is utilized more in the development and evaluation of systematic reviews and meta-analyses, the instrument will need to be updated to account for change. Because systematic reviews are increasingly used by all health care providers to inform clinical practice, utilization of this instrument is critical.

Appraisal Scales and Checklists for Diagnostic Accuracy

The **Standards for the Reporting of Diagnostic accuracy studies (STARD)** includes standard guidelines to improve the accuracy of reporting diagnostic research and was released in 2000. The 25-item checklist (Table 11-6) and flow diagram (Figure 11-5) are used to enhance completeness of reporting diagnostic methodology and findings to allow readers to assess the potential for bias in the study and to evaluate generalizability. The STARD is widely used as it is part of author guidelines of more than 200 biomedical journals. The STARD checklist is also located on the STARD website (www.stard-statement.org) and provides an opportunity for you to click on the description of the topic and a link to an example for that item. A flow diagram provides information about the method of recruitment of patients or samples (eg, based on a consecutive series of patients with specific symptoms or of cases and controls), the order of test execution, the number of patients undergoing the test under evaluation (index test), and the reference test or gold standard. An example of the utilization of the flow diagram for subject recruitment within a manual therapy assessment is provided in Figure 11-5B, which depicts comparisons between the reference standard and the clinical examination results.

The STARD checklist assists with the assessment of internal and external validity components and provides aid to authors who are putting together a diagnostic accuracy study. The major disadvantage in using the STARD is that it does not assess quality; therefore, use of another instrument (eg, Quality Assessment of Studies of Diagnostic Accuracy Included in Systematic Reviews [QUADAS]) may be necessary. The STARD, like all of the checklists and scales, is truly limited by the ability of authors to provide the details within their respective studies.

The QUADAS appraisal checklist was originally developed in 2003 as an evidence-based tool to determine the methodological rigor of systematic reviews pertaining to diagnostic accuracy studies. The original QUADAS checklist included 14 items assessing 3 main criteria: reporting of selection criteria, description of index test execution, and description of reference standard execution. Each item was in the form of a question and requires a response of yes, no, or unclear. The time taken to complete the QUADAS ranged from less than 10 minutes to longer than an hour, with efficiency of use increasing as an individual became more familiar with each question.

Anecdotal reports and feedback by users of the QUADAS indicated that they had problems rating certain items, that there was possible overlap among items, and that situations occurred in which the QUADAS was difficult to use. Therefore, the instrument was revised, and the QUADAS-2 was developed. The QUADAS-2 comprises 4 domains: patient selection, index test, reference standard, and flow and timing related to the flow of patients through the study and the timing of the index tests and reference standard. Each domain is assessed in terms of risk of bias, and patient selection, index test, and reference standard are also assessed in terms of concerns regarding applicability. The QUADAS-2 is applied in 4 phases: (1) summarize the review question, (2) tailor the tool to the review and produce review-specific guidance, (3) construct a flow diagram for the primary study, and (4) assess the risk of bias and concerns regarding applicability. Detailed information about the QUADAS-2 instrument can be found on the associated website (http://www.bris.ac.uk/quadas/quadas-2/).

Other Appraisal Scales and Checklists

The **Strengthening in the Reporting of Observations Studies in Epidemiology (STROBE)** is used for cohort, case-control, and cross-sectional studies and was developed through an initiative in 2004. Similar to the other appraisal checklists, the STROBE provides a checklist of items that should be included in observational research (ie, cohort, case-control, cross-sectional). Thus, this checklist does not evaluate research articles; it provides recommendations for standardized reporting of epidemiological studies. The fourth version of the checklist provides guidelines for observational studies in general and also provides specific information for each type of observation study being discussed. The general observational studies STROBE contains 22 items that relate to the following:

- Title and abstract

Table 11-6.
STARD Checklist for Reporting of Studies of Diagnostic Accuracy
(January 2003)

SECTION AND TOPIC	ITEM #		ON PAGE #
Title/abstract/keywords	1	Identify the article as a study of diagnostic accuracy (recommend MeSH heading "sensitivity and specificity").	
Introduction	2	State the research questions or study aims, such as estimating diagnostic accuracy or comparing accuracy between tests or across participant groups.	
Methods			
Participants	3	The study population: The inclusion and exclusion criteria, setting and locations where data were collected.	
	4	Participant recruitment: Was recruitment based on presenting symptoms, results from previous tests, or the fact that the participants had received the index tests or the reference standard?	
	5	Participant sampling: Was the study population a consecutive series of participants defined by the selection criteria in item 3 and 4? If not, specify how participants were further selected.	
	6	Data collection: Was data collection planned before the index test and reference standard were performed (prospective study) or after (retrospective study)?	
Test methods	7	The reference standard and its rationale.	
	8	Technical specifications of material and methods involved including how and when measurements were taken, and/or cite references for index tests and reference standard.	

(continued)

Table 11-6. (continued)

STARD Checklist for Reporting of Studies of Diagnostic Accuracy

(JANUARY 2003)

SECTION AND TOPIC	ITEM #		ON PAGE #
	9	Definition of and rationale for the units, cutoffs, and/or categories of the results of the index tests and the reference standard.	
	10	The number, training and expertise of the persons executing and reading the index tests and the reference standard.	
	11	Whether or not the readers of the index tests and reference standard were blind (masked) to the results of the other test and describe any other clinical information available to the readers.	
Statistical methods	12	Methods for calculating or comparing measures of diagnostic accuracy, and the statistical methods used to quantify uncertainty (eg, 95% confidence intervals).	
	13	Methods for calculating test reproducibility, if done.	
Results			
Participants	14	When study was performed, including beginning and end dates of recruitment.	
	15	Clinical and demographic characteristics of the study population (at least information on age, gender, spectrum of presenting symptoms).	
	16	The number of participants satisfying the criteria for inclusion who did or did not undergo the index tests and/or the reference standard; describe why participants failed to undergo either test (a flow diagram is strongly recommended).	

(continued)

Table 11-6. (continued)
STARD Checklist for Reporting of Studies of Diagnostic Accuracy
(January 2003)

SECTION AND TOPIC	ITEM #		ON PAGE #
Test results	17	Time-interval between the index tests and the reference standard, and any treatment administered in between.	
	18	Distribution of severity of disease (define criteria) in those with the target condition; other diagnoses in participants without the target condition.	
	19	A cross-tabulation of the results of the index tests (including indeterminate and missing results) by the results of the reference standard; for continuous results, the distribution of the test results by the results of the reference standard.	
	20	Any adverse events from performing the index tests or the reference standard.	
Estimates	21	Estimates of diagnostic accuracy and measures of statistical uncertainty (eg, 95% confidence intervals).	
	22	How indeterminate results, missing data, and outliers of the index tests were handled.	
	23	Estimates of variability of diagnostic accuracy between subgroups of participants, readers, or centers, if done.	
	24	Estimates of test reproducibility, if done.	
Discussion	25	Discuss the clinical applicability of the study findings.	

Reprinted from Bossuyt PM, Reitsma JB, Bruns DE, et al; Standards for Reporting of Diagnostic Accuracy. Toward complete and accurate reporting of studies of diagnostic accuracy: the STARD initiative. Standards for Reporting of Diagnostic Accuracy. *BMJ.* 2003;326:41-44.

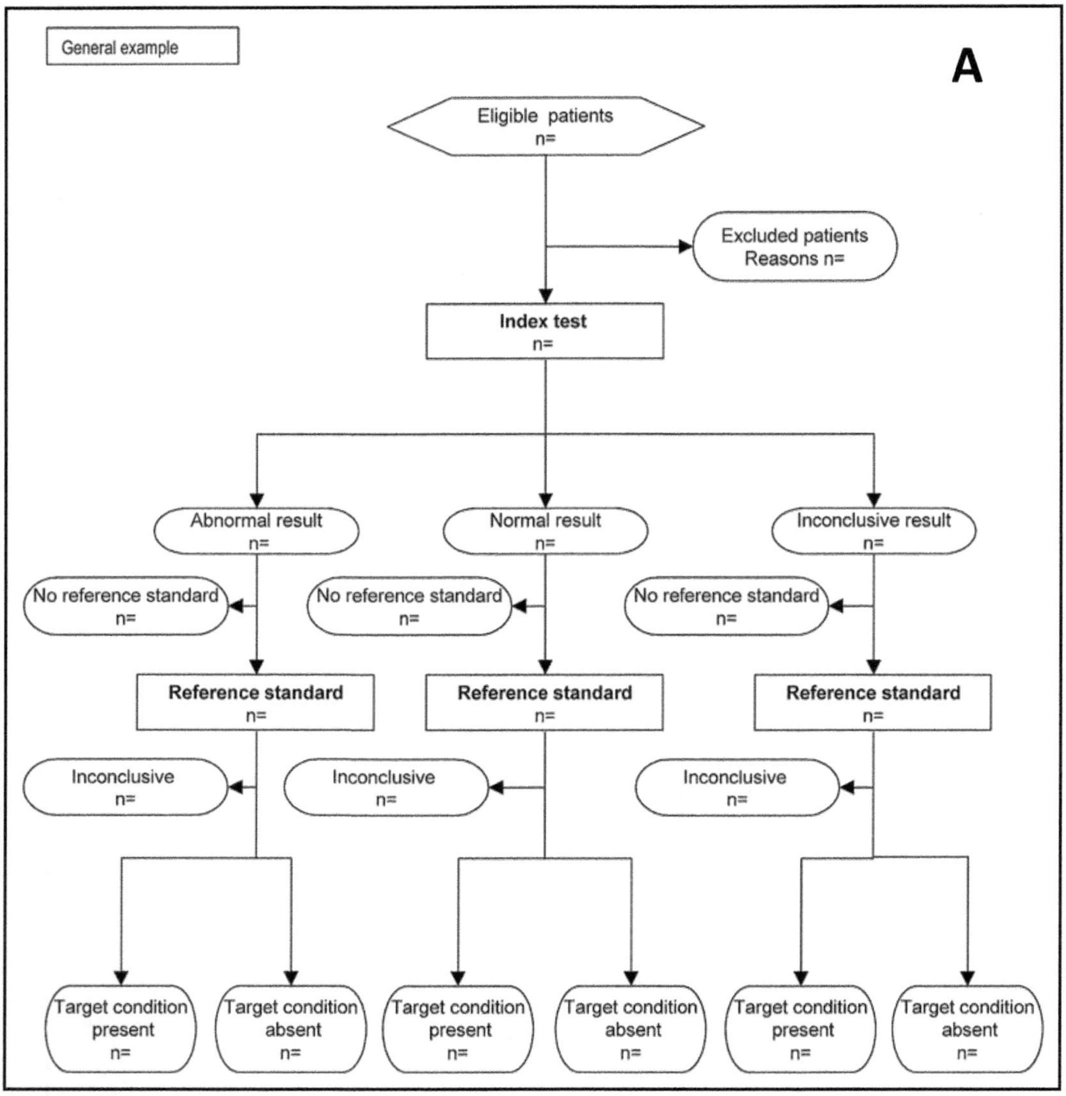

Figure 11-5. (A) Prototypical Standards for the Reporting of Diagnostic accuracy studies flow diagram of a diagnostic accuracy study. (Reprinted from Abbott JH, McCane B, Herbison P, Moginie G, Chapple C, Hogarty T. Lumbar segmental instability: a criterion-related validity study of manual therapy assessment. *BMC Musculoskelet Disord.* 2005,6:56.)

- Introduction (background/rationale, objectives)
- Methods (study design, setting, participants, variables, data sources/measurement, bias, study size, quantitative variables, statistical methods)
- Results (participants, descriptive data, outcome data, main results, other analyses)
- Discussion (key results, limitations, interpretation, generalizability)
- Other information (funding)
- Funding

Eighteen of the items are common to all 3 study designs and 4 items (participants, statistical methods, descriptive data, and outcome data) contain specific information for cohort, case-control, or cross-sectional studies (Table 11-7). The STROBE Statement was developed to assist authors when writing analytical observational studies, support editors and reviewers when considering

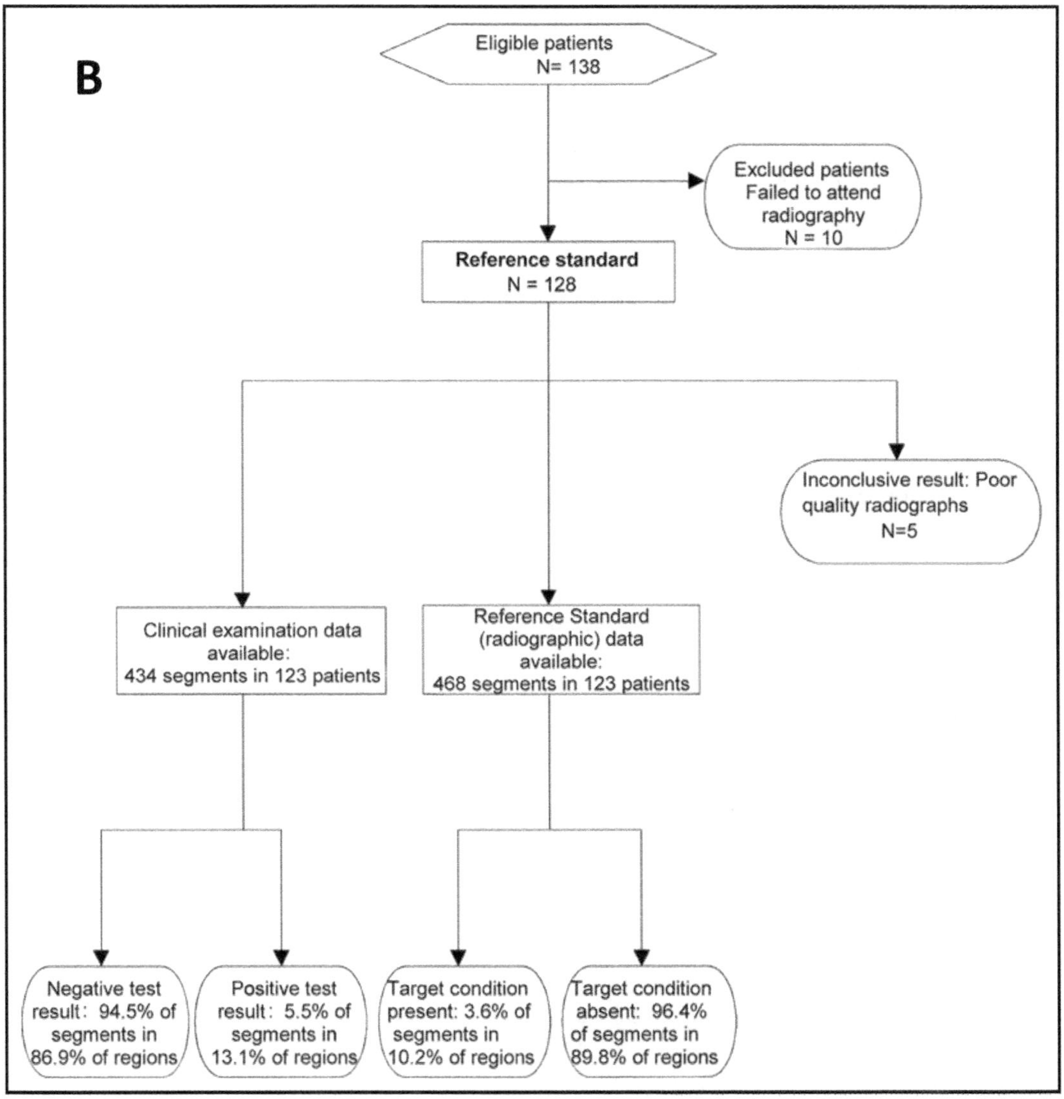

Figure 11-5. (B) Prototypical Standards for the Reporting of Diagnostic accuracy studies flow diagram of a diagnostic accuracy study. (Reprinted from Abbott JH, McCane B, Herbison P, Moginie G, Chapple C, Hogarty T. Lumbar segmental instability: a criterion-related validity study of manual therapy assessment. *BMC Musculoskelet Disord.* 2005,6:56.)

these types of articles for publication, and help readers when critically appraising published articles. The STROBE Statement was not developed as a tool for assessing the quality of published observational research; however, its use can assist with an improvement in methodological designs.

Systematic reviews are often concentrated on the review of RCTs; however, few of these types of studies exist in some areas. Establishing an instrument that could simultaneously examine randomized and nonrandomized trials was needed, so the **Downs and Black checklist** for randomized and nonrandomized studies of health care interventions was developed to do the following:

- Establish a valid and reliable checklist appropriate for assessing randomized and nonrandomized studies
- Provide an overall score for study quality and a profile of scores not only for the quality of reporting, internal validity and power, but also for external validity

- The Downs and Black checklist consists of 27 items that are broken down into various sections:
- Reporting (10 items)
- External validity (3 items)
- Internal validity—bias (7 items)
- Internal validity—confounding (selection bias) (6 items)
- Power (1 item)

The checklist requires that you score the item with a "yes," "no," or "unable to determine" answer. A higher score indicates that the article met more of the criteria for the checklist. The advantage in using this checklist is that you are able to use the same instrument for different types of study designs and compare scores. The reported disadvantage is that the external validity items had low reliability; therefore, the values may not provide information that you are seeking for applicability.

The **Appraisal of Guidelines, Research and Evaluation (AGREE) scale** is an international instrument for assessing the quality of the process and reporting of clinical practice guideline development that was formulated by an international group of researchers from 13 countries in 2002. It contains 23 items grouped into 6 quality domains with a 4-point Likert scale to score each item (scope and purpose, stakeholder involvement, rigor of development, clarity and presentation, applicability, editorial independence). Internal consistency of the scale ranges from 0.64 to 0.88 and is acceptable for most domains; however, the validity of the instrument has not been assessed. The AGREE instrument is designed to assess the process of guideline development and how well this process is reported. It does not assess the clinical content of the guideline or the quality of evidence that underpins the recommendations. These standards can be used for the planning, execution, and monitoring of guideline programs and for comparing guidelines internationally.

The original AGREE instrument has been refined and resulted in the AGREE II instrument, which includes a user's manual. The AGREE II has 23 items that are organized into the same previous domains. Information about the AGREE II instrument can be accessed at http://www.agreetrust.org/wp-content/uploads/2013/10/AGREE-II-Users-Manual-and-23-item-Instrument_2009_UPDATE_2013.pdf.

The **Grading of Recommendations Assessment, Development, and Evaluation (GRADE)** working group was established in 2000 to address the need for developing a single grading system that could be used in health care. This working group was established to develop an instrument to grade quality of evidence and provide a strength of recommendation for various types of study designs. The GRADE quality of evidence is divided into categories of high, moderate, low, or very low.

- High = Further research is very unlikely to change our confidence in the estimate of effect.
- Moderate = Further research is likely to have an important impact on our confidence in the estimate of effect and may change the estimate.
- Low = Further research is very likely to have an important impact on our confidence in the estimate of effect and is likely to change the estimate.
- Very low = Any estimate of effect is very uncertain.

The GRADE working group has developed a free software application that facilitates the use of the approach and allows the development of summary tables (www.gradeworkinggroup.org).

The GRADE has 2 levels of recommendation: strong and weak. To be classified as a strong recommendation, clinicians must be very certain that benefits do, or do not, outweigh risks and burdens based upon the available evidence. A weak recommendation is made if clinicians believe that benefits, risks, and burdens are finely balanced or appreciable uncertainty exists about the magnitude of benefits and risks based on the available evidence. Some of the factors associated

Table 11-7. STROBE Statement—Checklist of Items That Should Be Included in Reports of Observational Studies

	ITEM NO	RECOMMENDATION
Title and abstract	1	(*a*) Indicate the study's design with a commonly used term in the title or the abstract
		(*b*) Provide an informative and balanced summary of what was done and what was found
Introduction		
Background/ rationale	2	Explain the scientific background and rationale for the investigation being reported
Objectives	3	State specific objectives, including any prespecified hypotheses
Methods		
Study design	4	Present key elements of study design early in the paper
Setting	5	Describe the setting, locations, and relevant dates, including periods of recruitment, exposure, follow-up, and data collection
Participants	6	(a) *Cohort study*—Give the eligibility criteria and the sources and methods of selection of participants. Describe methods of follow-up *Case-control study*—Give the eligibility criteria and the sources and methods of case ascertainment and control selection. Give the rationale for the choice of cases and controls *Cross-sectional study*—Give the eligibility criteria and the sources and methods of selection of participants
		(b) *Cohort study*—For matched studies, give matching criteria and number of exposed and unexposed *Case-control study*—For matched studies, give matching criteria and the number of controls per case
Variables	7	Clearly define all outcomes, exposures, predictors, potential confounders, and effect modifiers. Give diagnostic criteria, if applicable
Data sources/ measurement	8*	For each variable of interest, give sources of data and details of methods of assessment (measurement). Describe comparability of assessment methods if there is more than one group
Bias	9	Describe any efforts to address potential sources of bias
Study size	10	Explain how the study size was arrived at

(continued)

Table 11-7. (continued)
STROBE Statement—Checklist of Items That Should Be Included in Reports of Observational Studies

	ITEM NO	RECOMMENDATION
Quantitative variables	11	Explain how quantitative variables were handled in the analyses. If applicable, describe which groupings were chosen and why
Statistical methods	12	(a) Describe all statistical methods, including those used to control for confounding
		(b) Describe any methods used to examine subgroups and interactions
		(c) Explain how missing data were addressed
		(d) *Cohort study*—If applicable, explain how loss to follow-up was addressed *Case-control study*—If applicable, explain how matching of cases and controls was addressed *Cross-sectional study*—If applicable, describe analytical methods taking account of sampling strategy
		(e) Describe any sensitivity analyses
Results		
Participants	13*	(a) Report numbers of individuals at each stage of study (eg, numbers potentially eligible, examined for eligibility, confirmed eligible, included in the study, completing follow-up, and analyzed)
		(b) Give reasons for nonparticipation at each stage
		(c) Consider use of a flow diagram
Descriptive data	14*	(a) Give characteristics of study participants (eg, demographic, clinical, social) and information on exposures and potential confounders
		(b) Indicate number of participants with missing data for each variable of interest
		(c) *Cohort study*—Summarize follow-up time (eg, average and total amount)
Outcome data	15*	*Cohort study*—Report numbers of outcome events or summary measures over time
		Case-control study—Report numbers in each exposure category,or summary measures of exposure
		Cross-sectional study—Report numbers of outcome events or summary measures

(continued)

Table 11-7. (continued)

STROBE Statement—Checklist of Items That Should Be Included in Reports of Observational Studies

	ITEM NO	RECOMMENDATION
Main results	16	(a) Give unadjusted estimates and, if applicable, confounder-adjusted estimates and their precision (eg, 95% confidence interval). Make clear which confounders were adjusted for and why they were included
		(b) Report category boundaries when continuous variables were categorized
		(c) If relevant, consider translating estimates of relative risk into absolute risk for a meaningful time period
Other analyses	17	Report other analyses done (eg, analyses of subgroups and interactions and sensitivity analyses)
Discussion		
Key results	18	Summarize key results with reference to study objectives
Limitations	19	Discuss limitations of the study, taking into account sources of potential bias or imprecision. Discuss both direction and magnitude of any potential bias
Interpretation	20	Give a cautious overall interpretation of results considering objectives, limitations, multiplicity of analyses, results from similar studies, and other relevant evidence
Generalisability	21	Discuss the generalizability (external validity) of the study results
Other information		
Funding	22	Give the source of funding and the role of the funders for the present study and, if applicable, for the original study on which the present article is based

*Give information separately for cases and controls in case-control studies and, if applicable, for exposed and unexposed groups in cohort and cross-sectional studies.

Note: An Explanation and Elaboration article discusses each checklist item and gives methodological background and published examples of transparent reporting. The STROBE checklist is best used in conjunction with this article (freely available on the Web sites of PLoS Medicine at http://www.plosmedicine.org/, Annals of Internal Medicine at http://www.annals.org/, and Epidemiology at http://www.epidem.com/).

Reprinted from von Elm E, Altman DG, Egger M, Pocock SJ, Gøtzsche PC, Vandenbroucke JP; STROBE Initiative. The Strengthening the Reporting of Observational Studies in Epidemiology (STROBE) statement: guidelines for reporting observational studies. *J Clin Epidemiol.* 2008;61(4):344-349.

with grading recommendations include the confidence in the best estimates of benefit and harm, importance of the outcome that the treatment prevents, the magnitude of the treatment effect, the precision of estimate of treatment effect, risks associated with therapy, burdens of therapy, and cost. All of these factors must also be considered within this system, as they vary from patient to patient. The GRADE provides you with one more option to examine available evidence, and you can then decide as to the usefulness of this information for your clinical practice.

Summary

To examine the available evidence that health care professionals and others have conducted, you need to be able to clearly delineate aspects of the research study that coincide with quality. However, it is the responsibility of researchers and the journals who publish the research to utilize the available guidelines, appraisal scales, and checklists to design and report their findings. Articles that are written based on the recommendations from these instruments are easier to interpret and appraise, and they will ultimately help you to make better decisions in clinical practice.

Key Points

- The Jadad scale is less utilized in athletic training research because it does not include items to assess the effects of treatments and interventions that are typically important in athletic training research.
- The CONSORT, QUORUM, and PRISMA checklists have flow diagrams associated with them that aid in the ease of use and comprehension of the articles they are appraising.
- The PRISMA is not intended to be a quality assessment tool; therefore, it should not be used in that manner.
- The CONSORT and PRISMA have Explanation and Elaboration documents associated with them that further explain the components and use for items in the checklists.
- The STARD and QUADAS are the only available checklists for analyzing diagnostic research; no appraisal scales are currently being circulated for diagnostic research.
- Many of the checklists and scales are limited by the ability of authors to provide the details within their respective studies.

Bibliography

Abbott JH, McCane B, Herbison P, Moginie G, Chapple C, Hogarty T. Lumbar segmental instability: a criterion-related validity study of manual therapy assessment. *BMC Musculoskelet Disord.* 2005,6:56.

AGREE Collaboration. Development and validation of an international appraisal instrument for assessing the quality of clinical practice guidelines: the AGREE project. *Qual Saf Health Care.* 2003;12(1):18-23.

Downs SH, Black N. The feasibility of creating a checklist for the assessment of the methodological quality both of randomised and non-randomised studies of health care interventions. *J Epidemiol Community Health.* 1998;52(6):377-384.

Jadad AR, Moore RA, Carroll D, et al. Assessing the quality of reports of randomized clinical trials: is blinding necessary? *Control Clin Trials.* 1996;17(1):1-12.

Liberati A, Altman DG, Tetzlaff J, et al. The PRISMA statement for reporting systematic reviews and meta-analyses of studies that evaluate health care interventions: explanation and elaboration. *Ann Intern Med.* 2009;151(4):W65-W94.

Maher CG, Sherrington C, Herbert RD, Moseley AM, Elkins M. Reliability of the PEDro scale for rating quality of randomized controlled trials. *Phys Ther.* 2003;83(8):713-721.

Moher D, Cook DJ, Eastwood S, Olkin I, Rennie D, Stroup DF. Improving the quality of reports of meta-analyses of randomized controlled trials: the QUOROM statement. *Lancet.* 1999;354(9193):1896-1900.

Moher D, Hopewell S, Schulz KF, et al. CONSORT 2010 explanation and elaboration: updated guidelines for reporting parallel group randomised trials. *BMJ.* 2010;340:c869.

Moher D, Liberati A, Tetzlaff J, Altman DG; PRISMA Group. Preferred reporting items for systematic reviews and meta-analyses: the PRISMA statement. *Ann Intern Med.* 2009;151(4):264-269.

PRISMA. www.prisma-statement.org. Accessed March 13, 2013.

Schulz KF, Altman DG, Moher D; CONSORT Group. CONSORT 2010 Statement: updated guidelines for reporting parallel group randomised trials. *BMC Med.* 2010;8:18.

Schulz KF, Altman DG, Moher D; CONSORT Group. CONSORT 2010 statement: updated guidelines for reporting parallel group randomized trials. *Ann Int Med.* 2010;152(11):726-732.

Schulz KF, Altman DG, Moher D; CONSORT Group. CONSORT 2010 statement: updated guidelines for reporting parallel group randomised trials. *BMJ.* 2010;340:c332.

Schulz KF, Altman DG, Moher D; CONSORT Group. CONSORT 2010 statement: updated guidelines for reporting parallel group randomised trials. *J Clin Epidemiol.* 2010;63(8):834-840.

STARD. www.stard-statement.org. Accessed March 13, 2013.

STROBE Statement. www.strobe-statement.org/index.php?id=available-checklists. Accessed March 13, 2013.

von Elm E, Altman DG, Egger M, et al. The Strengthening the Reporting of Observational Studies in Epidemiology (STROBE) statement: guidelines for reporting observational studies. *PLoS Med.* 2007;4(1):e296.

Whiting P, Rutjes AW, Dinnes J, Reitsma J, Bossuyt PM, Kleijnen J. Development and validation of methods for assessing the quality of diagnostic accuracy studies. *Health Technol Assess.* 2004;8(25):iii,1-234.

Whiting P, Rutjes AW, Reitsma JB, Bossuyt PM, Kleijnen J. The development of QUADAS: a tool for the quality assessment of studies of diagnostic accuracy included in systematic reviews. *BMC Med Res Methodol.* 2003;3:25.

Whiting PF, Rutjes AW, Westwood ME, et al. QUADAS-2: a revised tool for the quality assessment of diagnostic accuracy studies. *Ann Intern Med.* 2011;155(8):529-536.

Whiting PF, Weswood ME, Rutjes AW, Reitsma JB, Bossuyt PN, Kleijnen J. Evaluation of QUADAS, a tool for the quality assessment of diagnostic accuracy studies. *BMC Med Res Methodol.* 2006;6:9.

12

Application of Critical Appraisal

Throughout the last several chapters, we have introduced and discussed numerous concepts that are necessary for critical appraisal. It is understandable at this point that you may feel a bit overwhelmed with the critical appraisal process. As the most crucial step in the evidence-based practice (EBP) process, critical appraisal allows you to determine whether available research literature can be used to help you during the clinical decision-making process. In this chapter, we bring together the concepts of critical appraisal that have previously been discussed and identify some strategies you can use as you navigate your way through the appraisal process. Additionally, we discuss critical appraisal resources and how these resources can be incorporated during the clinical decision-making process for patient care.

To avoid feeling overwhelmed, it is sometimes helpful to remind yourself of the purpose of critical appraisal. Critical appraisal is the process of determining whether evidence from a viable source can be translated and applied to help you answer your clinical question. Globally, we identified that there are 3 general questions you should consider throughout the critical appraisal process:

1. Are the results of the study valid?
2. Are the results of the study reliable?
3. Are the findings of the study clinically relevant and applicable to your clinical question?

Now that you are more knowledgeable about the concepts that are involved in the critical appraisal process, we are going to return to each of these questions and discuss how they can be used as the foundation for critically appraising research evidence in a systematic manner. Remember, even though there are numerous concepts involved in critical appraisal, sometimes returning to the simplest questions will help you navigate this phase of the EBP process.

Van Lunen BL, Hankemeier DA, Welch CE.
Evidence-Guided Practice: A Framework for Clinical Decision Making in Athletic Training (pp 151-165).

Appraising the Validity of a Study

Now that you have an understanding of the concepts involved in validity, you can begin to answer the question of whether a study is valid. As we previously discussed, several factors that affect the internal and external validity of a study should be considered. However, to begin assessing a study's validity, you need to first identify the type of research design that was used for the investigation. The design of a study will dictate the types of validity questions you need to consider; therefore, it is important that the first step of appraising the validity of a study be to ensure the study design selected is appropriate. To help you determine if the study design is appropriate, you should establish the type of clinical question (ie, intervention, etiology, diagnosis, prognosis, meaning) the researchers were attempting to answer. Since each research design consists of different approaches for subject selection and assignment, the questions you need to consider as you assess the validity of the study will differ as well. For the purposes of this chapter, we will discuss the questions to consider for 3 common study designs seen in health care research: case-controls; cohorts; and randomized, controlled trials (RCTs).

If you are appraising the validity of a case-control study, you should assess if the selection methods used for the case participants and the control participants were appropriate. Remember, in a case-control study, the outcome has already occurred, and individuals are chosen for the study based on whether they have the condition of interest (eg, patellofemoral pain, no patellofemoral pain). Therefore, you should note if the authors reported inclusion or exclusion criteria for selecting their participants and if they matched the control participants with the case participants by any specific criteria. For example, if you wanted to examine what factors may be different between individuals with chronic ankle instability and those without, it would not be pertinent to include an individual in the control group who has had a history of ankle sprains. While participant matching is not always necessary, researchers may choose to match participants by age, sex, height, weight, limb dominance, or any other demographic information that is pertinent to the condition of interest. Finally, when appraising the validity of a case-control study, you should also assess whether the data collection methods for the participants of the separate groups (ie, case group, control group) were the same. Regardless of the group a participant is assigned to, the data should be collected in the same manner to ensure the information can accurately be compared. If you were collecting data on ankle dorsiflexion range of motion, you would not be able to compare data collected if you used a goniometer to collect range of motion data in one group and the weight-bearing lunge test to collect range of motion data in the other group. Overall, assessing participant selection and data collection methods will help you to assess whether the study you are appraising is valid.

Similar to case-control studies, cohort studies also assess differences between individuals with a condition of interest and individuals without that condition. However, when you appraise a cohort study, there are a few additional questions you need to consider. To begin, you should determine if the sample group included was representative of the population of individuals with that condition. For example, if the study you are appraising compared the outcomes of individuals who had a surgical intervention for shoulder instability and those with shoulder instability who did not have a surgical outcome, it may not be appropriate to include participants who previously had shoulder surgery since their outcomes may differ from the rest of the group. When appraising a cohort study, you should also determine if the outcome criteria were objective as well as whether the follow-up period was sufficient in duration to capture any changes in outcome measures. For example, if the outcome measured for the shoulder instability participants described above was pain, you should determine how pain was measured (eg, visual analog scale, numeric pain rating scale) and whether it was measured for a reasonable period of time. Finally, you should assess whether the researchers accounted for any cofounding variables during the analysis. Particularly for a prospective cohort study in which individuals are followed over a defined period of time to see if they incur the condition of interest, it is possible that other variables may influence the outcomes for the participant. In our shoulder instability example, since pain is being assessed as the outcome, it would be important to account for whether any of the participants were taking nonsteroidal anti-inflammatory drugs, which could cofound their perceived levels of pain.

Because RCTs involve randomization processes as well as the potential for blinding, there are several questions to consider when appraising the validity. When appraising the randomization procedures, it is important to assess if the individuals were randomly assigned. Additionally, you should assess if group assignment was concealed from the participants, as well as the individuals (eg, clinicians, researchers) who were enrolling participants into the study. Remember, while there are numerous ways participants can be randomized and allocated to groups, computer randomization is considered the most robust form of participant allocation. Along with the randomization processes, it is also important to appraise whether the participants and/or the providers were blinded to the study group. Blinding helps to remove any potential participant or researcher bias that may exist, which can enhance the validity of the study.

Once participants have been randomized to controls, it is also important to determine if the groups (ie, intervention group, control group) were homogenous prior to the intervention period. If groups were not similar at the beginning, it is difficult to know if any differences between groups following the intervention were actually due to the intervention itself or because the groups were different (ie, heterogeneous) from the start. Typically, you will be able to appraise a study if groups appear to be homogenous by reviewing the participant demographics (often presented in table form) reported by the authors. The authors of an RCT should also report if any participants dropped out of the investigation as well as indicate why any dropouts occurred.

Similar to the appraisal of a cohort study, it is necessary to assess if the outcome measures used for the RCT were appropriate (ie, were they valid and reliable instruments/tools), as well as if the outcomes were collected over a sufficient period of time. Particularly for an RCT, it is important to collect data over an adequate amount of time to be able to fully assess the effects of the intervention. For example, if an RCT was conducted to determine whether talocrural joint mobilizations were effective at increasing ankle dorsiflexion range of motion, you would expect the researchers to collect outcomes immediately following the intervention as well as several later time points to determine if ankle dorsiflexion range of motion immediately increased and if this increase in range of motion remained over time.

As you can see, there are a variety of questions you should consider depending on the type of study you are appraising. Just because a research study is published in a peer-review journal does not always guarantee that it is of high quality. Appraising the various aspects of how a study was conducted is important to ensure the study has good internal validity. If the methods of the study are not valid, it will be difficult to be confident in the results that are reported. While the approach to appraising the validity of a study can differ between individuals, Figure 12-1 shows the questions you should consider.

Appraising the Reliability of a Study

Along with appraising the validity of a study, it is also necessary to ensure that the study was reliable. In particular, you should address 3 main areas during your appraisal of the study's reliability. To begin, you should determine if the methodology used in the study is reproducible; that is, if the same study was conducted again, if it would be possible to reproduce the findings. If the methodology of a study was not reproducible, it would be difficult to conclude the accuracy of those results and how applicable they would be to clinical practice. For example, if the researchers of a study reported that a particular intervention was extremely effective at reducing pain following an acute ankle sprain but the methodology used was very intricate and was conducted in a laboratory setting, it is unlikely that another researcher would be able to reproduce the findings in a different environment. More importantly, it is also unlikely that you would be able to reproduce

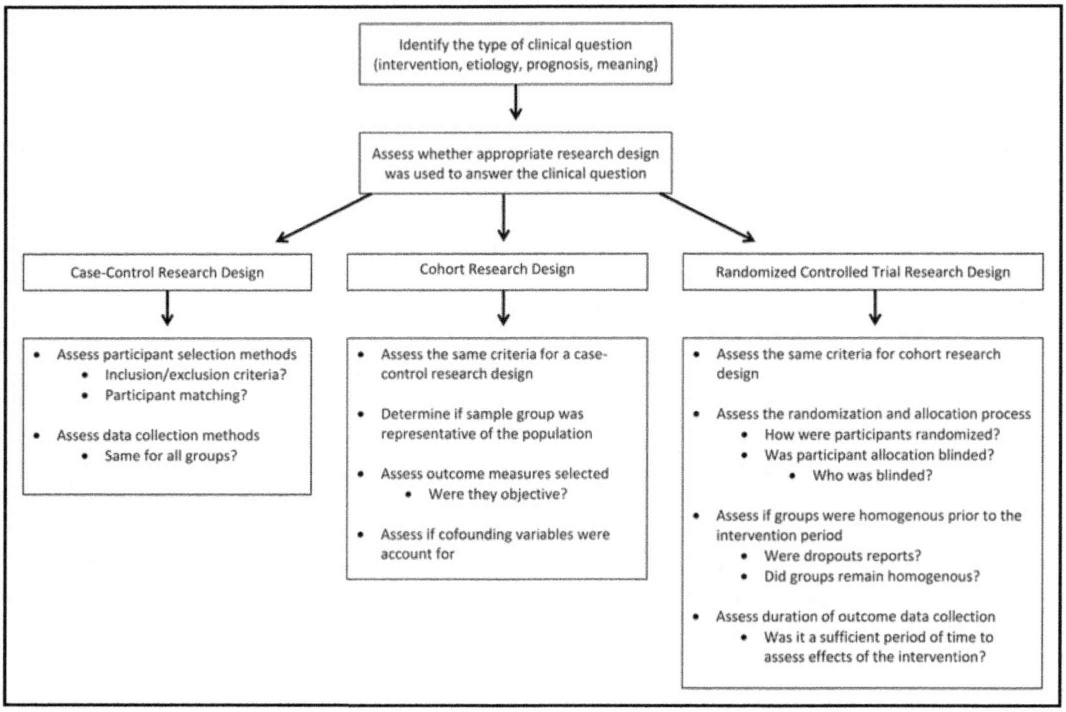

Figure 12-1. Appraising the validity of a study.

this intervention in your clinical practice setting. Therefore, if the methodology of a study or the intervention used cannot be reproduced, the results from that investigation may be irrelevant in helping you find an answer to your clinical question.

In addition to appraising whether the methodology and interventions of a study are reproducible, it is also necessary to assess if there was sufficient rater reliability. There are 2 types of rater reliability with which we are concerned: intrarater reliability, which refers to the consistency of data recorded by one individual, and interrater reliability, which refers to the consistency of data recorded by multiple individuals who measure the same group of subjects. If there is not good reliability within one individual or between a group of individuals collecting the data, it is difficult to trust the accuracy of the results of that particular study. For example, if a study that was conducted reported that the Functional Movement Screen (FMS) was effective at predicting musculoskeletal injuries, but there was poor intra- and interrater reliability of the raters collecting the data, you would be unsure if the results were accurate due to the participants' scores achieved on the FMS, or if the results occurred by chance because of the lack of reliability among the raters. Additionally, rater reliability is important to help you determine if you would be able to reproduce the assessment in your clinical practice. On the FMS, if a study reported that there was high intra- and interrater reliability between novice and expert FMS raters, you could feel confident that you would be able to accurately incorporate the FMS in your own clinical practice. To appraise the intra- and interrater reliability, you should assess whether the author of a study reported the intraclass correlation coefficient (ICC) values. Remember, ICC values range from 0.00 to 1.00, with higher values representing stronger reliability.

Finally, it is important to establish if the instruments used in the study you are appraising are reliable. If an instrument is not reliable, it is unlikely that the instrument will be able to capture the same data when reproduced. For example, if a survey was developed to assess individuals' knowledge of concussion best practices but the survey itself had poor reliability, you would not be able to be confident that the results collected on a sample of participants were accurate and representative of their true knowledge levels. To ensure the instruments used in a study are reliable, you should

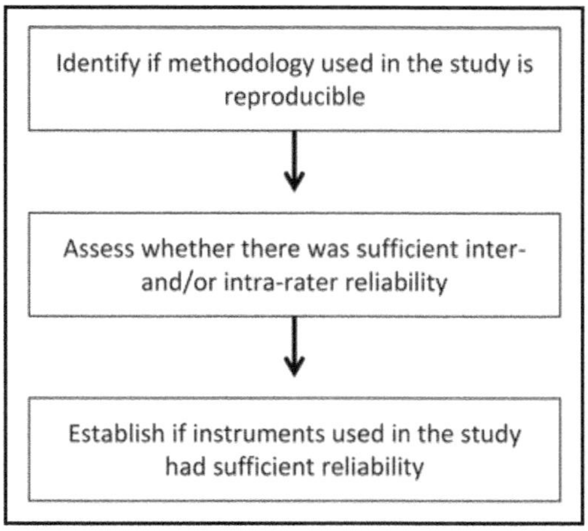

Figure 12-2. Appraising the reliability of a study.

look to see if the authors reported the internal consistency of the instrument, the test-retest reliability of the instrument, or both. Along with rater reliability, ICC values may also be reported for test-retest reliability. However, you may also see percent agreement reported for test-retest reliability of interval and ratio data or the kappa statistic reported for categorical data. Cronbach's alpha (α) is most often reported for the internal consistency of an instrument, and the values range from 0.0 to 1.0, with 0.90 considered to be highly reliable.

If a study methodology is not reproducible or if the raters or instruments used were not reliable, it is difficult to trust the results reported in the study and apply them within your own clinical practice. Unlike validity, the appraisal of a study's reliability does not necessarily depend on the type of research design used. Figure 12-2 provides the questions you should consider while you appraise the reliability of a study.

Appraising the Results of a Study

Appraising the results of a study may be one of the most challenging aspects of the critical appraisal process, particularly if you are not familiar with the various statistical concepts used in research. Although you are not expected to assess every statistical test conducted in a study and review all the data reported, there are a couple of questions to consider that will aid you in appraising the results. To begin, you should assess if the authors included confidence intervals (CIs) with the reported data. Confidence intervals are a range of values (minimum to maximum) that tell us how our estimates of sample statistics (eg, the mean value) are distributed in the population from which the sample is drawn. More specifically, the CI, which is usually reported at 95%, indicates how confident that researcher is that the population mean will fall within the calculated confidence range. Along with *P* values, CIs help you assess how precise the findings are.

If a study compares an intervention between 2 or more groups, such as in an RCT, it is also important to assess how large of an effect the intervention has. For example, if an author reports that significant differences exist between an intervention group and a control group, it is necessary to estimate how large that difference is. If the difference is small between the 2 groups, then the intervention may not be clinically meaningful for use in your clinical practice. Effectiveness of an intervention is typically measured by effect size, which can range from 0.00 to 3.00. However, relative risk or odds ratios, which are other measures used to assess effect, may also be reported. Regardless, CIs should also be reported with measures of effect to assess the amount of confidence as well.

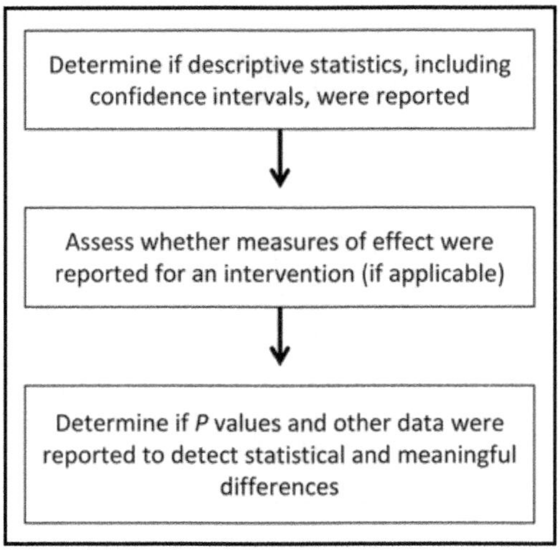

Figure 12-3. Appraising the results of a study.

While there are various aspects of the results that can be appraised, it is not necessary for you to be an expert in statistics to be able to appraise the results of a study. However, as a clinician, it is important that you have a general understanding of the commonly used statistical terminology so you can navigate through the results section of a research article. Primarily, you should not only be able to identify if actual differences between groups occurred, but also be able to assess the amount of confidence the researcher has regarding this difference as well as whether the differences are small or large. Remember, although there may be a statistical difference reported between 2 groups, if the difference is minimal, it might not be meaningful in clinical practice. For example, a research study you locate during your literature search reported a statistical significance between 2 groups regarding hamstring flexibility, indicating that the group that went through a 6-week lower-extremity stretching protocol had 2 degrees more hamstring flexibility than the control group. While this information tells us that the lower-extremity stretching protocol increased hamstring flexibility, in most instances a 2-degree increase is not clinically significant. Therefore, you may make the decision that it is not valuable to have patients complete the 6-week protocol because a 2-degree increase is not a meaningful change. Although there are numerous questions you could ask to appraise the results of a study, Figure 12-3 shows the basic questions you should always consider.

Appraising the Clinical Applicability of a Study

Along with appraising the validity, reliability, and results of a study, it is important to assess the clinical applicability of a study as well. It could be argued that appraising the clinical applicability is the most vital part of a critical appraisal. If the information from a study is not applicable to your population or clinical practice setting, then you will not be able to incorporate the findings from the study as part of your clinical decision-making process. Therefore, there are several questions you should consider to appraise the clinical applicability of a study.

First, you should assess whether the sample group included in the study is similar to the target population for which you provide care. For example, let us say you are trying to determine if incorporating a lower-extremity anterior cruciate ligament (ACL) prevention program is effective at reducing ACL injury rates among adolescent athletes. During your literature search, you come across 2 high-quality studies that report a lower-extremity ACL prevention program is effective at reducing ACL injury rates. However, you notice that the sample group in one study consisted of collegiate female soccer players and the other sample group included professional male basketball players. While these studies appear to have high validity and reliability, they include sample groups that are not similar to your population of interest (ie, adolescent athletes). Therefore, you must interpret the findings from these studies with caution, as it is unknown whether adolescent athletes will have the same outcomes with a lower-extremity ACL prevention program as collegiate female soccer players and professional male basketball players. While it is important to assess the internal validity of a study, it is also necessary to appraise the external validity (ie, how well the findings can be generalized to a larger population).

Next, you should consider if the results from a particular study can directly influence your clinical decision making. While a study may report that a particular intervention is effective at achieving a desired outcome (eg, a lower-extremity ACL prevention program to reduce ACL injuries), then you might be inclined to incorporate the intervention in your clinical practice. However, as you appraise research evidence, you must be cautious of the findings reported. More specifically, you should assess the type of research design that was used for the study. As you know, RCTs are often conducted in a rigorous manner to ensure potential biases are removed. Therefore, you might be more likely to use findings from this type of study to influence your clinical decision making. Conversely, other types of research designs (eg, case-control, cohort) are not as rigorous and, thus, the results are more likely to carry bias. As you appraise a research study, always remember to consider the type of research design as well as the level of evidence. Since systematic reviews make up the highest level of evidence, you should feel comfortable incorporating findings from this type of research to aid you in making informed clinical decisions.

Lastly, if you are appraising a study that includes an intervention that you are considering for your patients, you must ensure that all the potential risks and benefits for that intervention have been considered. Determining risks and benefits can particularly be supported if a research study includes the number needed to benefit or number needed to harm. The number needed to benefit represents the number of patients who need to be treated with the intervention to prevent a single injury, while the number needed to harm represents the number of patients who need to be treated with the intervention for 1 patient to experience an adverse event. You should discuss any potential risks and benefits of an intervention with your patient to ensure this intervention matches his or her goals and expectations of the desired outcome. For example, you are considering incorporating an 8-week lower-extremity ACL prevention program for your patient who has a history of ACL injury. This program has been found to be largely effective at reducing the recurrence of ACL injury. However, while there are no direct risks associated with the program, it is very intensive and requires 2 sessions a day for 8 weeks. As you discuss the program with your patient, she indicates that she does not want to commit that much time for the prevention program. Therefore, while this program may be effective at achieving the desired outcome (ie, reducing the recurrence of ACL injury), it does not match the patient's goals. As you appraise the clinical applicability of studies, you should consider your patient population, as well as individual patient goals. Moreover, it is important to discuss treatments you are considering with the patient and allow them to be a part of the decision-making process. Figure 12-4 provides the questions you should consider when appraising the clinical applicability of a study.

Critical Appraisal Resources

As a health care provider, you often seek tools and instruments that will help you gather important information to make a strong clinical decision. Generally, you may use valid and reliable tools to provide you with specific information about a patient or a condition. For example, you may use a scale to assess a patient's weight, a goniometer to assess a patient's range of motion at a particular joint, or a specific patient-reported outcome instrument to assess a patient's perceptions of his or her injury. Similarly, as part of the EBP process, you may seek available tools to help you gather information about a condition in a concise manner.

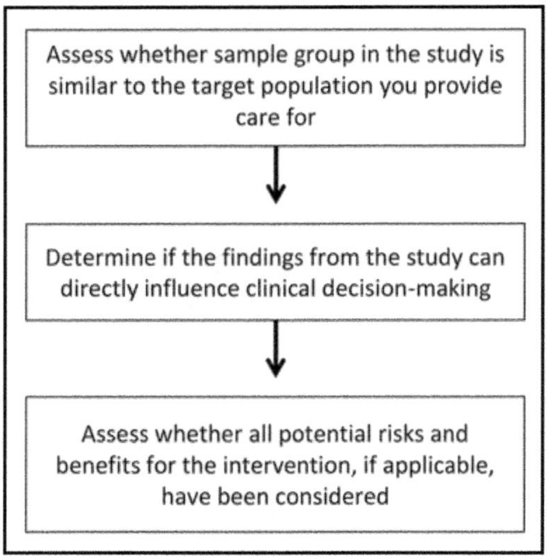

Figure 12-4. Appraising the clinical applicability of a study.

There are numerous critical appraisal scales and checklists to help you critically appraise research evidence. Generally, appraisal scales (eg, Physiotherapy Evidence Database, Jadad Scale) provide you with a score to objectively assess the methodological quality of the research article you are appraising. Appraisal checklists typically include a list of recommendations that authors should include to enhance the reporting of a research study. There are various checklists available, and each checklist is often developed to focus on a specific research design (eg, Consolidated Standards of Reporting Trials, Standards for the Reporting of Diagnostic accuracy studies). While appraisal scales and checklists are helpful for researchers and journals to ensure that the reporting of studies is of high quality, these tools may not provide you with the necessary in depth information you need to appraise research literature and incorporate it into your clinical decision-making process. Fortunately, there are other tools available that provide you with guidelines to ensure you are extracting and interpreting important information during the critical appraisal process. For example, **rapid critical appraisal worksheets** are available to help you navigate through the appraisal process. These worksheets often provide you with guiding questions related to validity, reliability, and clinical applicability to ensure you are collecting the necessary information to help you translate research literature into usable information. Several versions of rapid critical appraisal forms are available and can easily be obtained through a basic Internet search.

Critically Appraised Papers

Another appraisal tool you may consider using as you appraise a research study is a **critically appraised paper** (CAP). A CAP is a 1- to 2-page summary that focuses on appraising a single research study to help you determine if the reported results are valid, reliable, and clinically applicable. Although this critical appraisal tool is not frequently published in athletic training literature, a CAP is a great tool that provides you with a framework to guide you through the appraisal process of a single research study. While there are numerous versions of CAP templates available on the Internet, each template variation will likely include the following components:

- Clinical question
- Clinical bottom line
- Summary of key evidence
- Strengths/threats to internal validity
- Strengths/threats to external validity

Table 12-1.
Summary of Evidence Information

SUMMARY OF EVIDENCE SECTION	INFORMATION TO INCLUDE
Sample	The number of participants, subject characteristics (eg, sex, age ethnicity, years of clinical practice), inclusion/exclusion criteria
Procedures	A brief explanation of the procedure that highlights the key processes of the research investigation
Outcome Measures	The outcome measures (ie, dependent variables) identified along with frequency of collection
Results	A synopsis of the research findings to conclude the summary of key evidence; the author will present a brief write-up of distinguishing results

- Strength/threats to statistical validity
- Level of evidence
- Application

Clinical Question

The CAP typically begins by introducing the clinical question. As you know, the literature search that was conducted for this critical appraisal was based on this question; therefore, it is important that the question is written in a clear and concise manner.

Clinical Bottom Line

The **clinical bottom line** summarizes how the research study relates to the clinical question. In particular, this brief statement highlights what was accomplished in the research study and whether the use of the given intervention, if one was implemented, should be integrated into daily clinical practice. However, the clinical bottom line is determined from an appraisal of the validity of the study and its findings. Although the clinical bottom line of a CAP is often presented as one of the first sections, it is often the last portion of the CAP that is completed. The clinical bottom line may not be applicable to practice settings and populations outside of those referenced in the research study being appraised. Therefore, you should always keep in mind your patient or population of interest as you are appraising the research literature.

Summary of Key Evidence

The **summary of key evidence** identifies the study design, participants, procedures, outcome measures, and results. The primary goal of this section is to provide the reader of the CAP a brief overview of the study procedures. Table 12-1 provides some of the essential information that should be included in the summary of key evidence.

Strengths and Threats to Internal, External, and Statistical Validity

The strengths and threats to validity are the critical portion of the CAP. These 3 sections (ie, internal, external, and statistical) provide detailed information to help you determine if the findings from this research study could potentially be incorporated into your clinical decision making. The internal validity section helps you to determine if the study design was appropriately chosen for the research question the researchers intended to answer and highlights specific features of the study methodology that are considered a strength to the results produced, as well as components that may create a threat to the validity of the results. For example, if participants and/or clinicians were not blinded in an RCT, it may be considered a threat to the internal validity, whereas computerized randomization to ensure homogeneity of groups prior to the intervention may be considered a strength to internal validity.

As you now know, external validity is the degree to which the results from a sample can be generalized to a larger population. Therefore, it may be considered a threat to external validity if a research study only collected data on adolescent female field hockey players because the results will be difficult to generalize to a larger population (eg, collegiate athletes). Conversely, the lack of specific inclusion/exclusion criteria may be considered a strength to external validity because it makes it easier to generalize the results to the population.

Appraising the statistical validity of a research study includes assessing the degree to which a statistical procedure is appropriately used to draw valid conclusions about the relationship or differences of 2 variables. Generally, being able to highlight the strengths and threats to statistical validity requires a strong understanding of several statistical concepts. While you may not be required to interpret all of the results of a research study, you should still be able to assess if the researchers reported appropriate values (eg, *P* values, means, standard deviations, CIs) and used the appropriate type of statistical test for the type of data collected (eg, nonparametric test for ordinal data). For example, if a researcher does not report a power analysis, it could be considered a threat to statistical validity.

Level of Evidence and Application

The level of evidence indicates the strength of the methodological quality of the study being appraised. While there is no standardized level of evidence scale for CAPs, the Centre for Evidence-Based Medicine and Strength of Recommendation Taxonomy scales are most typically used. Finally, once the study design, sample group, study procedures, results, and validity have been closely assessed, you can construct a 1- to 2-sentence application summary addressing the feasibility of applying the study results to a broader spectrum of patients.

Unfortunately, CAPs relating to athletic training research are not frequently published. However, it is beneficial for you to understand the components of a CAP because you may choose to adopt a CAP template to help you organize and manage the research articles you read. Similar to managing your literature searches, it is also important to establish a consistent method of reviewing the literature and organizing the evidence you appraise in a manner that is most suitable to you.

Critically Appraised Topics

You should begin your literature search by searching relevant databases (eg, Cochrane Database) to determine whether a systematic review or meta-analysis is available on your topic of interest. Because systematic reviews and meta-analyses provide the highest level of evidence, it is important to search for this type of information. However, systematic reviews and meta-analyses may not be available for your topic, which may lead you to question whether there are any other tools available that present the information you need in a condensed manner. Although a systematic review would be most helpful to you when seeking information about your topic of interest, there are other resources available that provide you with appraised literature in a concise manner. Primarily, you may search to see if a **critically appraised topic** (CAT) is available.

A CAT is an appraisal tool used to synthesize numerous research articles that review the same general topic of interest. A CAT must contain no fewer than 3 articles on the same topic but typically does not contain more than 5. If more than 5 articles are available on 1 given topic, the likelihood that a systematic review has been conducted is high.

Although a CAT has some similar components of a CAP, this critical appraisal tool often includes multiple tables that identify the specific information from each study being appraised. Having a good understanding of the features of a CAT is beneficial to help you understand how to interpret the information being presented. Although there are different versions of CATs across health professions, a majority of CATs include the following main sections:

- Clinical scenario
- Focused clinical question
- Summary of search, best evidence appraised, and key findings
- Clinical bottom line
- Strength of recommendation
- Search strategy
- Inclusion and exclusion criteria
- Results of search
- Summary of best evidence
- Implications for practice, education, and future research

As you will notice, some of the sections included in the CAT are identical to the sections previously discussed for the CAP template.

Clinical Scenario

The **clinical scenario** provides you with an introduction to the topic being appraised in the CAT. While this introduction may offer varying types of information based on the type of clinical question it is focused around (eg, prognosis, diagnosis, therapy), the clinical scenario will give you the necessary information to understand the prevalence of the condition or why the clinical question is an important one to answer.

Focused Clinical Question

Following the clinical scenario, the clinical question is presented. Again, the clinical question guides the literature search to retrieve the research studies included in the CAT; therefore, it is important to ensure the clinical question is well developed. Examples of clinical questions in which CATs have been published are presented in Table 12-2.

Summary of Search, Best Evidence Appraised, and Key Findings

While it is important to know how the literature was appraised in a CAT, it is also valuable to have an understanding of how the search was conducted to find the articles included in the CAT. Having an understanding of the steps the authors took in searching for the literature helps you to ensure that they searched via the appropriate mechanism. This section of the CAT provides a brief overview of the literature search and the articles ultimately included, and the overall key findings from these individual studies are highlighted.

Clinical Bottom Line

Similar to the clinical bottom line of a CAP, this section provides a brief statement indicating whether the use of the given intervention might be worthwhile to integrate in clinical practice.

Table 12-2. Clinical Questions of Published Critically Appraised Topics

CLINICAL QUESTION	REFERENCE
Is a gastrocnemius-soleus stretching program, as a stand-alone treatment variable, effective in the treatment of plantar fasciitis?	Garrett TR, Neibert PJ. The effectiveness of a gastrocnemius-soleus stretching program as a therapeutic treatment of plantar fasciitis. *J Sport Rehabil.* 2013;22:308-312.
Does the use of joint mobilizations combined with a stretching protocol more effectively increase glenohumeral internal rotation ROM in adult physically active individuals who participate in overhead sports and are suffering from posterior shoulder tightness compared with a stretching protocol alone?	Harshbarger ND, Eppelheimer BL, McLeod TCV, McCarty CW. The effectiveness of shoulder stretching and joint mobilizations on posterior shoulder tightness. *J Sport Rehabil.* 2013;22:313-319.
Do prophylactic ankle braces reduce the incidence of acute ankle injuries in adolescent athletes?	Farwell KE, Powden CJ, Powell MR, Welch CE, Hoch MC. The effectiveness of prophylactic ankle braces in reducing the incidence of acute ankle injuries in adolescent athletes: a critically appraised topic. *J Sport Rehabil.* 2013;22:137-142.
How do clinical or field-based balance-assessment tools compare with laboratory-based balance measures in identifying deficits in postural stability among acutely concussed athletes?	Cripps A, Livingston SC. The value of balance-assessment measurements in identifying and monitoring acute postural instability among concussed athletes. *J Sport Rehabil.* 2013;22:68-71.
Is low-level laser therapy combined with an exercise program more effective than an exercise program alone in the treatment of adults with shoulder pain?	Thornton AL, Welch CE, Burgess M. Effectiveness of low-level laser therapy combined with an exercise program to reduce pain and increase function in adults with shoulder pain: a critically appraised topic. *J Sport Rehabil.* 2013;22:72-78.
Can lower extremity–injury prevention programs effectively reduce ACL injury rates in adolescent athletes?	Paszkewicz J, Webb T, Waters B, Welch CE, Van Lunen BL. The effectiveness of injury-prevention programs in reducing the incidence of anterior cruciate ligament sprains in adolescent athletes. *J Sport Rehabil.* 2012;21:371-377.
For individuals with acute lumbopelvic pain, is there evidence to suggest that muscle energy techniques are effective in reducing pain and disability scores?	Day JM, Nitz AJ. The effect of muscle energy techniques on disability and pain scores in individuals with low back pain. *J Sport Rehabil.* 2012;21:194-198.
In a healthy adult population, what lower extremity exercises produce the greatest mean gluteus medius activation, expressed as a percentage of maximum voluntary isometric contraction?	Hamstra-Wright KL, Bliven KH. Effective exercises for targeting the gluteus medius. *J Sport Rehabil.* 2012;21:296-300.

Since a CAT appraises findings from 3 to 5 research studies, the clinical bottom line may be more impactful than the clinical bottom line of a CAP.

Strength of Recommendation

Whereas a CAP reports the level of evidence of a single research study, a CAT reports the strength, or grade, of recommendation. Level of evidence (represented by a number) is only reported for a single study, whereas grades of recommendation (represented by letters) are reported for a grouping of studies. Since a CAT appraises 3 to 5 research studies on a similar topic, you will notice the strength of recommendation, which indicates the degree of confidence for the evidence to be incorporated into clinical practice.

Search Strategy

The search strategy section provides you with the exact search terms and databases used during the appraisal process. The search terms are classified by PICO component, and the Boolean operators are also identified. Additionally, multiple databases must be searched to ensure that all peer-reviewed articles relating to the clinical question are identified. Therefore, the search strategy section of the CAT also identifies all databases the authors of the CAT used to retrieve the research studies.

Inclusion and Exclusion Criteria

The inclusion and exclusion criteria portion of the CAT provides a list of information that the author(s) of the CAT used to decide on the articles included. This section also highlights the extent to which a particular level of evidence or type of research design was emphasized, search strategy limits, and subject characteristics that may have precluded the use of a particular research study.

Results of Search

The results of the search section provide a brief summary of the articles that were selected for the analysis within the CAT. Often, an author may choose to include a table of the selected articles for a clear summary of information.

Summary of Best Evidence

The summary of best evidence section provides you with a rationale as to why the selected articles were chosen. A table that summarizes the information from each individual research study, similar to the *Summary of Key Evidence* table in a CAP, also often follows this section. Table 12-3 provides a template of the type of information typically included in the table.

Implications for Practice, Education, and Future Research

Finally, the implications for practice, education, and future research provide a synthesis of the information included in the summary of best evidence section. More importantly, this portion of the CAT discusses the benefits and disadvantages of using the intervention (eg, balance training programs) within daily clinical practice. This section also highlights avenues for future research that would help to strengthen the conclusions made from this synthesis.

Overall, CAPs and CATs provide an excellent opportunity for you to review current research literature in a structured and concise manner. A CAP can provide a quick reference of information for a particular research study, while a CAT can provide a detailed synthesis of multiple research studies regarding a similar topic.

Over the past several years, several journals (eg, *Journal of Sport Rehabilitation*, *International Journal of Athletic Therapy and Training*) have begun to publish CATs on a regular basis. *Journal of Sport Rehabilitation* publishes CATs free of access, meaning you do not need to have a license to the journal to access the full text of published CATs. As more CAPs and CATs become available to the athletic training membership, you will be able to effectively remain up to date with

Table 12-3.
Template of Summary of Best Evidence Table

	STUDY 1 (AUTHOR AND YEAR)	STUDY 2 (AUTHOR AND YEAR)	STUDY 3 (AUTHOR AND YEAR)	STUDY 4 (AUTHOR AND YEAR)
Study design				
Participants				
Intervention investigated				
Outcome measures				
Main findings				
Level of evidence				
Validity score[a]				
Conclusion				

[a]Validity score refers to a score determined via an appraisal scale (eg, Physiotherapy Evidence Database, Quality Assessment of Diagnostic Accuracy Studies, Jadad, etc).

current research information without the hassle of conducting various literature searches and reading numerous journal articles to answer a clinical question. However, CATs are typically only relevant for a short period of time, and the results may shift in another direction as new research is conducted.

Summary

Critically appraising the evidence that is available for you to use within your clinical practice is a foundational component of being a clinician. Critical appraised papers and CATs are 2 methods whereby you can assess what is available, and they provide a mechanism for developing clinical bottom line statements for you to consider within your practice. Frequent examination of the literature is necessary for you to update your practice and clinical decision making. Locating sources that provide summarized information assists you within this process.

Key Points

- Critical appraisal allows you to determine whether available research literature can be used to help you during the clinical decision-making process.
- Critical appraisal is the process of determining whether evidence from a viable source can be translated and apply to help you answer your clinical question.

- When critically appraising a study, you should consider the validity, including study design, sampling methods, data collection methods, and outcome criteria, as well as reliability, including methodology, inter- and intrarater reliability, and instrument reliability.
- Critically appraised papers and CATs are ways to synthesize smaller amounts of available data.

BIBLIOGRAPHY

Barzilai DA, Weinstock MA. Accessible evidence-based medicine: critically appraised topics. *Arch Dermatol.* 2007;143(9):1189-1190.

Bennett S, McCluskey A, Wallen M. Introducing critically appraised papers: purpose and procedures. *Aust Occup Ther J.* 2003;50(3):178-179.

Dawes M. Critically appraised topics and evidence-based medicine journals. *Singapore Med J.* 2005;46(9):442-448.

Fetters L, Figueiredo EM, Keane-Miller D, McSweeney DJ, Tsao CC. Critically appraised topics. *Pediatr Phys Ther.* 2004;16(1):19-21.

Fineout-Overholt E, Melnyk BM, Schultz A. Transforming health care from the inside out: advancing evidence-based practice in the 21st century. *J Prof Nurs.* 2005;21(6):335-344.

Forrest JL, Miller SA. Evidence-based decision making in action: part 2—evaluating and applying the clinical evidence. *J Contemp Dent Pract.* 2003;4(1):42-52.

Lijmer JG, Mol BW, Heisterkamp S, et al. Empirical evidence of design-related bias in studies of diagnostic tests. *JAMA.* 1998;282(11):1061-1066.

Moher D, Cook DJ, Jadad AR, et al. Assessing the quality of reports of randomised trials: implications for the conduct of meta-analyses. *Health Technol Assess.* 1998;3(12):i-iv, 1-98.

Steves RS, Hootman JM. Evidence-based medicine: what is it and how does it apply to athletic training? *J Athl Train.* 2004;39(1):83-87.

Welch CE, Yakuboff MK, Madden MJ. Critically appraised papers and topics part 1: use in clinical practice. *Athl Ther Today.*2008;13(5):10-12.

Welch CE, Yakuboff MK, Madden MJ. Critically appraised papers and topics part 2: how to read and interpret a CAP. *Athl Ther Today.*2008;13(5):13-16.

Wingerchuk DM, Demaerschalk BM. Critically appraised topics: the evidence-based neurologist. *Neurologist* 2007;13(1);1.

13

Clinical Prediction Rules

Now that you have a good understanding of the research and appraisal process, it is time to discuss methods to incorporate evidence into your daily clinical practice. The amount of available research is significant, and it can be difficult to know how to incorporate all of that evidence into your patient care. Understanding the tools available to you to incorporate this research will make the task of evidence-based patient care more manageable. **Clinical prediction rules (CPRs)** are decision-making tools that can be used to help clinicians determine a diagnosis, prognosis, or a patient's response to a treatment. These decision-making tools often use algorithms that combine multiple variables (ie, patient characteristics, test results, disease characteristics) to indicate a potential successful outcome. Clinical prediction rules combine several clinically relevant findings and then use powerful statistics to determine the probability of a specific condition or the likelihood of a particular outcome. Most often, this combination of clinical findings or variables comes from information you typically would obtain in a patient history or physical examination. It is often the combination of variables that leads to a more powerful clinical decision tool. Clinical prediction rules have been used in medicine for many years; however, due to the development of more orthopedic diagnostic CPRs, there has been an increase in CPRs that are relevant to an active population often treated by athletic trainers (ATs).

There are 3 main types of CPRs used in health care: interventional, prognostic, and diagnostic. **Interventional CPRs** are used to determine how likely a person would be to respond to a particular intervention or combination of interventions. For example, there is an interventional CPR that assesses the likelihood that an individual with low back pain would respond favorably to lumbar manipulation techniques. A **prognostic CPR** is used to provide information about a likely outcome of patients with a specific condition. For example, a prognostic CPR can be used for individuals with shoulder pain by scoring symptoms to determine the percentage of risk the patient has for persistent shoulder pain after 6 weeks. **Diagnostic CPRs** are probably the most widely used decision-making tools by ATs, as they are used to help determine the probability that a patient has a particular condition of interest. The most widely known diagnostic CPR is the Ottawa Ankle

Van Lunen BL, Hankemeier DA, Welch CE.
Evidence-Guided Practice: A Framework for Clinical Decision Making in Athletic Training (pp 167-184).

Rules with Buffalo modification, which is used to determine if an individual needs a foot or ankle radiograph following an acute injury.

Development of Clinical Prediction Rules

To fully understand CPRs, it is important to understand how they are developed. The development of a CPR is a rigorous 3-step process (ie, derivation, validation, and impact analysis) that requires multiple patients with the condition of interest and should include a variety of settings (eg, multiple hospitals or clinics). Typically, CPRs are created through a research design or study. While any type of design can be used, prospective cohort studies are often used because they allow patients to be grouped based on specific criteria, and then their progress is tracked to determine the outcome.

Derivation

The first step in creating a CPR is the **derivation** process in which you identify factors that have predictive value. This often starts through a brainstorming process of all potential variables that are believed to have some predictive value. To explain the derivation process, we are going to use a hypothetical example for a CPR used to diagnose someone with medial epicondylitis. Table 13-1 shows how each step of the derivation process would be addressed. To develop your CPR, you decide that you are interested in active patients who have had medial elbow pain for at least 1 week. If you suspect someone has medial epicondylitis, you would then brainstorm the potential variables you think would help predict the outcome. These potential variables are called **predictor variables**, as they are examined to determine their relationship to the desired outcome. For medial epicondylitis, these could include strength deficits, range of motion decreases, or point tenderness. The table shows 7 predictor variables of interest that you would consider to be related to a medial epicondylitis diagnosis. While you want to include as many variables as possible, it is important to understand that for each predictor variable you want to test, it is recommended to have 10 to 15 participants enrolled in the study. This recommendation helps ensure that the derivation of the CPR is adequately powered for accurate statistical analysis.

Based on the predictor variables in the table, we would need 70 to 105 subjects. If we have 20 variables of interest, it is recommended that we should have at least 200 subjects to develop and test the CPR. Often, the number of subjects in CPR derivation studies is low or underpowered, so it is important to assess this aspect if you are evaluating a CPR to use in clinical practice. In addition to using the recommended number of participants per predictor variable, you should also evaluate a CPR in the context of its purpose by evaluating the risk and benefits of decision making on an underpowered study. For example, if our medial epicondylitis CPR derivation study only had 50 participants, it would be considered underpowered. Even though the study is underpowered, the risk of a severe or detrimental consequence related to misdiagnosing a patient with medial epicondylitis is relatively low. If the patient is misdiagnosed as having or not having the condition, there is little risk of having serious complications with the misdiagnosis. However, if a CPR is being used to determine if fracture is present (ie, ankle or cervical spine) or an individual has an illness (ie, strep throat), it would be important to make sure that the derivation study for the CPR is adequately powered with participants. An underpowered study could lead to missing fractures, which could lead to further complications. In many cases, studies used to derivate CPRs that have a higher risk for detrimental complications would enroll several hundred or thousands of participants to help ensure there would be no error in the decision-making process. When developing a CPR or evaluating CPRs for clinical use, you should consider the sample size in accordance with what the CPR is testing and consider the risks and benefits of having an adequately powered study.

Table 13-1.
Hypothetical Clinical Prediction Rule Derivation for the Diagnosis of Medial Epicondylitis

Target population	Active patients with medial elbow pain lasting longer than 1 week
Predictor variables of interest	• Pain with resisted wrist flexion • Pain with pronation • Point tender on the medial epicondyle • Point tender over wrist flexor muscle group • Numbness or tingling in ulnar nerve distribution • Decreased grip strength bilaterally • History of overhead throwing
Sample size determination	70 to 105 subjects
Reference criterion	Magnetic resonance imaging
Application of statistics	Potential statistics • Logistic regression model for prediction variables • Forward stepwise selection procedure used to enter the variables of those who were in the treatment success group only • Sensitivity, specificity, and likelihood ratios
Identified predictor variables of interest	• Pain with resisted wrist flexion • Point tender over medial epicondyle • Decreased grip strength • Absence of tingling in ulnar nerve distribution

Once you have determined your variables of interest and sample size, then each subject that is enrolled in the study is examined based on all of the predictor variables. You would keep track of which variables were present or absent. Typically, the researcher collecting the data is blinded to the study to eliminate potential bias during the data collection process. In our case, the same researcher or clinician would collect data on each of the 7 predictor variables. The researcher would record the presence or absence of pain with wrist flexion and pronation, measure grip strength, document the history of overhead throwing, and where the participants had point tenderness or numbness and tingling. Since the researcher is blinded to the study and because this individual is often the treating clinician, they may collect more information than the predictor variables. Each participant should be evaluated in the same manner by the same individual to help increase the internal validity of the study. Once all of the predictor variables are measured, the clinical findings need to be compared with a reference criterion, which is more often called a gold standard. A **reference criterion** is a well-established and accepted diagnostic test for diagnostic CPRs or a previously determined level of improvement in an interventional CPR. The reference criterion should be applied by a different researcher than the individual collecting data on the predictor variables to reduce bias. In our case, the use of magnetic resonance imaging would be the reference criterion used to determine tendon degeneration or inflammation. This would be used to determine if the patient actually has medial epicondylitis. All participants would be evaluated clinically for the predictor variables, and then each participant would receive magnetic resonance imaging.

Once all of the predictor variables are collected and the subject has been tested by the reference criterion, all of the data collected need to be analyzed. There are several statistical operations that can be used to assess the data, and the methods used will largely depend on the type and amount of data. The intricacies of applying the statistical analyses are beyond the scope of this book, but many CPR derivation studies use logistical regression, sensitivity, specificity, receiver operating characteristic curves, and likelihood ratios (LRs). These statistics are used to determine if there are variables or groups of variables that predict the outcomes. Positive LRs (LR+) express the change in odds favoring a potential outcome or diagnosis. This means that the subject in the study would meet the criteria for the CPR and essentially confirm the diagnosis. A negative LR (LR–) expresses the change in odds when the subject does not meet the CPR criteria and would rule out the diagnosis. A group of variables with a large (> 5.0) LR+ and one with a small (< 0.20) LR– would be considered moderately accurate, and an LR+ of greater than 10.0 and LR– less than 0.10 is considered to be substantially accurate. Understanding the LRs of the variables or grouping of variables is another tool you can use to assess the accuracy of a CPR.

When the statistical analysis is complete, there may be a variable or small set of variables that can be used to determine the correct diagnosis. Some CPRs look at these variables on a point scale in which the patient would receive a set number of points for each variable present and the total number of points corresponds to a probability percentage that the condition is present. For example, the Walsh Criteria to assess for streptococcal pharyngitis has 5 variables that are assessed. One point is awarded for the presence of 4 of the variables, and a negative point is awarded for the presence of the fifth variable. The total score possible is a 4, and the corresponding score of the variables assessed relates to the probability of a positive result. If a patient scored –1, they would have a 4.6% probability of a positive streptococcal pharyngitis test, whereas a score of 3 would indicate that they had an 83.3% probability of a positive streptococcal pharyngitis test. The presence of more variables often equates to a higher probability of the condition being present or the treatment being accurate. Other CPRs examine the group of variables as a whole; if all are present, it is recommended that the patient get further testing or treatment. For example, the Pittsburgh Knee Rule has a group of 3 variables of interest. If the patient had the specified mechanism and was in the designated age range, they should be sent for a radiograph. If the patient did not fit in the age range but was unable to walk immediately following the incident, they were also referred to a radiograph. If we go back to the table and our hypothetical example for the diagnosis of medial epicondylitis, a statistical analysis may show that 4 variables of interest (pain with resisted wrist flexion, point tenderness of the medial epicondyle, decreased grip strength, and an absence of tingling in the ulnar nerve distribution) were key in determining the correct diagnosis. These variables could be scored so that each variable received 1 point, like the Walsh Criteria, or they could be looked at together so that all would need to be present to reach the diagnosis. Since the statistical analysis of each CPR is extremely detailed and often complex because of the number of initial predictor variables, there can also be multiple groups of variables that are successful. Due to the differences in statistical analyses, you want to pay particular attention to how each variable factored into the CPR when assessing derivation studies. There may be 1 variable that was highly predictive (ie, 90% of each positive case had this variable present), or there may be a group of 3 variables that showed high probability of the CPR being accurate. Each CPR has specific criteria on how the variables should be applied, so you should always carefully read the derivation studies associated with the CPR to ensure that you are applying your clinical findings appropriately.

Table 13-2.
Levels of Validation

LEVEL OF VALIDATION	PURPOSE	RESEARCH METHOD	CLINICAL IMPACT
Level I	Determine the impact the CPR has on outcomes and clinical practice	Prospective study with variety of patients and clinicians that evaluates the impact on clinical practice	Use in a variety of settings with confidence that it improves outcomes
Level II	Determine if the CPR can be used with a variety of patients	Prospective study with a variety of patients and clinicians	Use CPR with confidence in a variety of settings
Level III	Determine stability of CPR	Prospective study with similar patients and clinicians to derivation study	Use with caution and only in settings similar to those used in study
Level IV	Confirm findings of original CPR	Original derivation study or often uses retrospective data	Should not be used until further validation occurs

Abbreviation: CPR, clinical prediction rule.

Validation

Just because a CPR has been derived does not mean that it should be widely used and accepted in clinical practice. **Validation** of the CPR in a different patient sample or different clinical setting helps to confirm that the variables in the CPR did not result due to chance or a fluke. Since derivation of the CPR typically happens in one setting or with a homogenous group of individuals, it is important to ensure that the CPR can be reproduced in different settings. Validation studies can be completed using different clinicians, treatment settings, or patient populations. Table 13-2 shows 4 levels of validation that have been proposed by various researchers. Level 4 validation is the lowest level and is often accomplished by using retrospective data to confirm the findings of the derived CPR. The next highest level of validation, Level 3, is often completed through a prospective cohort study with a similar patient sample and similar clinicians. Completing this type of validation helps to confirm the stability of the CPR and provides cautionary evidence that supports the CPR. To fully implement widespread change, Level 2 validation is needed. This level of validation includes a variety of patients and clinicians implementing the rule. For example, Flynn et al[1] derived an interventional CPR to determine short-term improvements with spinal manipulation in patients with low back pain. The study was conducted using 71 patients at 2 outpatient clinics. When the validation study was conducted, Childs et al[2] evaluated 131 patients at 8 clinics across the United States. The validation study confirmed the findings of the original study, thus increasing the confidence that this interventional CPR can be used with individuals with low back pain. Using different clinicians to apply the CPR helps determine if the rule can be applied consistently. Also, when different clinicians are utilized, it is important to train the clinicians on how the rule should be applied to help increase the external validity. The highest level of validation is Level 1, which means that, in addition to being tested with a variety of patients and clinicians, it must undergo an impact analysis.

Impact Analysis

Completing an impact analysis on the CPR is the final step in the CPR development process. This process needs to be completed to reach the highest level of validation. An **impact analysis** is a study that demonstrates that the CPR has led to change in behavior, improved patient outcomes, reduced the cost of care, or improved the cost-effectiveness of treatment. Impact analyses are typically conducted in 1 of 3 ways. The best methodological manner is through a randomized, controlled trial in which patients would randomly receive care based on the CPR or standard practice. While this is the most robust in terms of methods, it would be difficult for clinicians to bounce back and forth between 2 treatment plans. It may be more logical to randomize patient settings so that 5 clinics apply the CPR and 5 clinics do not apply the CPR but instead treat the patient based on their historical plan of care. This would allow comparison of the outcomes of the different sites and could be a more feasible alternative to a true patient-based randomized, controlled trial. The final method is a nonrandomized option and, thus, is not as strong of an approach. In this model, you could complete a before and after design that looks at the data before the CPR was implemented and then compares it to the outcomes after the CPR was implemented. When a CPR has been validated and an impact analysis has shown to change clinical practice, it is often then referred to as a **clinical decision rule** (CDR). Few CPRs have gone through an impact analysis. The Ottawa Ankle Rules is one CPR that is considered to be a Level 1 due to the impact analysis. This CPR has been shown to decrease the number of unnecessary radiographs, decrease the patient's time spent in the emergency room, and decrease the cost to the patient, but it does not decrease patient outcomes or satisfaction. This shows that this CPR has made an impact on clinical practice without diminishing the care the patient receives.

Appraisal of Clinical Prediction Rules

The use of the validation scale is the most common way to assess the quality of a CPR. The level of validation, sometimes called the level of evidence, should always be assessed when considering a CPR for clinical implementation. Unfortunately, several CPRs have been derived that have not reached the Level 1 status. Several CPRs are derived annually, but they often never move beyond Level 4. In addition to understanding the level of the CPR, it is important to consider the methodological quality of the derivation study. This is of extreme importance when the CPR has not been validated with other patient populations or clinical settings. Similar to the appraisal scales and checklists discussed in Chapter 11, there have been methodological assessment tools designed to assess CPRs. An appraisal tool was developed to assess the quality of prognostic studies by determining the quality of 18 statements.[3] While this tool was specifically developed to be used with shoulder disorders, the concepts could be applied to other conditions. Statements are scored based on being positive, which achieves 1 point, and 0 points are awarded for neutral or negative responses to the statement. Statements assess the quality of methods, participant criteria, follow-up, statistical analysis, descriptive statistics, and participant response. A percentage is then determined by taking the total score (out of 18) and multiplying it by 100. It is recommended that percentages of greater than 60% indicate high-quality studies. For interventional studies, the appraisal tool for prognostic studies was modified to include statements related to patient outcomes and clinicians providing the treatment.[4] This tool is scored in the same manner, with the same 60% indicator of high quality. There is no formalized methodological assessment for diagnostic CPRs, but you could use the appraisal scales and checklists previously discussed in this text to help you determine the rigor of the derivation studies of these CPRs. Regardless of the type of CPR you are using, it is important that you assess the quality of the derivation study before implementing the CPR into practice unless it has already been validated in other studies.

Application of Clinical Prediction Rules

To better understand the whole CPR process, let us take a look at one of the most commonly implemented CPRs in athletic training. The Ottawa Ankle Rules was developed to determine the necessity of ankle or midfoot radiographs. When the CPR was developed, the following variables were determined to increase the probability of a positive radiograph: inability to bear weight for 4 steps immediately after injury or in the emergency department and tenderness in the distal 6 cm of the inferior pole or posterior border of either malleolus or tenderness on the navicular or base of the fifth metatarsal. The Ottawa Ankle Rules has shown to have a high sensitivity of 100% and a low specificity of 37%. Through impact analyses, it was determined that implementation of the Ottawa Ankle Rules reduced unnecessary radiographs by 30% to 40%, decreased the time spent waiting in the emergency room by approximately 36 minutes, and resulted in decrease medical costs for patients. The CPR was derived, validated at the highest level, and shown to change clinical practice. Due to this, the Ottawa Ankle Rules can be called a CDR. This CDR was being implemented more widely, and researchers began to investigate additional ways to improve the original Ottawa Ankle Rules. The Buffalo modification of the CDR was used to enhance the specificity of the CDR. The original rules stayed the same, with the exception that the palpation of the malleolus changed from the inferior and posterior edge to the midline of the malleolus. This change was implemented because researchers wanted to eliminate the areas of ligamentous attachments. This variation improved the specificity up to 59% while not changing the sensitivity. Another impact analysis showed that this slight change further reduced the number of unnecessary radiographs to 54%. The use of validation and impact analyses studies can improve existing CPRs. It is important that when reading a derivation study, you also search the literature for corresponding validation studies, as they may show small changes that improve the accuracy and probability of the CPR.

By having an understanding of the derivation and assessment process of CPRs, you can better implement them into your clinical practice. As stated, there are several published CPRs available at a variety of levels of validation. As an AT, it can be overwhelming to find CPRs that could be used in your clinical practice. Table 13-3 through Table 13-5[3,5-38] show examples of each of the 3 types CPRs that may be relevant to your athletic training practice. The CPRs are listed by level and should be used in accordance with the level of validation. With the rapid evolving literature in this area, the list may not be the most up to date or comprehensive, but it will give you a starting point. The specifics of each CPR can be obtained by looking at the referenced study.

If you are relatively new to CPRs, it is important not to try to implement all of these CPRs at once. Take a look at the lists to determine which 1 or 2 are most relevant to your patient setting and then implement them on a smaller scale. Once you get comfortable with a CPR, you can start implementing more or encourage your colleagues to also use the CPRs. With the growing call for the implementation of evidence-based practice, CPRs are an easy and useful tool that clinicians can use to support their clinical decisions with evidence. By integrating CPRs into your clinical practice, you can often help reduce health care costs and also improve patient satisfaction.

Summary

Clinical prediction rules must undergo full development throughout the 3 steps of derivation, validation, and impact analysis before they can be used with confidence. Although most CPRs are at the derivation level, or Level 4, the findings can still be used to guide decision making when limited research exists. All CPRs must be thoroughly examined before they are implemented within clinical practice.

Table 13-3.
Diagnostic Clinical Prediction Rules Relevant to Athletic Trainers

NAME OF CPR	PURPOSE	LEVEL OF VALIDATION	DERIVATION REFERENCE
Ottawa Ankle Rules	Determines if ankle or foot radiograph is necessary	Level I	Stiell IG, Greenberg GH, McKnight RD, Nair RC, McDowell I, Worthington JR. A study to develop clinical decision rules for the use of radiography in acute ankle sprains. *Ann Emerg Med.* 1992;21(1):384-390.
Buffalo Modification to the Ottawa Ankle Rules	Determines if ankle or foot radiograph is necessary	Level I	Leddy JJ, Smolinski RJ, Lawrence J, Snyder JL, Priore RL. Prospective evaluation of the Ottawa ankle rules in a university sports medicine center, with a modification to increase specificity for identifying malleolar fractures. *Am J Sports Med.* 1998;26:158-165.
Ottawa Knee Rules	Determines if knee radiograph is necessary	Level I	Stiell IG, Greenberg GH, Wells GA, et al. Derivation of a decision rule for the use of radiography in acute knee injuries. *Ann Emerg Med.* 1995;26(4):405-413.
Wells Score-Lower Extremity Deep Vein Thrombosis	Determines if further testing is necessary to determine potential LE DVT	Level I	Wells PS, Hirsh J, Anderson DR, et al. A simple clinical model for diagnosis of deep-vein thrombosis combined with impedance plethysmography: potential for an improvement in the diagnostic process. *J Intern Med.* 1998;243(1):15-23.
Pittsburgh Knee Rules	Determines if knee radiograph is necessary after a fall or blunt trauma	Level II	Seaberg DC, Yealy DM, Lukens T, Auble T, Mathias S. Multicenter comparison of two clinical decision rules for the use of radiography in acute, high-risk knee injuries. *Ann Emerg Med.* 1998;32(1):8-13.

(continued)

Table 13-3. (continued) Diagnostic Clinical Prediction Rules Relevant to Athletic Trainers

NAME OF CPR	PURPOSE	LEVEL OF VALIDATION	DERIVATION REFERENCE
Canadian C-Spine Rules	Determines if a cervical spine radiograph is necessary	Level II	Canadian CT Head and Spine (CCC) Study Group. Canadian C-spine rule study for alert and stable trauma patients: II. study objectives and methodology. *CJEM*. 2002;4(3):185-193.
Canadian CT Head Rules	Determines if a CT scan is necessary after blunt head trauma	Level II	Stiell IG, Wells GA, Vandemheen K, et al. The Canadian CT Head Rule for patients with minor head injury. *Lancet*. 2001;357(9266):1391-1396.
New Orleans Criteria for Head Injuries	Determines if a CT scan is necessary after acute/blunt head trauma	Level II	Haydel MJ, Preston CA, Mills TJ, Luber S, Blaudeau E, DeBlieux PM. Indications for computed tomography in patients with minor head injury. *N Engl J Med*. 2000;343(2):100-105.
Walsh Criteria – Strep Throat	Determines need for throat culture	Level II	McGinn TG, Deluca J, Ahlawat SK, Mobo BH Jr, Wisnivesky JP. Validation and modification of streptococcal pharyngitis clinical prediction rules. *Mayo Clin Proc*. 2003;78(3):289-293.
Wells Score – Pulmonary Embolism	Categorizes patients with low, moderate, or high risk of a pulmonary embolism and the need for referral	Level II	Wells PS, Anderson DR, Rodger M, et al. Derivation of a simple clinical model to categorize patient's probability of pulmonary embolism: Increasing the model's utility with the SimpliRED D-dimer. *Thromb Haemost*. 2000;83(3):416-420.

(continued)

Table 13-3. (continued)
Diagnostic Clinical Prediction Rules Relevant to Athletic Trainers

NAME OF CPR	PURPOSE	LEVEL OF VALIDATION	DERIVATION REFERENCE
Upper Extremity Deep Vein Thrombosis	Determines if further testing is necessary to determine potential UE DVT	Level II	Constans J, Salmi LR, Sevestre-Pietri MA, et al. A clinical prediction score for upper extremity deep venous thrombosis. *Thromb Haemost.* 2008;99(1):202-207.
NEXUS – National Emergency X-Radiography Utilization Study	Determines if a cervical spine radiograph is necessary	Level II	Hoffman JR, Schriger DL, Mower WR, Luo JS, Zucker M. Low-risk criteria for cervical-spine radiography in blunt trauma: a prospective study. *Ann Emerg Med.* 1992;12(12):1454-1460.
NEXUS II for Head Injuries	Determines if a CT scan is necessary after blunt head trauma	Level II	Mower WR, Hoffman JR, Herbert M, Wolfson AB, Pollack CV Jr, Zucker MI. Developing a decision instrument to guide computed tomographic imaging of blunt head injury patients. *J Trauma.* 2005;59(4):954-959.
Revised Geneva Score – Pulmonary Embolism	Categorizes patients with low, intermediate, or high probability of a pulmonary embolism and the need for referral	Level II	Le Gal G, Righini M, Roy PM, et al. Prediction of pulmonary embolism in the emergency department: the revised Geneva score. *Ann Intern Med.* 2006;144(3):165-171.
Rotator Cuff Tear Diagnosis	Determines probability of a rotator cuff tear	Level III	Litaker D, Pioro M, Bilbeisi HE, Brems J. Returning to the bedside: using the history and physical examination to identify rotator cuff tears. *J Am Geriatr Soc.* 2000;48(12):1633-1637.

(continued)

Table 13-3. (continued) Diagnostic Clinical Prediction Rules Relevant to Athletic Trainers

NAME OF CPR	PURPOSE	LEVEL OF VALIDATION	DERIVATION REFERENCE
Diagnosis of Lumbar Spinal Stenosis	Screens patients with symptoms lumbar spinal stenosis	Level III	Sugioka T, Hayashino Y, Konno S, Kikuchi S, Fukuhara S. Predictive value of self-reported patient information for the identification of lumbar spinal stenosis. *Fam Pract.* 2008;25(4):237-244.
American College of Rheumatology Criteria for Classification of Osteoarthritis of the Hip	Determines probability that patients have evidence of clinical osteoarthritis when compared with physician diagnosis through radiographs, lab results, and history	Level III	Altman R, Alarcón G, Appelrouth D, et al. The American College of Rheumatology criteria for the classification and reporting of osteoarthritis of the hip. *Arthritis Rheum.* 1991;34(5):505-514.
American College of Rheumatology Criteria for Classification of Osteoarthritis of the Knee	Determines probability that patients with knee pain will have clinical osteoarthritis	Level III	Altman R, Asch E, Bloch D, et al. Development of criteria for the classification and reporting of osteoarthritis. Classification of osteoarthritis of the knee. *Arthritis Rheum.* 1986;29(8):1039-1049.

(continued)

Table 13-3. (continued)

Diagnostic Clinical Prediction Rules Relevant to Athletic Trainers

NAME OF CPR	PURPOSE	LEVEL OF VALIDATION	DERIVATION REFERENCE
Subacromial Impingement and Full-Thickness Rotator Cuff Tears	Determines if patients with shoulder pain have impingement syndrome or a rotator cuff tear	Level IV	Park HB, Yokota A, Gill HS, El Rassi G, McFarland EG. Diagnostic accuracy of clinical tests for the different degrees of subacromial impingement syndrome. *J Bone Joint Surg Am.* 2005;87(7):1446-1455.
Carpal Tunnel Syndrome Diagnosis	Determines probability that a patient will test positive for carpal tunnel with needle electromyography	Level IV	Wainner RS, Fritz JM, Irrgang JJ, Delitto A, Allison S, Boninger ML. Development of a clinical prediction rule for the diagnosis of carpal tunnel syndrome. *Arch Phys Med Rehabil.* 2005;86(4):609-618.
Diagnosis of a Medial Collateral Ligament Tear	Determines probability that clinical findings would suggest a medial collateral ligament tear as diagnosed through MRI	Level IV	Kastelein M, Luijsterburg PA, Wagemakers HP, et al. Diagnostic value of history taking and physical examination to assess effusion of the knee in traumatic knee patients in general practice. *Arch Phys Med Rehabil.* 2009;90(1):82-86.

Abbreviations: CT, computed tomography; DVT, deep vein thrombosis; LE, lower extremity; MRI, magnetic resonance imaging; UE, upper extremity.

Table 13-4. Interventional Clinical Prediction Rules Relevant to Athletic Trainers

NAME OF CPR	PURPOSE	LEVEL OF VALIDATION	DERIVATION REFERENCE
Lumbar Manipulation for Acute Back Pain	Determines probability that individuals with acute low back pain will experience at least 50% improvement in function after lumbopelvic manipulation	Level II	Flynn T, Frtiz J, Whitman J, et al. A clinical prediction rule for classifying patients with low back pain who demonstrate short-term improvement with spinal manipulation. *Spine (Phila Pa 1976)*. 2002;27(24):2835-2843.
Trigger Point Treatment for Chronic Tension Headaches	Determines probability that individuals with chronic tension headaches will receive a moderate global improvement or a 50% reduction in headache frequency, intensity, or duration after 3 weeks of trigger point therapy	Level IV	Fernández-de-las-Peñas C, Cleland JA, Cuadrado ML, Pareja JA. Predictor variables for indentifying patients with chronic tension-type headache who are likely to achieve short-term success with muscle trigger point therapy. *Cephalalgia.* 2008;28(3):264-275.
Cervical Traction in the Treatment of Mechanical Neck Pain	Determines probability that individuals with neck pain would experience a perceived benefit or change in symptoms after 3 weeks of cervical traction	Level IV	Raney NH, Peterson EJ, Smith TA, et al. Development of a clinical prediction rule to identify patients with neck pain likely to benefit from cervical traction and exercise. *Eur Spine J.* 2009;18(3):382-391.
Mobilization With Movement for Lateral Epicondylagia	Determines probability that individuals will feel improved after 3 weeks of mobilization with movement and exercises	Level IV	Vincenzino B, Smith D, Cleland J, Bisset L. Development of a clinical prediction rule to identify initial responders to mobilization with movement and exercise for lateral epicondylalgia. *Man Ther.* 2009;14(5):550-554.

(continued)

Table 13-4. (continued)
Interventional Clinical Prediction Rules Relevant to Athletic Trainers

NAME OF CPR	PURPOSE	LEVEL OF VALIDATION	DERIVATION REFERENCE
Lumbar Stabilization for Low Back Pain	Determines probability of success or nonsuccess after lumbar stabilization after 8 weeks	Level IV	Hicks GE, Fritz JM, Delitto A, McGill SM. Preliminary development of a clinical prediction rule for determining which patients with low back pain will respond to a stabilization exercise program. *Arch Phys Med Rehabil.* 2005;86(9):1735-1762.
Prone Mechanical Lumbar Traction in Treatment of Single Nerve Root Compression	Determines likelihood of patients experiencing 50% improvement after 6 weeks of manual therapy and lumbar traction	Level IV	Fritz JM, Lindsay W, Matheson JW, et al. Is there a subgroup of patients with low back pain likely to benefit from mechanical traction? Results of a randomized clinical trial and subgrouping analysis. *Spine (Phila Pa 1976).* 2007;32(26):E793-E800.
Supine Mechanical Lumbar Traction for Low Back Pain	Determines likelihood of patients experiencing 50% improvement after 3 sessions of intermittent traction	Level IV	Cai C, Pua YH, Lim KC. A clinical prediction rule for classifying patients with low back pain who demonstrate short-term improvement with mechanical lumbar traction. *Eur Spine J.* 2009;18(4):554-561.
Response to Exercise in Patients With Ankylosing Spondylitis	Determines probability that patients will experience improved function of a moderate global improvement after 15 sessions of an exercise program	Level IV	Alonso-Blanco C, Fernández-de-las-Peñas C, Cleland JA. Preliminary clinical prediction rule for identifying patients with ankylosing spondylitis who are likely to respond to an exercise program: a pilot study. *Am J Phys Med Rehabil.* 2009;889(6):445-454.

(continued)

Table 13-4. (continued)
Interventional Clinical Prediction Rules Relevant to Athletic Trainers

NAME OF CPR	PURPOSE	LEVEL OF VALIDATION	DERIVATION REFERENCE
Patellar Taping for Patellofemoral Pain Syndrome	Determines global improvement immediate benefit and/or a reduction of pain by 50% after medial patellar taping	Level IV	Lesher JD, Sutlive TG, Miller GA, Chine NJ, Garber MB, Wainner RS. Development of a clinical prediction rule for classifying patients with patellofemoral pain syndrome who respond to patellar taping. *J Orthop Sports Phys Ther.* 2006;36(11):854-866.
Prefabricated Orthotics as Treatment for Patellofemoral Pain Syndrome	Determines improvement in patients with patellofemoral pain syndrome after 3 weeks of orthotic use and activity modification	Level IV	Sutlive TG, Mitchell SD, Maxfield SN, et al. Identification of individuals with patellofemoral pain whose symptoms improved after a combined program of foot orthosis use and modified activity: a preliminary investigation. *Phys Ther.* 2004;84(1):49-61.
Hip Mobilization for Knee Osteoarthritis	Determines probability of global improvement or pain with functional tests in individuals with knee osteoarthritis after hip mobilizations and exercise	Level IV	Currier LL, Froehlich PJ, Carow SD, et al. Development of a clinical prediction rule to identify patients with knee pain and clinical evidence of knee osteoarthritis who demonstrate a favorable short-term response to hip mobilization. *Phys Ther.* 2007;87(9):1106-1119.
Manual Therapy and Exercise for Inversion Ankle Sprains	Determines probability of moderate improvement from 2 treatment session of manual therapy in individuals with inversion ankle sprains	Level IV	Whitman JM, Cleland JA, Mintken P, et al. Predicting short-term response to thrust and nonthrust manipulation and exercise in patients post inversion ankle sprain. *J Orthop Sports Phys Ther.* 2009;39(3):188-200.

Table 13-5.
Prognostic Clinical Prediction Rules Relevant to Athletic Trainers

NAME OF CPR	PURPOSE	LEVEL OF VALIDATION	DERIVATION REFERENCE
Prediction of Persistent Shoulder Pain	Determines percentage risk of having persistent shoulder pain at 6 weeks	Level III	Kuijpers T, van der Windt DA, van der Heijden GJ, Bouter LM. Systematic review of prognostic cohort studies on shoulder disorders. *Pain.* 2004;109(3):420-431.
Predicting Short-Term Outcomes With Cervical Radiculopathy	Determines probability of improvement at 4 weeks in patients with cervical radiculopathy	Level IV	Cleland JA, Fritz JM, Whitman JM, Heath R. Predictors of short-term outcome in people with a clinical diagnosis of cervical radiculopathy. *Phys Ther.* 2007;87(12):1619-1632.
Diagnosis of Ankylosing Spondylitis	Determines probability that low back pain is due to ankylosing spondylitis	Level IV	Rudwaleit M, Metter A, Listing J, Sieper J, Braun J. Inflammatory back pain in ankylosing spondylitis: a reassessment of the clinical history for application as classification and diagnosing criteria. *Arthritis Rheum.* 2006;54(2):569-578.

Key Points

- Clinical prediction rules combine several clinically relevant findings and then use powerful statistics to determine the probability of a specific condition or the likelihood of a particular outcome.
- While you want to include as many variables as possible, it is important to understand that for each predictor variable you want to test, it is recommended to have 10 to 15 participants enrolled in the study.
- When developing a CPR or evaluating CPRs for clinical use, you should consider the sample size in accordance with what the CPR is testing and consider the risks and benefits of having an adequately powered study.
- The highest level of validation is Level 1, which means that, in addition to being tested with a variety of patients and clinicians, it must undergo an impact analysis.
- Regardless of the type of CPR you are using, it is important that you assess the quality of the derivation study before implementing the CPR into practice unless it has already been validated in other studies.

- With the growing call for the implementation of evidence-based practice, CPRs are an easy and useful tool that clinicians can use to support their clinical decisions with evidence.

References

1. Flynn T, Frtiz J, Whitman J, et al. A clinical prediction rule for classifying patients with low back pain who demonstrate short-term improvement with spinal manipulation. *Spine (Phila Pa 1976)*. 2002;27(24):2835-2843.
2. Childs JD, Cleland JA. Development and application of clinical prediction rules to improve decision making in physical therapist practice. *Phys Ther*. 2006;86(1):122-131.
3. Kuijpers T, van der Windt DA, van der Heijden GJ, Bouter LM. Systematic review of prognostic cohort studies on shoulder disorders. *Pain*. 2004;109(3):420-431.
4. Beneciuk JM, Bishop MD, George SZ. Clinical prediction rules for physical therapy interventions: a systematic review. *Phys Ther*. 2009;89(2):114-124.
5. Stiell IG, Greenberg GH, McKnight RD, Nair RC, McDowell I, Worthington JR. A study to develop clinical decision rules for the use of radiography in acute ankle sprains. *Ann Emerg Med*. 1992;21(4):384-390.
6. Leddy JJ, Smolinski RJ, Lawrence J, Snyder JL, Priore RL. Prospective evaluation of the Ottawa ankle rules in a university sports medicine center, with a modification to increase specificity for identifying malleolar fractures. *Am J Sports Med*. 1998;26:158-165.
7. Stiell IG, Greenberg GH, Wells GA, et al. Derivation of a decision rule for the use of radiography in acute knee injuries. *Ann Emerg Med*. 1995;26(4):405-413.
8. Wells PS, Hirsh J, Anderson DR, et al. A simple clinical model for diagnosis of deep-vein thrombosis combined with impedance plethysmography: potential for an improvement in the diagnostic process. *J Intern Med*. 1998;243(1):15-23.
9. Seaberg DC, Yealy DM, Lukens T, Auble T, Mathias S. Multicenter comparison of two clinical decision rules for the use of radiography in acute, high-risk knee injuries. *Ann Emerg Med*. 1998;32(1):8-13.
10. Canadian CT Head and C-Spine (CCC) Study Group. Canadian C-spine rule study for alert and stable trauma patients: II. study objectives and methodology. *CJEM*. 2002;4(3):185-193.
11. Stiell IG, Wells GA, Vandemheen K, et al. The Canadian CT Head Rule for patients with minor head injury. *Lancet*. 2001;357(9266):1391-1396.
12. Haydel MJ, Preston CA, Mills TJ, Luber S, Blaudeau E, DeBlieux PM. Indications for computed tomography in patients with minor head injury. *N Engl J Med*. 2000;343(2):100-105.
13. McGinn TG, Deluca J, Ahlawat SK, Mobo BH Jr, Wisnivesky JP. Validation and modification of streptococcal pharyngitis clinical prediction rules. *Mayo Clin Proc*. 2003;78(3):289-293.
14. Wells PS, Anderson DR, Rodger M, et al. Derivation of a simple clinical model to categorize patient's probability of pulmonary embolism: increasing the model's utility with the SimpliRED D-dimer. *Thromb Haemost*. 2000;83(3):416-420.
15. Constans J, Salmi LR, Sevestre-Pietri MA, et al. A clinical prediction score for upper extremity deep venous thrombosis. *Thromb Haemost*. 2008;99(1):202-207.
16. Hoffman JR, Schriger DL, Mower W, Luo JS, Zucker M. Low-risk criteria for cervical-spine radiography in blunt trauma: a prospective study. *Ann Emerg Med*. 1992;12(12):1454-1460.
17. Mower WR, Hoffman JR, Herbert M, Wolfson AB, Pollack CV Jr, Zucker MI. Developing a decision instrument to guide computed tomographic imaging of blunt head injury patients. *J Trauma*. 2005;59(4):954-959.
18. Le Gal G, Righini M, Roy PM, et al. Prediction of pulmonary embolism in the emergency department: the revised Geneva score. *Ann Intern Med*. 2006;144(3):165-171.
19. Litaker D, Pioro M, Bilbeisi HE, Brems J. Returning to the bedside: using the history and physical examination to identify rotator cuff tears. *J Am Geriatr Soc*. 2000;48(12):1633-1637.
20. Sugioka T, Hayashino Y, Konno S, Kikuchi S, Fukuhara S. Predictive value of self-reported patient information for the identification of lumbar spinal stenosis. *Fam Pract*. 2008;25(4):237-244.
21. Altman R, Alarcón G, Appelrouth D, et al. The American College of Rheumatology criteria for the classification and reporting of osteoarthritis of the hip. *Arthritis Rheum*. 1991;34(5):505-514.
22. Altman R, Asch E, Bloch D, et al. Development of criteria for the classification and reporting of osteoarthritis. Classification of osteoarthritis of the knee. Diagnostic and Therapeutic Criteria Committee of the American Rheumatism Association. *Arthritis Rheum*. 1986;29(8):1039-1049.
23. Park HB, Yokota A, Gill HS, El Rassi G, McFarland EG. Diagnostic accuracy of clinical tests for the different degrees of subacromial impingement syndrome. *J Bone Joint Surg Am*. 2005;87(7):1446-1455.
24. Wainner RS, Fritz JM, Irrgang JJ, Delitto A, Allison S, Boninger ML. Development of a clinical prediction rule for the diagnosis of carpal tunnel syndrome. *Arch Phys Med Rehabil*. 2005;86(4):609-618.

25. Kastelein M, Luijsterburg PA, Wagemakers HP, et al. Diagnostic value of history taking and physical examination to assess effusion of the knee in traumatic knee patients in general practice. *Arch Phys Med Rehabil.* 2009;90(1):82-86.
26. Fernández-de-las-Peñas C, Cleland JA, Cuadrado ML, Pareja JA. Predictor variables for identifying patients with chronic tension-type headache who are likely to achieve short-term success with muscle trigger point therapy. *Cephalalgia.* 2008;28(3):264-275.
27. Raney NH, Peterson EJ, Smith TA, et al. Development of a clinical prediction rule to identify patients with neck pain likely to benefit from cervical traction and exercise. *Eur Spine J.* 2009;18(3):382-391.
28. Vincenzino B, Smith D, Cleland J, Bisset L. Development of a clinical prediction rule to identify initial responders to mobilization with movement and exercise for lateral epicondylalgia. *Man Ther.* 2009;14(5):550-554.
29. Hicks GE, Fritz JM, Delitto A, McGill SM. Preliminary development of a clinical prediction rule for determining which patients with low back pain will respond to a stabilization exercise program. *Arch Phys Med Rehabil.* 2005;86(9):1735-1762.
30. Fritz JM, Lindsay W, Matheson JW, et al. Is there a subgroup of patients with low back pain likely to benefit from mechanical traction? Results of a randomized clinical trial and subgrouping analysis. *Spine (Phila Pa 1976).* 2007;32(26):E793-E800.
31. Cai C, Pua YH, Lim KC. A clinical prediction rule for classifying patients with low back pain who demonstrate short-term improvement with mechanical lumbar traction. *Eur Spine J.* 2009;18(4):554-561.
32. Alonso-Blanco C, Fernández-de-las-Peñas C, Cleland JA. Preliminary clinical prediction rule for identifying patients with ankylosing spondylitis who are likely to respond to an exercise program: a pilot study. *Am J Phys Med Rehabil.* 2009;88(6):445-454.
33. Lesher JD, Sutlive TG, Miller GA, Chine NJ, Garber MB, Wainner RS. Development of a clinical prediction rule for classifying patients with patellofemoral pain syndrome who respond to patellar taping. *J Orthop Sports Phys Ther.* 2006;36(11):854-866.
34. Sutlive TG, Mitchell SD, Maxfield SN, et al. Identification of individuals with patellofemoral pain whose symptoms improved after a combined program of foot orthosis use and modified activity: a preliminary investigation. *Phys Ther.* 2004;84(1):49-61.
35. Currier LL, Froehlich PJ, Carow SD, et al. Development of a clinical prediction rule to identify patients with knee pain and clinical evidence of knee osteoarthritis who demonstrate a favorable short-term response to hip mobilization. *Phys Ther.* 2007;87(9):1106-1119.
36. Whitman JM, Cleland JA, Mintken PE, et al. Predicting short-term response to thrust and nonthrust manipulation and exercise in patients post inversion ankle sprain. *J Orthop Sports Phys Ther.* 2009;39(3):188-200.
37. Cleland JA, Fritz JM, Whitman JM, Heath R. Predictors of short-term outcome in people with a clinical diagnosis of cervical radiculopathy. *Phys Ther.* 2007;87(12):1619-1632.
38. Rudwaleit M, Metter A, Listing J, Sieper J, Braun J. Inflammatory back pain in ankylosing spondylitis: a reassessment of the clinical history for application as classification and diagnosing criteria. *Arthritis Rheum.* 2006;54(2):569-578.

Bibliography

Bruce SL, Wilkerson GB. Clinical prediction rules, part 1: conceptual overview. *Athlet Ther Today.* 2010;15(2):4-9.

Bruce SL, Wilkerson GB. Clinical prediction rules, part 2: data analysis procedures and clinical applications. *Athlet Ther Today.* 2010;15(2):10-13.

Childs JD, Fritz JM, Flynn TW, et al. A clinical prediction rule to identify patients with low back pain most likely to benefit from spinal manipulation: a validation study. *Ann Intern Med.* 2004;141(12):920-928.

Cook CE. Potential pitfalls of clinical prediction rules. *J Man Manip Ther.* 2008;16(2):69-71.

Glynn PE, Weisbach PC. *Clinical Prediction Rules: A Physical Therapy Reference Manual.* Sudbury, MA: Jones and Bartlett Publishers; 2011.

McGinn TG, Guyatt GH, Wyer PC, Naylor CD, Stiell IG, Richardson WS. Users' guide to the medical literature: XXII: how to use articles about clinical decision rules. *JAMA.* 2000;284(1):79-84.

Reilly BM, Evans AT. Translating clinical research into clinical practice: impact of using prediction rules to make decisions. *Ann Intern Med.* 2006;144(3):201-209.

Vesci BJ. Current evidence guiding clinical practice in athletic training. *Athl Train Sport Health Care.* 2010;2(2):57-60.

Wallace E, Smith SM, Perera-Salazar R, et al. Framework for the impact analysis and implementation of clinical prediction rules (CPRs). *BMC Med Inform Decis Mak.* 2011;62(11):1-7.

Wasson JH, Sox HC, Neff RK, Goldman L. Clinical prediction rules. Applications and methodological standards. *New Engl J Med.* 1985;313(13):793-799.

14

Epidemiological Measures

Sports injury epidemiology, the study of injury occurrence in athletic populations, is important for your clinical practice because it provides information regarding the injury trends that occur in the athletes or patients that you encounter on a daily basis. Understanding the trends associated with injury occurrence in athletic populations is also the foundation for one of your primary roles as an athletic trainer (AT): injury prevention. In this chapter, we review basic concepts in injury surveillance and many of the measures that you can use to understand injury trends and make evidence-based decisions for implementing injury prevention strategies.

Injury surveillance is the documentation of injuries. Injury surveillance systems can be as large scale as the National Collegiate Athletic Association Injury Surveillance System (NCAA ISS), which is the most comprehensive database on sports-related injuries at the collegiate level. The NCAA ISS has kept record of injury information on thousands of intercollegiate athletes in several sports and divisions for longer than 2 decades. These databases may include information on athlete exposures, injury occurrences, and potentially modifiable risk factors that would be used to develop injury prevention strategies. The benefit to databases such as the NCAA ISS is that a large number of participants can be tracked from many institutions over several years. Clinicians and researchers can use NCAA ISS data to make strong inferences regarding expected injury trends for certain sports, levels of competition, and types of exposure.

Injury surveillance can also be small-scale (eg, by consistently and accurately completing injury documentation records). Recording the numbers of participants and the injuries that occur is a part of basic clinical documentation and standard practice. The information that you gather can be used in much the same way as information collected for the NCAA.

In either case, injury epidemiology is important for understanding injury rates, injury risk, and making evidence-based decisions regarding injury prevention strategies in your clinical practice. It can also be used to evaluate injury trends in different groups (eg, in comparing injury rates between a group that performs an injury prevention program and a group that does not). These types of studies will facilitate evidence-based decision making as you plan whether to implement

Van Lunen BL, Hankemeier DA, Welch CE.
Evidence-Guided Practice: A Framework for Clinical Decision Making in Athletic Training (pp 185-192).

an injury-prevention strategy. To understand how epidemiological information can be used in your clinical practice, some basic concepts must be examined.

When beginning to understand injury epidemiology methods and statistics, you should consider what constitutes an **injury** and a unit of exposure. It might appear that injury is easily defined, but it is of utmost importance that the definition is consistent across all injuries that will be documented. For example, the NCAA ISS defined an injury by the following criteria: (1) occurred during organized intercollegiate practice or competition, (2) required medical attention by an AT or physician, and (3) resulted in a participation restriction for at least 1 day. Injury may be defined by different criteria for other documentation systems, but consistency is the key. With inconsistent or nonexistent documentation, injury surveillance (and injury epidemiology) is impossible.

An **exposure** is an opening up to the chance of an incident (in this case a sports injury) occurring. An individual does not have the chance to incur a sports injury (ie, is not exposed) when sitting at home watching television. However, if that individual is participating in a practice or game, then that individual is exposed to the chance of getting injured. Again, exposure can be defined differently depending on the documentation system. The NCAA ISS defined an exposure as "the participation in a NCAA-sanctioned practice or competition."[1] To clarify, as long as the individual was "suited up" and prepared to play, even if that individual did not get on the field, that individual was considered "exposed." Like *injury*, other systems may have a different definition for exposure; the crucial part is keeping the definition consistent.

Once injury and exposure have been defined, you can examine injury prevalence and injury incidence. While these terms may seem synonymous, the way they are calculated enables different aspects of the injury problem to be described. As discussed in previous chapters, **prevalence** is the segment of a group that is currently injured at a given time point. For example, if you have a football team of 80 individuals and you know that 16 currently have ankle sprains, you can calculate the prevalence of ankle sprains on your team. Prevalence is typically expressed as a fraction (a proportion or percentage).

The following is the typical equation for prevalence:

$$Prevalence = \frac{Number\ of\ Injured\ Participants}{Number\ of\ Total\ Participants} \times 100$$

To return to the football team example, if there are 80 participants on the team and 16 had an ankle sprain at that moment in time, the prevalence would be (16/80), or 0.20. To express this as a percentage, you would multiply by 100, giving you 20%. Expressing prevalence either by using the proportion (16/80) or the percentage (20%) is correct.

Prevalence is used in your clinical practice to answer the question, "What is the proportion of participants who currently have an injury right now?" It is a measure of the injury problem you currently have to manage. The larger the prevalence, the bigger the injury problem you have. To examine if the injury prevalence is greater in 1 sample than another, you may choose to use the **prevalence ratio**. For this, you divide the prevalence in one group by the prevalence in another group.

The following is the equation for prevalence ratio:

$$Prevalence\ Ratio = \frac{Prevalence\ Group\ 1}{Prevalence\ Group\ 2}$$

If the prevalence ratio is greater than 1, then the prevalence in group 1 is higher. If the prevalence ratio is less than 1, the prevalence in group 2 is higher. For the football example, we can add a second team with 70 players and 12 have ankle sprains.

Prevalence for team 1 = 16/80 = 20%

Prevalence for team 2 = 12/70 = 17%

Prevalence Ratio = team 1/team 2 = 20/17 = 1.18 ≈ 1.2

This indicates that the prevalence of ankle sprains on team 1 is about 1.2 times greater (or 120% of, 20% larger than) than the prevalence on team 2. This is a slight increase for team 1, and if you decide that is an important amount of increase, you may begin to study why that might be occurring. Conversely, if team 1's prevalence was 17 and team 2's prevalence was 20, the prevalence ratio would be 85%, indicating that there is 15% lower prevalence for team 1 than team 2.

Incidence refers to the number of new injuries occurring in a sample over a defined time interval. The primary difference between prevalence and incidence is that prevalence refers to the proportion of injuries at a specific time point, while incidence refers to the number of new injuries that occur within a specified time period. Furthermore, incidence will require prospective injury tracking of participants over that specified time period (eg, over one sports season).

For **incidence rate**, we use the number of injuries that occur per a given time frame. We also have to come back to exposure. As defined previously, exposure is the opening up to the chance of injury, and it is typically defined in sports as participation in a practice or competition. As an example, 1 individual might participate in 5 practices and 1 game per week for a 15-week season: that is 6 exposures per week for 15 weeks, which equals 90 exposures. That 1 athlete had 90 exposures for the season (ie, that individual had 90 chances to get injured). However, we do not typically track just 1 athlete; we have an entire team. If the team has 20 athletes and each athlete has 90 exposures, then we have an accumulation of 1800 athlete exposures, the total exposure for the team for the whole season. The incidence rate is the number of new injuries that occurs during the total exposure time.

In athletic training, incidence rate is sometimes referred to as injury rate. The injury rate value is often expressed as injuries per 1000 athlete exposures to increase the size of the injury rate to a whole number, which is easier to interpret. For example, if you observed 10 injuries during 450 athlete exposures, the injury rate would be 10/450 = 0.022 injuries per athlete exposure. This is somewhat difficult to interpret, so you can multiply it by 1000, and you have 22.2 injuries per 1000 athlete exposures. You can get 1000 athlete exposures using any multiplicative combination; by having 20 athletes participate for 50 exposures or 100 athletes participate for 10 exposures, you can expect a new injury rate of about 22.

Incidence rates are used in your clinical practice when asking, "How many participants are expected to acquire a new injury over the course of a season?" This is useful information if you want to compare your injury rate problems between years, practice/competitions, coaches, teams, etc. If you see a dramatic increase in incidence rate from year to year, you might choose to investigate possible causes for that increase in injuries.

The following is the equation for incidence rate:

$$Incidence\ Rate = \frac{Number\ of\ New\ Injuries}{Total\ Exposure\ Time}$$

To make these comparisons, we use an extension of incidence (or injury) rate known as the **incidence rate ratio (IRR)**. The IRR informs you of the magnitude of an increased or decreased rate of injury between groups. The IRR is calculated by dividing 1 incidence rate by another. The interpretation for IRR follows the same premise as prevalence ratio: values of 1.0 indicate no difference in incidence rates between groups. Incidence rate ratios greater than 1 indicate greater incidence rate in group 1, while IRRs less than 1 indicate a greater incidence rate in group 2.

The following is the equation for IRR:

$$Incidence\ Rate\ Ratio = \frac{Incidence\ Rate\ 1}{Incidence\ Rate\ 2}$$

For example, if you determined that the incidence rate during competition was 10.6 injuries per 1000 athlete exposures and the incidence rate during practices was 5.3 injuries per 1000 athlete exposures, the IRR = 10.6/5.3 = 2.0. This indicates that you observed a rate of injury during competition exposures that was 100% (or 2 times) greater than during practice exposures.

Thus far, the discussion has centered on determining the magnitude of the injury problem and how to interpret it. There is also value to calculating the chance that an athlete will get an injury (ie, the risk of injury). We assess the risk of an adverse event every day and make determinations on whether the risk is worth the benefit. In sports, athletes take a risk of getting injured every time they participate (are exposed). As a clinician, there are ways that you may be able to mitigate that risk, or perhaps, make the decision to accept the risk as it stands. The ability to objectively quantify risk is essential to making clinical decisions.

The **incidence proportion** (IP; ie, cumulative incidence) is a first step in quantifying risk and is a measure of the probability of injury. It is determined by dividing the number of athletes who sustained an injury by the total number of participants.

The following is the equation for IP:

$$\textit{Incidence Proportion} = \frac{\textit{Number of Newly Injured Participants}}{\textit{Number of Total Participants}} \times 100$$

The equation for IP is slightly different than incidence rate; the IP includes the number of participants as the denominator, whereas the incidence rate has the total exposure time (number of participants × exposures) as the denominator.

The following is an example of calculating IP: if there are a total of 80 participants on the football team and 32 sustained a lower-extremity injury throughout the season, the IP would be (32/80), or 0.40. To express this as a percentage, you multiply by 100. In this scenario, you would have determined that the probability of lower-extremity injury for a football participant during 1 season was 40%.

The IP by itself informs you of the individual risk of injury for your sample. An extension of IP is the **risk ratio** (ie, relative risk), a comparison of risk between 2 groups. This comparison allows you to contrast risk of injury between seasons, teams, etc, and is a powerful tool to evaluate clinical interventions. For example, you can use the risk ratio to compare the risk of sustaining an injury in a group that received an intervention versus the risk of sustaining an injury in another group that did not receive an intervention.

The following is the equation for risk ratio:

$$\textit{Risk Ratio} = \frac{\textit{Incidence Proportion Group 1}}{\textit{Incidence Proportion Group 2}}$$

The risk ratio is calculated by dividing 1 IP by another. Again, with risk ratio, a value of 1.0 indicates no increased risk of injury for either group. A risk ratio greater than 1 signifies increased risk for group 1, and a value less than 1 indicates decreased risk for group 1. For example, to compare the risk of injury between a set of men's and women's basketball players, you need the IP for each group. If the IP for men's basketball was 0.40 (40%) and the IP for women's basketball was 0.32 (32%), the risk ratio would be (0.40/0.32), or 1.25. This would indicate that the risk of sustaining an injury in men's basketball is 25% greater.

For all ratios, confidence intervals (CIs) are an important part of interpreting these point estimates. A CI is a measure of variability based on a statistical z-score and indicates precision of the point estimate. A 95% CI is most commonly used in social sciences. The CI is a range of values within which the true (population) value will probably be found in a replication of the same study. You can be 95% confident that the population value falls within that CI. Similar to a standard deviation around a mean, a wide CI indicates that there is less precision, while a narrow CI indicates greater precision. For CIs that are built around a ratio, the smallest limit you can have for a ratio CI is less than 0 (you cannot actually have a 0, just approaching toward 0); however, your upper limit is infinity. There is a marker of uncertainty as to the difference between groups; that

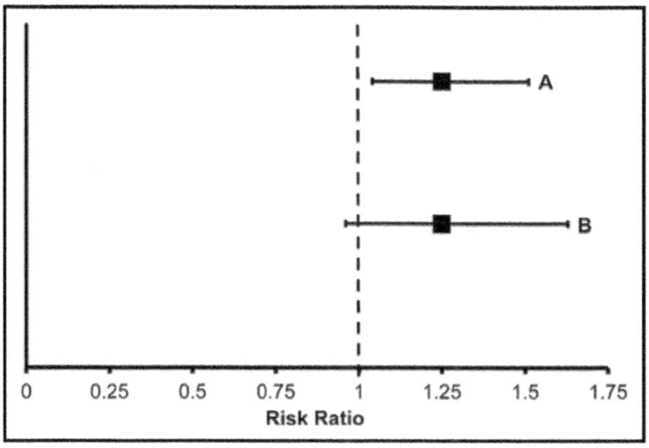

Figure 14-1. Risk ratio forest plot that provides a visual depiction of the risk ratios and their corresponding 95% confidence intervals (CIs). When interpreting risk ratio forest plots, it is important to examine the magnitude of the risk ratio point estimates and their corresponding 95% CIs. In this example, the CI for point estimate A does not cross 1 (the vertical dashed line), which indicates you should be more confident there is a difference in injury risk between groups. However, the CI for point estimate B does not cross 1, which indicates you should be less confident there is a difference in injury risk between groups.

value is 1. That is, there is a chance that the ratio between your 2 groups is 1:1, indicating that they are the same. If the range of values for your CI includes 1, you cannot be completely sure that there is actually no difference between your groups and a level of caution would need to be used when interpreting the risk ratio point estimate.

If the 95% CI in our fictitious example had a lower bound of 1.04 and an upper bound of 1.51, you can be confident that the probability of sustaining an injury in men's basketball is greater than women's basketball because the lower bound of the CI does not cross 1.0. Conversely, if the 95% CI in our example had a lower bound of 0.96 and an upper bound of 1.63, you cannot be confident that the probability of sustaining an injury in men's basketball is greater than women's basketball because the CI does cross 1.0 (Figure 14-1). As with all measures, CIs will likely be narrower and more precise in studies with larger sample sizes.

There are additional measures, including relative risk reduction and absolute risk reduction, that provide more interpretation for comparing injury risks. **Relative risk reduction (RRR)** represents the percentage that injury risk is reduced in an intervention group compared with a control group. Essentially, it is a measure of how well the treatment worked to decrease the chance of injury. Relative risk reduction is calculated by taking 1 minus the risk ratio and multiplying by 100 to get the percentage of difference.

The following is the equation for RRR:

$$\textit{Relative Risk Reduction}\ (\%) = (1 - \textit{Risk Ratio}) \times 100$$

Interpreting RRR is slightly more straightforward to interpret than risk ratio; an RRR value of 0% indicates no risk reduction for the intervention group. Anything other than 0% represents a decrease in injury risk for the intervention group. For example, we have 2 groups of athletes: group 1 (n = 250) does an injury-prevention program and sustains 25 injuries, while group 2 (n = 300) does not perform an injury-prevention program and sustains 55 injuries.

To determine RRR, we must first calculate the IP for both teams:

Group 1 IP = 25/250 = 0.10

Group 2 IP = 55/300 = 0.18

Next, we determine the risk ratio between these teams:

Risk ratio = group 1 IP/group 2 IP = 0.10/0.18 = 0.56

Finally, we will determine the RRR between group 1, the intervention group, and group 2, the control group:

RRR (%) = (1 – .56) × 100 = 44%

Since we calculated the IP of the intervention group to be 10% and the IP of the control group to be 18%, the risk ratio is 0.56. In this case, the RRR would be (1 – 0.56) × 100, or a 44% decrease in risk in the intervention group. An RRR that is greater than 25% is considered potentially beneficial, and an RRR greater than 50% is considered clinically meaningful. In this case, the RRR of 44% indicates that the intervention was probably beneficial to preventing the injury of interest.

In cases in which the injury risk is greater in the intervention group and the RRR is negative, the sign is changed to positive and expressed as relative risk increase. When applying 95% CIs to RRR or relative risk increase, you are now examining if the CI encompasses 0%. For example, if the lower bound of the 95% CI in our example was 15%, you can be confident that the intervention group decreased risk compared with the control group because the CI does not cross 0%.

Absolute risk reduction (ARR) is used to represent the risk difference between an intervention group and a control group. Absolute risk reduction is calculated by subtracting the control group injury risk from the intervention group.

The following is the equation for ARR:

$$\textit{Absolute Risk Reduction} = IP\ 1 - IP\ 2$$

For example, if you determined the IP of the control group to be 18% and the IP of the intervention group to be 10%, the ARR would be 8%. This indicates that there are 8 fewer injuries per 100 athletes in the intervention group compared with the control group. In cases in which the injury risk is heightened in the intervention group and the ARR is negative, the sign is changed to positive and expressed as an absolute risk increase (ARI). A 95% CI should also be examined when interpreting ARR or ARI following the same guidelines previously discussed with RRR.

Perhaps the most meaningful assessment of risk comes as an extension of ARR known as **numbers needed to treat to benefit (NNTB)**. The NNTB represents the number of participants who need to be treated with the intervention to prevent a single injury compared with receiving no intervention and is calculated by finding the inverse of the ARR (1/ARR). Using the example with an ARR of 8%, you can calculate the NNTB:

$$\text{NNTB} = 1/\text{ARR} = 1/0.08 = 12.5$$

Since the NNTB represents a number of people, and in this example is not a whole number, we need to round it up. This means that you would need to treat approximately 13 individuals to prevent 1 injury. Numbers needed to treat to benefit values can range from 1 (most desirable) to infinity (least desirable). The ideal situation, an NNTB of 1, indicates that if you treat 1 patient with the intervention, you would prevent 1 injury from occurring, and you would have the perfect treatment against injury. The worst case scenario, an NNTB of infinity, indicates that you could treat patients forever and never prevent that 1 injury from occurring.

However, neither is typically the case of most of the injury-prevention programs used in clinical practice. It is up to you to decide whether the decreased chance of injury from the intervention is worth the cost of implementing the intervention. For example (in a completely hypothetical situation), we can consider taping an ankle to prevent an ankle sprain. You must consider the clinical cost of taping an ankle: the cost of the roll of tape and the time it takes to tape that ankle. If you could tape 13 athletes and prevent 1 ankle sprain, you might consider those 13 athletes a reasonable cost to prevent that sprain. However, if the NNTB was 350, that might be too cost-prohibitive in certain situations to prevent that 1 ankle sprain.

If the intervention is beneficial, this measure is usually referred to as NNTB. Conversely, if the intervention is harmful, this measure is often referred to as **numbers needed to treat to harm (NNTH)** and is interpreted similarly: the number of individuals you would treat with an intervention to harm 1. Although clinicians would not think of intentionally harming their patients, NNTH can be used to assess potential side effects or adverse events associated with an intervention. When applying 95% CIs to NNTB or NNTH, you are examining if the CI encompasses or crosses infinity (Figure 14-2). If the 95% CI encompasses infinity, you should have less confidence in the ability of the intervention to prevent an injury in even a very large number of participants; some individuals may be harmed.

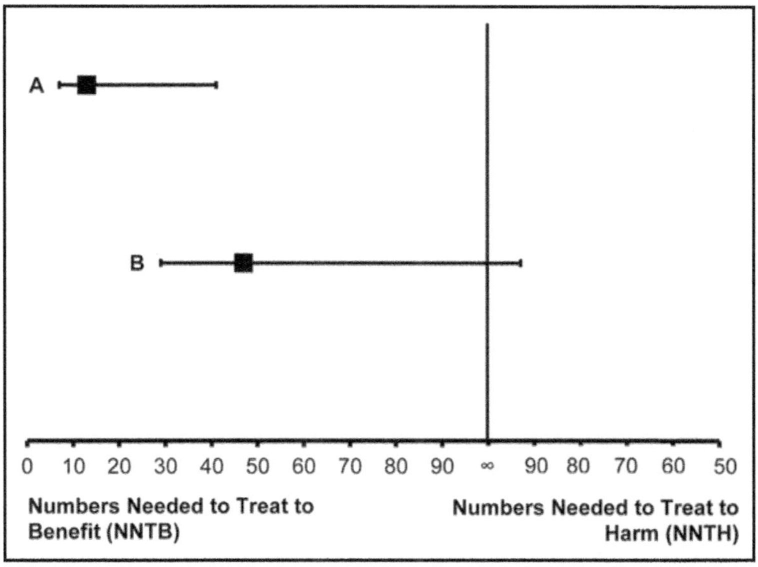

Figure 14-2. Numbers needed to treat forest plot that provides a visual depiction of numbers needed to treat and their corresponding 95% confidence intervals (CIs). When interpreting this plot, it is important to examine the magnitude of the numbers needed to treat point estimates and their corresponding 95% CIs. In this example, the CI for point estimate A does not cross ∞ (the vertical solid line); therefore, you can be more confident the intervention may prevent an injury. However, the CI for point estimate B does cross ∞, which indicates you should be less confident the intervention can prevent injuries.

Finally, you may commonly see within injury epidemiology studies or hear other clinicians refer to the **odds of being injured**. Odds are a somewhat tricky concept; it is the probability of an injury occurring compared with the probability of it not occurring. Remember, IP is the probability of injury; to calculate odds, you divide the probability of getting injured (the IP) by the probability of not getting injured (1 – IP).

The following is the equation for odds:

$$Odds = \frac{Incidence\ Proportion}{1 - Incidence\ Proportion}$$

Odds are typically expressed in comparison to another number, such as 2:1 or 100:1. For an example of calculating the odds of sustaining an injury, we will use the previously calculated IP of 0.40 and divide it by 1 – 0.40. In this case, the odds of sustaining an injury are (0.40/0.60) or 0.67:1 that an injury will occur. When the first number is less than 1, you may see the inverse of the odds presented. In this case, the inverse (1/0.67) would result in an odds of 1.50:1 (or 3/2) that an injury will not occur.

In some cases, we may want to compare the odds of being injured in an intervention group vs a control group. Again, you would use a ratio to compare these odds—the **odds ratio**—which represents the odds of injury for an individual who received an intervention compared with the odds of injury for an individual who did not receive the intervention. To calculate the odds ratio, you would divide the odds of the control group by the odds of the intervention group.

The following is the equation for the odds ratio:

$$Odd\ Ratio = \frac{Control\ Group\ Odds}{Intervention\ Group\ Odds}$$

An odds ratio of 1.0 would indicate that the odds are identical for both groups. Odds ratios greater than 1.0 would indicate that there is an increased odds of sustaining an injury in the control group. Odds ratios less than 1.0 would be associated with increased odds of sustaining an injury in the intervention group, for example:

Control group odds = 0.24:1

Intervention group odds = 0.12:1

Odds ratio = 0.24/0.12 or 2.0.

Therefore, the odds of sustaining an injury in the control group compared with sustaining an injury in the intervention group is 2:1 in this scenario. A 95% CI should also be examined when interpreting the odds ratio point estimates following the same guidelines previously discussed with all other measures that used 1.0 as a critical value.

Summary

Injury documentation has a place beyond that of just keeping track of injuries. We presented some clear examples in which standard injury documentation, combined with some fairly simple calculations, can provide you with a wealth of information that you can use for your own clinical practice.

Key Points

- Understanding the trends associated with injury occurrence in athletic populations is also the foundation for one of your primary roles as an AT: injury prevention.
- Incidence rates provide useful information if you want to compare your injury rate problems between years, practice/competitions, coaches, teams, etc, and to use this information to make evidence-based determinations about the injury prevention strategies that you might use.
- In addition to determining the magnitude of the injury problem, there is also a value to calculating the chance that an athlete will get an injury (ie, the risk of injury).
- Using NNTB or NNTH allows clinicians to decide whether the decreased chance of injury from the intervention or the potential adverse side effect of an intervention is worth the cost of implementing the intervention.
- Consistent and accurate documentation is a standard of clinical practice and can greatly assist you in a decision-making process.

Reference

1. Dick R, Agel J, Marshall SW. National Collegiate Athletic Association Injury Surveillance System commentaries: introduction and methods. *J Athl Train.* 2007;42(2):173-182.

Bibliography

Barratt A, Wyer PC, Hatala R, et al. Tips for learners of evidence-based medicine: 1. relative risk reduction, absolute risk reduction and number needed to treat. *CMAJ.* 2004;171(4):353-358.

Dick R, Agel J, Marshall SW. National Collegiate Athletic Association Injury Surveillance System commentaries: introduction and methods. *J Athl Train.* 2007;42(2):173-182.

Hootman JM, Dick R, Agel J. Epidemiology of collegiate injuries for 15 sports: summary and recommendations for injury prevention initiatives. *J Athl Train.* 2007;42(2):311-319.

Knowles SB, Marshall SW, Guskiewicz KM. Issues in estimating risks and rates in sports injury research. *J Athl Train.* 2006;41(2):207-215.

Sistrom CL, Garvan CW. Proportions, odds, and risks. *Radiology.* 2004;230(1):12-19.

15

Disablement Models

Evidence-based practice (EBP) incorporates the best available evidence, clinical expertise, and patient values and beliefs during patient care. The EBP process is integral in the treatment of your patients in the clinical setting. However, for EBP to be fully implemented, outcomes that demonstrate the effectiveness of the treatments you may utilize in clinical practice must be collected, synthesized, and made available. **Outcomes research** is evidence that is made available to you that demonstrates the final result of a treatment, most often incorporating the patient's values and experiences throughout the course of treatment and into the final outcome. Outcomes research can further be described as **patient-oriented evidence (POE)**. Patient-oriented evidence is the collection of outcomes that demonstrates the effectiveness of treatments utilized in the clinical setting from the patient's perspective. Patient-oriented evidence is said to be the most valuable outcomes evidence for you to utilize in clinical practice because it demonstrates outcomes related to the treatments of injuries from the patient's perspective. The collection and dissemination of POE is what fuels the EBP process for you and other health care professionals.

Disablement models provide the structure needed to advance the collection and dissemination of POE, thus improving EBP in your clinical practice. These models are available to help guide you in asking the appropriate clinical question and to help you in selecting the appropriate outcomes to answer your questions, which will strengthen the collection and dissemination of POE. These models are also available to ensure whole-person health care rather than impairment-focused health care, thus shifting focus away from the impairment and toward the person and enhancing patient care. Additionally, these models assist you in whole-person health care by giving you the ability to incorporate the patient's values and experiences into your clinical decision making, often through the use of patient-based outcome measures. Patient-oriented outcomes are patient-based outcomes that are able to capture the patient's values and experiences and will be discussed in great detail in the next chapters. Finally, these models provide consistent terminology that you and other health care professionals can utilize when collecting, synthesizing, and disseminating POE and also when communicating across professions.

Van Lunen BL, Hankemeier DA, Welch CE.
Evidence-Guided Practice: A Framework for Clinical Decision Making in Athletic Training (pp 193-201).

The Evolution of Disablement Models

Disablement refers to the impact of a health condition on your patient's body, as well as their ability to participate in meaningful activities and to perform their desired roles in society. Disablement models are frameworks that are used to help describe the relationship between your patient's health condition and the consequences of the health condition. In addition, these frameworks allow you to examine the influence that other factors, such as societal and environmental factors, have on your patient's health condition. The disablement models that are currently used in clinical practice and outcomes research are multidimensional and have numerous interactions amongst the concepts to properly identify your patient's disablement and provide a framework for treatment. However, there were previous perspectives of disablement, such as the medical and social perspectives, that did not allow for whole-person health care. For you to better understand and appreciate the current biopsychosocial perspectives, such as the Nagi disablement model and the World Health Organization's (WHO's) International Classification of Functioning, Disability and Health (ICF) model, it is important for you to understand the medical and social perspectives of disablement.

Medical Perspective

The **medical perspective** of disability views the patient's disability as a problem specific to the patient, caused by their health condition or injury. The health care professional then treats the health condition or injury with the hope of curing the injury, thus improving the patient's disability. For example, let us envision a college student who sustained an injury to his right knee while working and has to use crutches when ambulating. The elevator in the building where one of his classes is held is unavailable due to maintenance; therefore, the student reports that he is unable to get to his class on the third floor. Under the medical model, the health care professional would focus on the knee injury and continue to treat the knee injury rather than attempt to modify the patient's environment. The problem is attributed to the individual and not to the environment, which in this case is the lack of an elevator to get to class. Under the medical perspective, once the patient is off of the crutches or his injury is cured, he will be able to get to his class, thus improving his disability. As you are able to interpret, the medical perspective primarily focuses on returning the patient to his or her normal state of health. What this traditional perspective does not allow for is the interaction of other factors associated with the injury, such as societal factors. In addition, the medical perspective allows for very little interaction between you and your patient and does not allow you to take into account the patient's experiences and values during their treatment because the focus is on the injury and not the entire person.

Social Perspective

The **social perspective** of disability views society and/or the patient's environment as the creator of the person's disability. This perspective primarily focuses on what the environment or society does to promote or create your patient's disability. Therefore, for your patient to overcome his or her disability, the environment and society must adapt to create accessibility for your patient. For example, let us revisit the college student who sustained a knee injury while working. Recall that this student is on crutches and unable to get to his class on the third floor of the building. When applying the social perspective to this patient, the health care professional would realize the impact that the environment (ie, a building with unavailable elevators) is having on the student's injury, resulting in his inability to fulfill important roles, like being a student. In this example, the health care professional may recommend the student contacts the professor and asks that the class session be videotaped so the student could view the materials covered in class rather than miss the information entirely. A limitation of this model is that it does not allow for the interaction of the disease (knee injury), impairments (decreased knee flexion), limitations (unable to walk), and societal and personal factors (student, employee, etc), as this model focuses on societal limitations and remediating the situation based on the current abilities of the person.

Biopsychosocial Perspectives

The **biopsychosocial perspectives** are a combination of the medical and social perspectives. Biopsychosocial perspectives allow you to examine the influence of the health condition or injury on physical limitations or impairments, as well as environmental factors and social factors. This perspective is grounded in the theory that it is the interaction of the health condition or injury, limitations, impairments, and environmental and social factors that result in disablement. Therefore, the different models formed using this perspective allow you to develop all-encompassing treatment choices and provide a whole-person approach to health care. In addition, this perspective takes into consideration the patient's values and beliefs through the use of patient-reported outcomes when assessing limitations and restrictions, which are also imperative for whole-person health care and POE. For example, let us envision a senior collegiate soccer athlete who sustains a severe ankle injury near the end of the season. During your evaluation, you determine that the patient has limited and painful dorsiflexion range of motion and is unable to run and kick a soccer ball; therefore, she is unable to participate in soccer practices or games. The patient reports a history of ankle sprains and understands the playing time that will be missed. However, the injury has occurred so late in the season that it appears she will miss the final 2 games. The biopsychosocial perspective not only addresses the ankle sprain but also allows you to further understand the influences of the environment and social factors on the person's health status. For our patient, the impairment is limited dorsiflexion range of motion, but the environmental and social factors that may affect her recovery are you, the athletic trainer, her medical history, her role on the soccer team, and her teammates and coaches. From there, you are able to identify the interactions of the limited dorsiflexion range of motion and societal and environmental factors, such as her medical history, her role on the team, her coach's influence, and the effects these have on your patient's ability to participate in soccer-related activities. In addition, the models that utilize this perspective provide you with a framework in which you are able to measure levels of impairment, activity limitations, and participation restrictions through clinician- and patient-reported outcomes.

To better understand the components of each of the models that utilize the biopsychosocial perspective, each component will be described from the origin, organ, person, and societal levels, which are overarching, broad categories in which the various model components can be grouped. The **origin level** is where you determine the pathology or health condition. For this level, you would use diagnostic tests to confirm the pathology or health condition. In the case of the soccer athlete with the ankle sprain, the ankle sprain is the pathology or the health condition. The **organ level** is where you determine the impairment. In the case of the soccer athlete with the ankle sprain, the loss of dorsiflexion range of motion is the impairment at the organ level. For this level, you would use clinician-based outcome measures to assess the level of impairment, such as the weight bearing lung test or range of motion measures with a goniometer. The **person level** is where you assess the patient's ability to participate in meaningful activities. In the case of the soccer patient, she is unable to kick a soccer ball. For this domain, you would use patient-reported outcome measures, such as the Foot and Ankle Ability Measure (FAAM), and clinician-based outcomes, such as a timed T-test, to assess the extent of the impact of the patient's health condition on the ability to participate in meaningful activities. Finally, the **societal level** is where you can assess the patient's ability to fulfill their desired role in society. For the soccer patient, she is unable to participate in soccer practice and games. Like with the person level, the societal level is evaluated through the use of patient-reported outcome measures to assess the extent of the impact of the patient's health condition on the ability to fulfill his/her role in society. Some models have domains that do not fall within the categories of origin, organ, person, or societal levels. For these

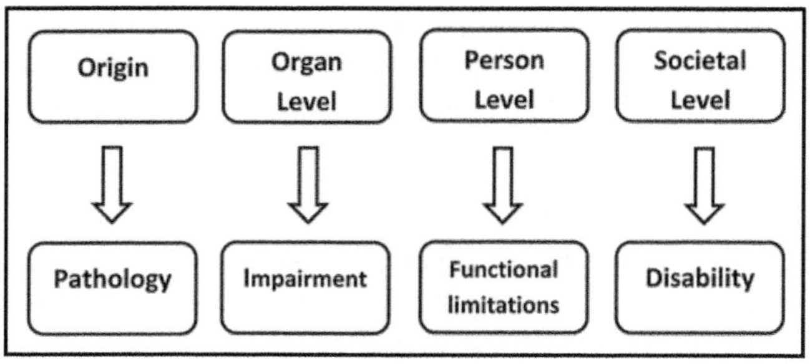

Figure 15-1. Disablement model components: Nagi disablement model.

domains, such as environmental or social factors, you may be able to use patient-reported outcomes to measure health-related quality of life in addition to continued conversation with your patient and a thorough understanding of the patient's medical history. The next sections present 2 disablement models that utilize the biopsychosocial perspective: the Nagi disablement model, which was the first disablement model that utilized this biopsychosocial perspective and laid the foundation for subsequent models, and the ICF model. Numerous models utilize this perspective; however, we have chosen 2 to present that are currently utilized in health care.

Nagi Disablement Model

The **Nagi disablement model** is a disablement model that describes the interaction between a health condition and your patient's environment. The Nagi model consists of 4 domains: active pathology, impairment, functional limitation, and disability (Figure 15-1). To best illustrate the concepts of the Nagi model, let us go back to the previous example of the collegiate soccer player who sustained an ankle sprain that has limited her ability to kick a soccer ball and participate in soccer practices and games. In addition, let us assume that this patient is the team captain and rarely misses practices or games.

The Nagi model begins with **active pathology** at the origin level, which is defined as the disruption of normal cellular processes and the simultaneous homeostatic efforts of the organism to regain a normal state. For our patient example, the active pathology at the origin level is a tear of the anterior talofibular ligament (ATFL). To determine the active pathology in this case, you would use clinical tests, such as the Anterior Drawer, possibly a standard radiograph to rule out a fracture, and possibly magnetic resonance imaging to confirm diagnosis (Figure 15-2).

The next domain in the Nagi model is **impairment**, or a loss or abnormality at the tissue, organ, and body system level. For our patient, the impairment associated with a partial tear of the ATFL could be decreased dorsiflexion range of motion. To determine the level of impairment, you may use clinician-based assessment tools, such as the weight-bearing lunge test to measure dorsiflexion (see Figure 15-2).

At the person level, **functional limitations** are restrictions in the patient's performance specifically related to the patient's ability to complete their activities of daily living and other meaningful activities to them. Functional limitations for our patient are her inability to kick a ball and run. To determine the extent of functional limitations, you may use patient-based outcomes (eg, patient-reported outcome measures) or clinician-based outcomes. An example of these for our patient would be the FAAM-Sport and Timed T-test (Figure 15-3).

Finally, at the societal level, Nagi defines **disability** as the inability of your patient to fulfill her necessary, desired, or expected social or personal roles. Disability for our patient would be her inability to play in the upcoming soccer game or participate in soccer practice. Since she is a captain, she may feel as if she is letting her teammates down, thus impacting her overall well-being. Nagi did not intend for functional limitations to be the direct result of impairments; the model was designed for functional limitations to be distinct from impairments at the organ or body systems

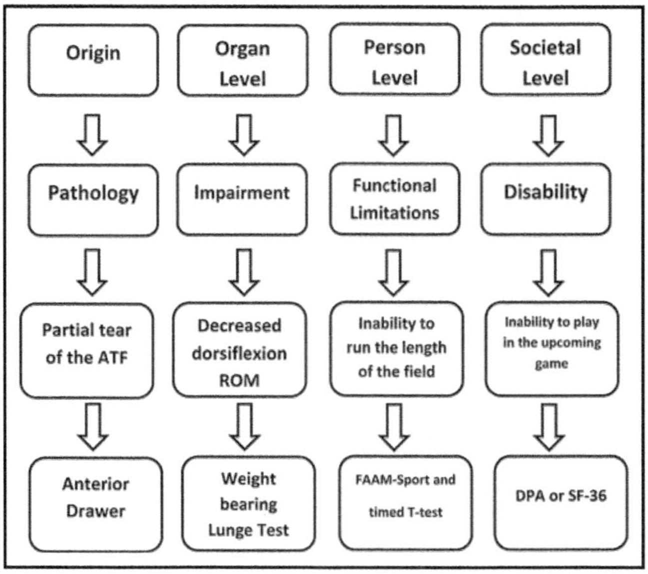

Figure 15-2. Example using the Nagi disablement model. Abbreviations: ATF, anterior talofibular; DPA, Disablement in the Physically Active; FAAM, Foot and Ankle Ability Measure; ROM, range of motion; SF-36, Short Form 36.

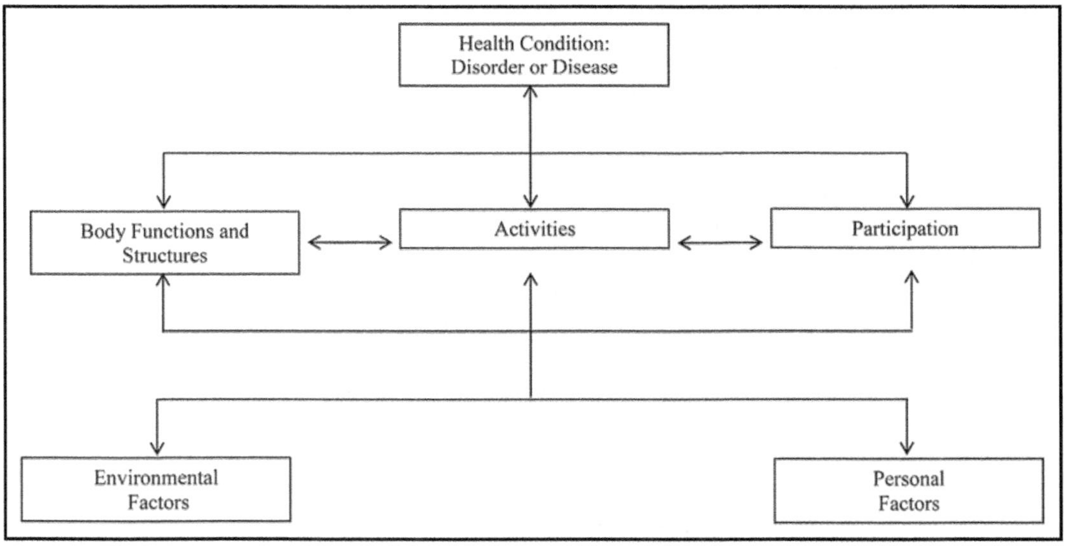

Figure 15-3. The International Classification of Functioning, Disability and Health (ICF) model: interaction between ICF components. (Reprinted with permission from World Health Organization. *How to Use the ICF: A Practical Manual for Using the International Classification of Functioning, Disability and Health [ICF].* http://www.who.int/classifications/drafticfpracticalmanual2.pdf?ua=1. Accessed July 7, 2014.)

level. This means that the patient could exhibit other functional limitations, which are not necessarily associated with the impairment but are limiting the patient from participating in activities.

The Nagi model was the first to define key concepts of disability in a disablement model utilizing the biopsychosocial perspective. This model provided the framework that influenced other models of disablement, such as the WHO's ICF model.

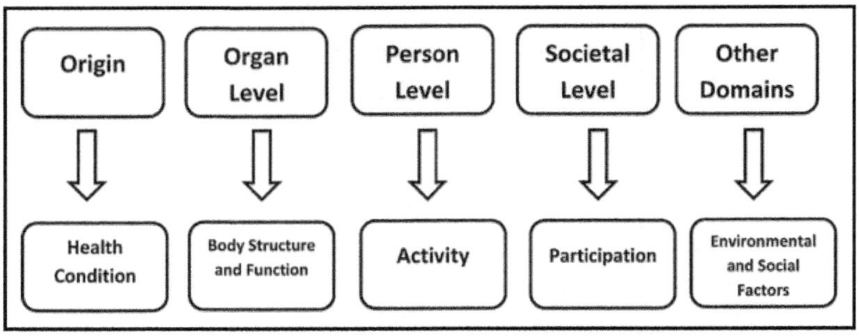

Figure 15-4. Disablement model domains: International Classification of Functioning, Disability and Health.

The World Health Organization's International Classification of Functioning, Disability and Health

The WHO's **International Classification of Functioning, Disability and Health (ICF)** model was designed to depict decreases in function on 3 health domains (body function and structure, activity, and participation) as the result of a dynamic interaction between the health condition and environmental and personal factors (see Figure 15-3). Furthermore, this model has been said to represent disability in a positive fashion: describing the patient's ability to function as opposed to the patient's disability.

To best illustrate the concepts of the ICF model, let us go back to the female collegiate soccer player that we used as an earlier example. The ICF model begins with a **health condition** at the origin level, which is a global term used to represent a disease or injury. In the case of the soccer player, the health condition is the ankle sprain, specifically, an injury to the ATFL.

The ICF model then has 3 health domains of function: body function and structure, activity, and participation (Figure 15-4). At the organ level, **body function** refers to the physiological functions of the body systems, whereas **body structure** refers to the anatomical parts of the body. Therefore, impairment in body function or structure is a decrease in, problem with, or deviation from the norm. Similar to the Nagi model, you would use clinician-based outcomes to assess the level of impairment. For our patient with the ankle sprain, an example of impairment to the body function and structure domain would be decreased dorsiflexion range of motion, and this could be assessed using the weight bearing lunge test (Figure 15-5).

Activity and participation are the other 2 health domains of function that can be affected by the health condition (see Figure 15-4). At the person level, **activity** is described as the execution of a specific task or action by an individual, with no social involvement. For example, an activity for a soccer athlete would be kicking a ball. If the patient was participating in a team drill to kick a ball, this would be considered a social involvement (see Figure 15-4). A health condition that affects a patient's ability to execute a task or action is said to result in **activity limitation**. An activity limitation for our patient would be the inability of the patient to kick a ball (see Figure 15-5). Please keep in mind that an activity limitation for a patient who participates in another sport, such as basketball, may be different. An activity limitation for a basketball player would be the inability of the player to execute a layup during an individual drill.

At the societal level, **participation** is described as involvement in life situations. For example, participation for a soccer athlete would be kicking the ball during a team drill or in a game (see Figure 15-5). When a patient is unable to participate in life situations, they are said to have **participation restriction**. An example of participation restrictions related to our patient would be her inability to compete in the soccer game or practice. To assess activity limitations and participation restrictions, you can use patient- and clinician-based outcomes. For the example of our patient

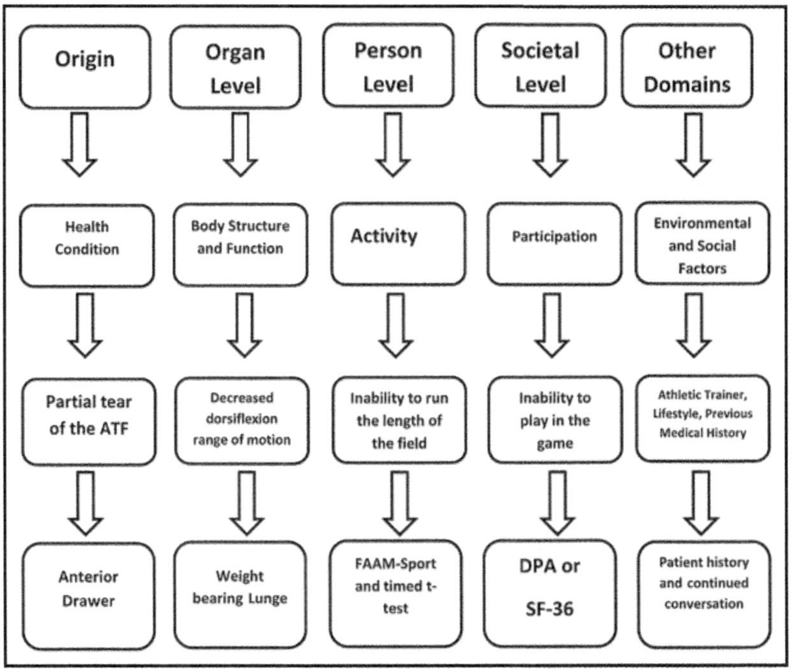

Figure 15-5. Example using the International Classification of Functioning, Disability and Health. Abbreviations: ATF, anterior talofibular ligament; DPA, Disablement in the Physically Active; FAAM, Foot and Ankle Ability Measure; SF-36, Short Form 36.

with the ankle sprain, we may use the FAAM-Sport and a Timed T-test (see Figure 15-5). Keep in mind that a participation restriction for a patient who participates in another sport, such as basketball, may be different. For example, a participation restriction for the basketball player may be the inability to participate in the upcoming basketball game.

To further make the ICF model a unique model of disablement, there are 2 additional contextual factors, or health-related domains: environmental factors and personal factors (see Figures 15-3 and 15-4). **Environmental factors** are the physical, social, and attitudinal environments in which the patient lives and conducts their life. The subdomains of environmental factors include alterations to the environment, technology, support and relationships, attitudes, and public services and policies. Our patient with the ankle sprain may view you, the AT providing treatment, as an environmental factor that may influence activity limitations and participation restrictions through patient care. For our example, let us say you have been with the women's soccer team for 4 years and have previously treated the patient. The patient may view you as a part of their support system given your previous relationship and experiences together. This relationship would be a positive factor related to the patient's health care.

Personal factors are defined as the background of the patient's life, which are composed of features of the patient that are not specific to the health condition. Personal factors include sex, race, age, prior health conditions, fitness, lifestyle, habits, upbringing, coping styles, social background, and past and current experiences. For our patient with the ankle sprain, a personal factor that may influence her health condition is her history of ankle sprain. Since the patient has a history of ankle sprain, she may be able to cope better with her current situation as she understands the injury process and the rehabilitation that must occur for her to return to participation (see Figure 15-5). However, this personal factor may negatively influence her health condition. For example, let us envision that this patient's previous ankle injury recovery period took much longer than expected. Because of this extra-long recovery period, the patient became quite agitated and irritated because she missed so many practices and games. Therefore, when this current injury occurred, she may not be able to cope as well as she did not enjoy the length of time it took to get back to activity following her last injury.

The ICF model (see Figure 15-3) is a dynamic disablement model that represents a health condition across multiple domains of function, which is contextually dependent in nature. While it is logical that activity and participation may improve once the impairment is addressed, this model views these as 3 separate domains that need to be individually assessed. Because the ICF model outlines multiple contextual factors, activity limitations and participation restrictions may persist as the result of other factors beyond impairment. Through constant interaction and influence of environmental and personal factors, you are able to use the model for not only patient evaluation and treatment, but also to enhance patient-centered care and overall patient outcomes following injury.

Summary

A standardized language across all disciplines will ensure effective communication when treating our patients. More importantly, these models provide the framework for you to enhance patient-centered care, a central piece to EBP, as they provide the framework necessary for the collection of POE. Patient-oriented evidence is vitally important to the EBP process, as it incorporates the patient's values and experiences into their treatment and final outcome. In addition, you and other clinicians can use disablement models to provide a framework for treating patients in your clinical practice. These frameworks assist you in evaluating each individual health and health-related domains and ensure you capture not only clinician-oriented outcomes but also patient-oriented outcomes through the use of patient-reported outcomes. The use of patient- and clinician-based outcomes throughout the treatment process ensures you are treating the whole person and providing patient-centered health care. Finally, disablement models allow for a common language across health care disciplines, which is essential in promoting interprofessional health care for the care of our patients.

Key Points

- Disablement models assist you in whole-person health care by providing you the ability to incorporate the patient's values and experiences into your clinical decision making, often through the use of patient-based outcome measures.
- The Nagi model was the first to define key concepts of disability in a disablement model utilizing the biopsychosocial perspective.
- The ICF model has been said to represent disability in a positive fashion; it describes the patient's ability to function as opposed to the patient's disability.
- A participation restriction for a patient that participates in another sport, outside of the sport specified for the disablement model, may be different.
- The ICF model is a dynamic disablement model that represents a health condition across multiple domains of function, which is contextually dependent in nature. While it is logical that activity and participation may improve once the impairment is addressed, this model views these as 3 separate domains that need to be individually assessed.
- These models provide the framework for you to enhance patient-centered care, a central piece to EBP, as they provide the framework necessary for the collection of POE.

- The use of patient- and clinician-based outcomes throughout the treatment process ensures you are treating the whole person and are providing patient-centered health care.
- Disablement models allow for a common language across health care disciplines, which is essential in promoting interprofessional health care for the care of our patients.

Bibliography

Clancy CM, Eisenberg JM. Outcomes research: measuring the end results of health care. *Science.* 1998;282(5387):245-246.

Engel GL. The need for a new medical model: a challenge for biomedicine. *Science.* 1977;196(4286):129-136.

Jette AM. Outcomes research in physical therapy. *Phys Ther.* 1995;75(11):965-970.

Jette AM. Physical disablement concepts for physical therapy research and practice. *Phys Ther.* 1994;74(5):380-386.

Jette AM. The changing language of disablement. *Phys Ther.* 2005;85(2):118-119.

Jette AM. Toward a common language for function, disability, and health. *Phys Ther.* 2006;86(5):726-734.

Jette AM. Toward a common languate of disablement. *J Gerontol A Biol Sci Med Sci.* 2009;64(11):1165-1168.

Masala C, Petretto DR. From disablement to enablement: conceptual models of disability in the 20th century. *Disabil Rehabil.* 2008;30(17):1233-1244.

McKeon PO, Medina McKeon JM, Mattacola CG, Lattermann C. Finding context: a new model for interpreting clinical evidence. *Int J Athl Ther Train.* 2011;16(5):10-13.

Parsons JT, Valovich McLeod TC, Snyder AR, Sauers EL. Change is hard: adopting a disablement model for athletc training. *J Athl Train.* 2008;43(4):446-448.

Sackett DL, Rosenberg WM, Gray JA, Haynes RB, Richardson WS. Evidenced based medicine: what it is and what it isn't. *BMJ.* 1996;312(7023):71-72.

Snyder AR, Parsons JT, Valovich McLeod TC, Bay R, Michener L, Sauers EL. Using disablement models and clinical outcomes assessment to enable evidence-based athletic training practice, part I: disablment models. *J Athl Train.* 2008;43(4):428-436.

Stucki G, Cieza A, Melvin J. The International Classification of Functioning, Disability and Health: a unifying model for the conceptual description of the rehabilutation strategy. *J Rehabil Med.* 2007;39(4):279-285.

Valovich McLeod TC, Snyder AR, Parsons JT, Curtis Bay R, Michener LA, Sauers EL. Using disablement models and clinical outcomes assessment to enable evidence-based athletic training practice, part II: clinical outcomes assessment. *J Athl Train.* 2008;43(4):437-445.

Verbrugge LM, Jette AM. The disablement process. *Soc Sci Med.* 1994;38(1):1-14.

Whiteneck G. Conceptual models of disability: past, present, and future. In: Field MK, Jette AM, Martin L, eds. *Workshop on Disability in America: A New Look.* Washington, DC: National Academics Press; 2006:50-66.

World Health Organization. Towards a Common Language for Functioning, Disability, and Health: ICF. Geneva, Switzerland: World Health Organization; 2002.

16

Patient-Oriented Outcomes Assessments

Health care outcomes have been defined as the end results of health care services that consider unique patient experiences and values. The evaluation of health care outcomes and the emphasis on patient-oriented outcomes is not new. Health care outcomes assessment started in the 1900s by Ernest Codman, a surgeon who was instrumental in evaluating the end results of health care services for the purpose of quality improvement. Dr. Codman believed that patients should be followed over time to determine whether the treatment received had been successful. Living was frequently the indicator of a successful outcome, and an unsuccessful outcome was indicated by death. Additionally, Dr. Codman made his outcomes public so that potential patients could determine the quality of his care. Ultimately, he worked to find ways to prevent poor health care outcomes. Dr. Codman was influential in terms of bringing attention toward quality improvement as well as the value of assessing health care outcomes. In addition to the efforts of Dr. Codman to encourage a health care system that valued outcomes, other events within health care influenced interest in this area.

One influencing factor was the advancement of health care. As health care advanced, the costs of health care services grew at a much higher rate than the rest of the economy. Treatments and services grew in number and the costs of care kept rising, but there was little understanding about the outcomes of different treatment options. The changing health care environment sparked the era of assessment and accountability in which there was a need to know more about costs, safety, and effectiveness of medical services. Outcomes related to patients (eg, **health-related quality of life [HRQOL]**, reinjury rate, patient satisfaction), providers (eg, treatment effectiveness, provider satisfaction), and service (eg, referral rates, reimbursement patterns) were all important. Assessment of quality once looked quite different than it does now. For example, a traditional approach to quality emphasized professional judgment and technical quality. Quality care, from this approach, was validated by ensuring quality decision making and high performance in delivering the treatment. Emphasis on professional judgment and skill tended to position the value of quality more from the perspective of the clinician than from the patient. At the time, this approach was reasonable because of the limited knowledge attributed to patients and the difficulty in measuring the patient

Van Lunen BL, Hankemeier DA, Welch CE.
Evidence-Guided Practice: A Framework for Clinical Decision Making in Athletic Training (pp 203-226).

perspective of health status in an accurate way. However, this traditional approach to quality was limited because a clinician-based focus tends to emphasize measures, such as strength, changes in radiographs, range of motion, and laxity as opposed to what really matters to the patient (eg, getting back to sport, ability to dress, fulfilling life roles). Furthermore, clinician-based measures are typically not the primary reason that patients seek care. When evaluating quality, other perspectives matter. Slowly, with the evolution of health care, the value of the patient's perspective has increased. Patient opinions of care have become indicators of quality, and the general sense that care should respond to patient values and preferences has been accepted. Furthermore, patients are changing in that they have become consumers of health care services and want to know more about the treatment options available to them and subsequent outcomes for those treatments as they pertain to them personally. Today, we are also better at capturing patient perspectives than we were before because of improved methodologies. Improved ability to measure patient perspective assists in making the patient an integral component in the care process. These historical perspectives are important because they have contributed to the path to where we are in health care today.

Over the past several years, there have been numerous calls for clinicians from all health care backgrounds to deliver care in a patient-centered manner. **Patient-centered care** can be described as care that respects differences in patients and appreciates their uniqueness. Respecting the unique values and needs of patients is important because what matters most to one patient may be different from what matters most to another patient, even if they have the same health condition. A patient-centered approach to care has been presented as the ideal way to practice because this approach should lead to better patient outcomes, create more compliant patients, integrate patients into the care process, and assist in establishing a therapeutic partnership between clinician and patient. The value of patient-centered care to health care in general is illustrated by the introduction of the **Patient-Centered Outcomes Research Institute (PCORI)**, which was created by the government through the 2010 Patient Protection and Affordable Care Act for the purpose of providing patients with information to make better decisions about their health and to improve the outcomes of health care services. Patient-Centered Outcomes Research Institute's efforts center around funding patient-centered outcomes research and assisting in disseminating findings from these studies to the broader health care community, which includes patients and clinicians. An essential perspective to all of their work is that patients are unique; therefore, one option in health care may not fit all patients the same. More information about PCORI and its emphasis on patients' unique needs can be found on their website (http://www.pcori.org). As health care continues to evolve, the inclusion of the patient into the health care process will remain a priority.

To practice in a patient-centered manner requires that there is an avenue for gathering the patient perspective in a systematic and objective way. The idea of patient-centered care aligns well with the definition of evidence-based practice, which includes patient values and circumstances as essential ingredients to successful practice. Moreover, it has been suggested that integration of unique values and circumstances into the clinical decision-making process is necessary to best serve the patient. The challenge, when considering a more traditional delivery of patient care, is identifying a method to gather that unique patient information systematically and objectively. As athletic trainers, we do a great job of knowing our patients, taking histories, and listening to our patients. Asking these questions and collecting this information helps us create a relationship, or therapeutic partnership, with our patients, which is an essential component of patient-centered care. However, loosely gathering information through general conversation does not produce a reliable mechanism by which we can identify improvements or decrements in health. For example, if you ask a patient how he/she is doing, responses might include "feeling pretty good," or "little pain, but better than yesterday," or "great." Verbal responses are helpful in getting a general sense of how a patient perceives his/her health, but they do not provide a metric from which to determine whether subsequent responses (eg, in the days following the previous report) indicate improvement, no change, or deterioration in health. Therefore, we must use a system that allows for an evaluation of health from the patient's perspective in a meaningful and measurable way.

A revisit of the disablement model helps remind us that patients can be viewed from a variety of different perspectives, from the health condition all the way to the resulting social and role changes that occur as a result of the health condition. This spectrum highlights the role of patient outcomes in the care process. Let us consider a high school soccer player who has an anterior cruciate ligament (ACL) injury and will soon be undergoing reconstructive surgery, with the hopes of returning to competitive athletics at some point. According to disablement models, we should be able to view our patient from any of the domains within the model. For example, our typical evaluation of impairments may lead us to measure changes in swelling, strength, and range of motion with our various clinician-based tools, such as a tape measure, manual muscle testing, and goniometer. Attention toward functional limitations would provide opportunity to measure improvements in walking, ascending and descending stairs, and getting up from a seated position. Finally, a view from the perspective of disability would allow us to look at things such as role functioning (eg, being a soccer athlete, friend, or student) and overall quality of life. Function can be measured with functional assessments, but you can also evaluate function through the perspective of the patient. We are quite good at evaluating the impairments and functional limitations within disablement, but we are less accustomed to evaluating disability. Recall that **disability** refers to a person's ability to fulfill necessary, desired, or expected roles in society. Measuring patient perspective is essential when evaluating disability since disability occurs as a result of change in the relation between the patient and his/her environment and measures what is important to the patient. Thus, if you do not use tools to get at the patient perspective, you likely limit your ability, and perhaps your opportunity, to evaluate disability and provide patient-centered care.

Clinical Outcomes Assessment

Most basically, **health care outcomes** are meaningful results following an episode or period of intervention and can be related to the patient, clinician (or provider), and service provided. While provider and service outcomes are important, the primary focus of this chapter is on patient outcomes. When considering patient outcomes, some have refined the basic definition of health care outcomes to indicate the end result of care that also considers patient experiences, preferences, and values. Like the definitions of EBP and patient-centered care, health care outcomes also highlight the central role of the patient. Health care outcomes can be classified as clinician or patient based. **Clinician-based outcomes** are outcomes that are rated by, and of most value to, the clinician. If we consider the International Classification of Functioning, Disability, and Health disablement model, clinician-based outcomes are typically related to body structures and functions (ie, impairments) and include common measurements, such as joint range of motion, muscular strength, and joint or limb swelling. While clinician-based outcomes provide valuable information to clinicians about the state of tissue healing, they typically do not address the health domains that are of most interest to the patient. For example, a patient is more likely to seek help based on the inability to complete an activity of importance to him/her, such as kicking a soccer ball, throwing a baseball, or reaching for objects overhead, than based on a loss of some joint range of motion or strength. Patients think more in terms of the activity or participation restriction they are experiencing as opposed to the impairment that may be contributing to the problem. As a result, clinician-based outcomes generally produce **disease-oriented evidence**, which is more related to the pathology and mechanisms of disease development and progression than to what matters most to patients. When considering a patient-centered approach to care, clinician-based measures may be viewed as less valuable to the care process because of their lack of attention toward what is important to patients.

In contrast, patient-based outcomes, also commonly referred to as **patient-rated outcomes (PRO)** instruments, are surveys or questionnaires that a patient completes about his/her health status. Patient-based outcomes, when compared with clinician-based outcomes, are most valuable to the patient and include measures such as mortality and morbidity, HRQOL, function, satisfaction, and cost. Additionally, patient-based outcomes result in patient-oriented evidence that matters and, as a result, produce the type of evidence that is needed for EBP and has the strongest ability to change clinical practice. Considering the International Classification of Functioning, Disability, and Health disablement model, patient-based outcomes are categorized in the health and health-related domains of activities and participation (eg, kicking a soccer ball, throwing a baseball, being a soccer player, and being a friend). With a focus on patient-based outcomes, it is possible to create goals related to function and HRQOL, evaluate treatment effectiveness, and direct care toward areas of disablement that matter to patients. It could be argued that if you do not include patient-based outcomes into the care process, you never really offer yourself the chance to care for a patient across all disablement model domains. Furthermore, without using a PRO instrument, it is difficult to gather the patient perspective in a meaningful, systematic way, which makes it more challenging to include them as part of the care process. Patient-based outcomes are the clinical outcomes or endpoints that, as a clinician, you should be most interested in because they highlight the end goals that you will be focusing your treatment and intervention toward achieving. A criticism of PRO instruments is that they gather subjective information, or information based on a person's opinions or emotions, which can be biased. Because the information is subjective in nature, some people have considered PRO instruments as less trustworthy than other, more objective methods of measurement. While PRO instruments gather information from patients that is reflective of their opinions, these instruments can be thought of as objective if measurement properties, such as reliability, validity, and responsiveness, have been established.

Patient-rated outcome measures are generally categorized according to their applicability (ie, generic or specific) and their length (ie, single- or multi-item). **Generic outcome measures** are global in scope and applicable to a wide range of people, including healthy, injured, or ill populations. Some examples of generic PRO instruments are the Short Form (SF) family of instruments (eg, SF-12 and SF-36), the Pediatric Quality of Life Inventory (PedsQL), and the Disablement in the Physically Active (DPA) Scale. The questions in generic instruments tend to be broad in nature and, together, all of the questions cover several domains of health. An example of a generic measure question comes from the SF-12 and reads, "In general, would you say your health is: excellent, very good, good, fair, or poor?" Another example reads, "Have you felt calm and peaceful?" Using a generic PRO instrument allows for a global assessment of health status and may provide insight into areas impacted by an event, such as an injury or illness that is unanticipated. One benefit of generic measures is that they can be used to compare health status across patients who have different conditions (eg, musculoskeletal injury vs concussive injury), which could help in better understanding the different, yet important, impacts of particular conditions on health. A disadvantage of generic measures is that because they are broad in scope, they are not highly relevant to any one illness or health condition. As a result, generic measures have fewer relevant items to any one illness or health condition and, thus, may respond less to changes that result from specific treatment and interventions.

In contrast to generic PRO instruments, **specific outcome** measures are narrower in scope and typically relate to specific body regions, diseases, or injuries. Specific PRO instruments can also relate to psychological conditions, such as depression, kinesiophobia, and fear avoidance. For example, the **Foot and Ankle Ability Measure (FAAM)** is a specific PRO instrument targeted toward individuals who have foot and ankle conditions. The FAAM would not be a good fit for those who have a knee injury because the questions within the instrument are specific to people with foot and ankle issues. Another example is the **Lower Extremity Functional Scale (LEFS)**, which is a specific scale that primarily addresses functional issues in people with injuries to the lower extremity. It is important to remember that because the questions in specific PRO instruments are narrowly focused to a particular condition, injury/illness, or body region, they do not apply to all people and are relevant only to those people who fit the focus of the instrument. Additionally, because specific instruments are built for a particular condition, they should

Overall since your first athletic training visit, has there been any change in your injury status?

Please check only one answer.

___ A very great deal better
___ A great deal better
___ A good deal better
___ Moderately better
___ Somewhat better
___ A little better
___ About the same, no change
___ A little worse
___ Somewhat worse
___ Moderately worse
___ A good deal worse
___ A great deal worse
___ A very great deal worse

Figure 16-1. Global Rating of Change.

include questions that are expected to change as a result of improvements or decrements in health. For example, the **International Knee Documentation Committee Knee Form (IKDC)**, a knee-specific instrument, asks patients to identify the highest level of activity that can be performed without significant swelling in the knee. Additionally, questions on the IKDC ask patients to rate the level of impact the injured knee has on their difficulty in performing tasks, such as going up and down stairs, squatting, and rising from a chair. All of these questions would be important to people who have knee injuries. Furthermore, as a patient with a knee injury recovers, their amount of swelling with activity should decrease, and their difficulty with tasks, such as ascending and descending stairs, squatting, and rising from a chair, should decrease. The relevance of the questions to the condition of interest makes a specific instrument better able to detect small, but important, changes over time when compared with a generic instrument. We call this ability to capture small and meaningful change **instrument responsiveness**. The concept of instrument responsiveness is important to understand when considering PRO instruments. A useful PRO instrument must be responsive to change; if it is not, it will not capture changes in health status as a result of improved, deteriorated, or unchanged health status.

In addition to a PRO instrument being generic or specific, another characteristic that differentiates PROs is instrument length. Some PRO instruments are composed of a single item, such as the Global Rating of Change, which is a single question that asks a person to rate how much change he/she has experienced since some previous point in time (eg, the initial visit; Figure 16-1). Other PROs are composed of many questions, such as the FAAM or the LEFS, and provide a more comprehensive evaluation of a health construct or constructs. **Single-item PROs** are appealing because of their ease of use. In general, single-item PRO instruments are quick to score, quick to complete, and require no training for use, which is a benefit when considering their implementation into patient care in busy athletic training facilities.

While there are many benefits to single-item PROs, they are not without limitations. Perhaps the biggest drawback of single-item outcome measures is that you gain only a little information from a single question, limiting the richness of the information obtained. One question also creates a narrow focus and does not allow for the evaluation of more complex health constructs, such as HRQOL. What matters most to patient can change, and these global questions do not give us much more insight into health status other than a perceived positive or negative change or neutral perception of health from one time point to another. Even given these limitations, the single-item outcome measures should be considered when implementing routine assessment of PROs in clinical practice because these outcomes are quick and easy to use and provide some guidance on aspects of health important to patients. The GROC is a single-item outcome measure that evaluates a patient's perceived change in one point in time (eg, therapy discharge) to another (eg, initial therapy visit). Other single-item PRO instruments are related to constructs, such as pain, satisfaction, function, and disability.

Multi-item PRO instruments capitalize on the limitations of single-item measures by asking patients several questions about various aspects of their health and providing a more comprehensive assessment of the construct(s) of interest. Because multi-item measures consist of many questions, it is possible to gather information on more than one disablement domain (eg, activity and participation) and potentially even the construct of HRQOL. The comprehensiveness of multi-item measures can provide a better understanding of the impact of an injury or illness on a patient's life. Studies have reported differing impacts of sport-related injuries on athlete quality of life based on the type of injury. For example, athletes who have sustained concussions tend to report a bigger impact on mental health than athletes who have sustained musculoskeletal injuries. Like single-item measures, multi-item measures are not without limitations. More time is needed to complete and score multi-item measures when compared with single-item measures, and this may translate to a larger burden to the patient and the clinician. However, there are multi-item PRO instruments that consist of relatively few questions, and those could be considered when administration of the measures is in busy athletic training rooms. Additionally, the clinician should consider the balance between the purpose of using the instrument with the quantity of information desired and the time burden associated with completing and scoring the instrument. In general, the value of a multi-item PRO instrument outweighs the time it takes to put the measure into practice. Additionally, the quality and quantity of information gathered from multi-item PRO instruments makes them desirable when measuring patient outcomes over time.

Now that we have the basic information about clinical outcomes assessments, it is important to take a closer look at 2 commonly reported patient outcomes as well as provide some examples of PRO instruments used in athlete health care. The next sections of this chapter focus on a basic introduction to HRQOL and patient satisfaction, which are 2 common patient outcomes. Following these introductory sections, a variety of examples of PRO instruments will be presented, which will be categorized as generic, specific, single-item, and multi-item. While it is beyond the scope of this chapter to introduce you to all available PRO instruments, these examples should give you a starting point as you begin to implement them into your clinical practice. Additionally, it may be helpful to review the development articles about these PRO instruments prior to using them to ensure that you follow any usage guidelines (eg, license fees) established by the instrument developers.

Health-Related Quality of Life

The evaluation of HRQOL has received increased attention over the years. Emphasis on HRQOL emerged through cancer and chronic disease research because these conditions had a lasting impact on patient lives as well as the lives of their families. The evaluation of HRQOL has become a standard endpoint in clinical research (eg, clinical trials) in part because many treatments do not result in a cure and some treatments are terribly unpleasant with little benefit. In addition, the value of assessing HRQOL has strengthened because there have been changes in health care, including with patients. Patients have become an increasingly important part of care. They are more interested in their treatment options, in obtaining information about the benefits and harms of particular interventions (eg, surgery vs no surgery), and also have a general desire to express their own opinions. Furthermore, patients tend to place a great emphasis on the nonclinical results of health care services, such as the impact on HRQOL. Because of this emphasis on HRQOL in health care, it is important to understand what HRQOL is and how it can be measured.

By definition, HRQOL is a multidimensional construct that includes physical, psychological, social, spiritual, and economic domains of health. Each domain of HRQOL is made up of different attributes. For example, the social domain can include the attributes of family, friendships, social interactions, and recreational activities. If we consider the psychological domain, the attributes may include emotional behaviors, happiness, stress, or depression. The number of available attributes is large, and there is no specific makeup when considering individual people. Together, these domains, as well as their attributes, are influenced by personal experiences, perceptions, and values, which makes HRQOL unique to individuals. Additionally, because HRQOL is the combination of interacting health-related dimensions and personal beliefs and experiences, it is a patient-centered construct. Recall that patient-centered care is care that respects patient differences and values individual needs and preferences. As a result, by measuring HRQOL, it is possible to generate meaningful patient-oriented evidence, or **patient-oriented evidence that matters (POEM)**, which is useful in justifying treatments, determining treatment effectiveness, and changing clinical practice. In addition to being individualized and patient-centered, HRQOL is also variable in that it can change based on many different influencing factors, such as patient experiences, the perception of others, and injuries and illnesses. Therefore, HRQOL is not static. The variability of HRQOL makes it an important variable to routinely evaluate because decreases in HRQOL may indicate the need for a review of the treatment protocol, changes in care, or referral to other health care professionals.

One of the values in measuring HRQOL is capturing the changing scores (high scores and low scores) as a result of events, such as injury. Recall that we measure HRQOL through PRO instruments, and this evaluation can be done with generic and specific measures. Generic PRO instruments are likely more comprehensive in capturing HRQOL than specific PROs because their emphasis tends to be more on global health in comparison to specific instruments. However, this may not always be the case. When you select a PRO for the purpose of measuring HRQOL, it is important to remember that the questions in the instruments dictate the domains of HRQOL captured. Not all PRO instruments measure HRQOL in its entirety. For example, a PRO focused on function, such as the LEFS, emphasizes the domain of function. Therefore, you may select the LEFS if you are interested in the function of a patient with a lower-extremity injury, but you would likely not select the LEFS if you were interested in the psychological health of this patient. Furthermore, a PRO instrument focused on one domain, such as the physical domain, may address a very narrow or very broad range of that health area. Therefore, to determine the scope of the domain, a review of all the questions within the instrument is needed. Once you have selected a PRO instrument for the purpose of measuring HRQOL, the instrument can be administered at various time points along a patient's recovery. We call the repeat administration of the PRO instrument serial administration. **Serial administration** allows you to capture the peaks and valleys in HRQOL and to adjust care accordingly. Additionally, demonstrating that you have made a positive impact on your patients, through documentation of improved HRQOL at the time of discharge may go a long way in showing your value to your patients, employers, and other health care stakeholders. That is, you have evidence to show that your care made your patient's health status better. As clinicians, we often receive positive feedback about our impact on the lives of patients from them, but we do not often objectively measure this information. An objective assessment will provide more value than anecdotal stories about your patient care.

While emphasis on HRQOL in athlete health care is relatively new, there is a body of literature available that has provided us with some helpful information regarding HRQOL and healthy and injured athletes. For example, studies have demonstrated that HRQOL differs between athletes and nonathletes, with athletes tending to report higher HRQOL than the general population. Additionally, we have learned a little about the impact of events, such as musculoskeletal and concussive injury, on athlete HRQOL. Research suggests that injury negatively impacts HRQOL, and this impact may be different depending on the type of injury experienced. For example, athletes with musculoskeletal injuries may report more deficits in the physical dimension of HRQOL than those who suffer concussive injuries. Those with concussions may feel a greater deficit in health in relation to the psychosocial domains of HRQOL. Much more study on the HRQOL of athletes as a result of injuries is needed, but these initial examples are helpful in seeing the value of the quality of life outcome.

The following example also may assist in understanding how the evaluation of HRQOL can be applied to patient care. Let us consider that you have a soccer athlete who has sustained a second-degree ankle sprain and will not be able to play soccer for the next month or more. Initially, this soccer athlete may present in fairly good spirits, even given the injury, but as time in recovery continues and time out of play increases, this soccer athlete may have a decrease in his/her health status. The impact could be measured with a PRO instrument, such as the FAAM, and areas of deficit likely would initially include physical health. With a longer time out of play, it is possible that this soccer athlete may also demonstrate a decrease in emotional or psychological health, again, which could be measured with a PRO instrument. The decrease in emotional or psychological health could result because the soccer athlete misses being in sport, does not feel like part of the team, and/or worries that the injury will not heal, which may translate to decreased mood and perhaps depression. To best measure emotional health, it may be necessary to use a generic PRO, such as the DPA scale, PedsQL, or SF-12. Again, generic PRO instruments tend to capture a broader health perspective and may include more questions related to the various domains of HRQOL, such as emotional health, than specific PROs.

As the emphasis on the patient as a central piece to the care process continues to grow, it will be increasingly important to ensure that we measure HRQOL as a standard part of patient care. A variety of generic and specific PRO instruments will be discussed later in this chapter to give you a starting point when beginning to add these assessments to your practice.

Satisfaction

Just like HRQOL, satisfaction is a valuable patient-based health care outcome to assess. Satisfaction can be examined from the perspective of the patient, clinician or provider, and the service organization (eg, hospital, clinic, secondary school). **Patient satisfaction** typically comes from 2 angles, as follows: (1) the satisfaction a patient has with the recovery of his/her injured body part, and (2) the satisfaction a patient has with the overall care experience. Clinicians may find it beneficial to know whether a patient is satisfied with the recovery of the injured body part because this information will help direct care. For example, if someone is satisfied with the progress of recovery, then it may lead a clinician to continue the course of care because the care strategy appears to be working. If, in contrast, a patient is not satisfied with the recovery of the injured body part, then the clinician may consider altering the course of care to better address the patient's needs with the hopes of improving satisfaction.

Clinicians may also be interested in how satisfied patients are with their care experience. Information related to satisfaction with care can be used to demonstrate value (eg, patients enjoy their experience with you), which is of interest to many people, including employers and new patients. Documented information about patient satisfaction with the care experience can also be great for marketing. Clinicians often feel undervalued and overworked. Objective information that is related to how satisfied patients feels after the health care they receive can go a long way in demonstrating value and worth.

Another reason that it is important to measure patient satisfaction is because satisfied patients tend to be different than unsatisfied patients. Satisfied patients may be more likely to adhere to treatments, maintain use of health care services, establish and continue relationships with clinicians, and participate in their care. Fostering an experience for patients that creates satisfaction is beneficial for positive health outcomes. Unsatisfied patients tend to make the care experience less effective because unsatisfied patients may not seek care when care is needed, and they have the potential to become noncompliant patients who do not follow their treatment prescription.

Satisfaction PRO instruments can be single- or multi-item and may be generic (related to people of various conditions) or specific (related to people with a specific injury or condition). Multi-item satisfaction outcome measures can cover multiple dimensions as well, meaning that these instruments can address different aspects of satisfaction. Often, satisfaction questionnaires will be generic in nature so that they have broad application to populations and are relevant to many types of patients. Having a satisfaction questionnaire with broad applicability allows for comparisons to be made between people with different injuries. For example, with a generic satisfaction questionnaire, it would be possible to compare the satisfaction of people who received ankle injury rehabilitation with those who received knee injury rehabilitation. These types of comparisons are valuable for quality monitoring and improvement.

Common Generic PRO Instruments

Short Form 12

The Medical Outcome Study **Short Form** family of instruments, such as the SF-12 and SF-36, are some of the most widely used generic measures of HRQOL in health care. These measures were designed for use in a wide variety of people with different conditions, injuries, and diseases. The SF-12 and the SF-36 function similarly and allow for the calculation of 8 dimensions of HRQOL and 2 composite scores that are scored with a response format ranging from 0 (poorer health) to 100 (better health). Scores on the SF-12 and the SF-36 can also be presented as normative scores, where 50 is the average score and scores higher than 50 indicate better than average health and scores less than 50 represent less than average health. The 8 subscales of the SF instruments include physical functioning, role physical, bodily pain, general health perception, vitality, social functioning, role emotional, and mental health. Composite scores are generated for physical and mental health. The primary difference between these 2 instruments is that the SF-36 has 36 questions and the SF-12 has 12 questions. In busy athletic training facilities, the shorter SF-12 may be desired to reduce patient burden. Using the short form instruments is helpful in capturing a global assessment of health, but one limitation in clinical practice is that scoring these instruments can be challenging. The company that regulates the SF instrument (Optum: http://www.optum.com/optum-outcomes.html) provides scoring software at a fee. Additionally, depending on the purpose of use (eg, research vs clinical practice), there may be associated licensing fees that permit use of the instruments.

Disablement in the Physically Active Scale

The **Disablement in the Physically Active (DPA) scale** was developed to measure disability in athletes through evaluation of 3 disablement model domains, including impairments, functional limitations, and disability. There are 16 questions on the DPA, which are rated using an adjectival response format from 1 (no problems) to 5 (severe problem), with a range of scores from 0 to 64. Higher scores are indicative of more disablement. One advantage of the DPA over some of the other available generic outcomes instruments is that it was developed specifically for an athletic population. As a result, many of the questions on the instrument relate to things that matter to athletes. For example, there are questions related to muscular function, skill performance, overall fitness, and participation in activities, which suggests that the instrument may relate more to an athletic population than some of the generic instruments not designed for athletes.

Pediatric Quality of Life Inventory

The **Pediatric Quality of Life Inventory (PedsQL)** is a generic PRO instrument tailored specifically for younger patient populations. With 23 questions in the instrument, the PedsQL can be used to evaluate physical, emotional, school, and social functioning. Additionally, a summary score can be calculated to address psychosocial health, taking into consideration scores from the emotional, social, and school functioning subscales. Questions on the PedsQL are in Likert style response format, with scores ranging from 0 to 100. Higher scores suggest better health. The PedsQL does not take long to administer, but scoring can take some time depending on whether a hand-scoring or electronic scoring system is used. There are versions of the PedsQL for children, teens, and parents. The parent form is called a proxy report. Proxy reporting is when someone other than the patient completes the questionnaire. In the case of a parent proxy report, the parent completes the instrument on the child's behalf. Typically, proxy reports are used when someone does not have the capacity to answer the questions for him/herself (eg, health condition that limits ability to read and answer the questions, cognitive limitations, age too young to read). While the PedsQL was not designed specifically for athletes, it does contain subscales that may be of interest for secondary school athletes. For example, school functioning is a subscale that might be impacted should an athlete be removed from athletics or school for a period of time as a result of injury. A decrease in score may prompt the clinician to focus in on this finding and consider the reason for the lower score as well as get assistance, perhaps in the form of academic accommodation, should that be needed. The PedsQL, like the SF family of instruments, may require a license fee prior to use.

Patient-Reported Outcomes Measurement Information System

The **Patient-Reported Outcomes Measurement Information System (PROMIS) outcome measures** are a family of instruments that were developed through funding from the National Institutes of Health for the purpose of creating an advanced, reliable system for measuring health outcomes from the patient perspective, with emphasis on physical, mental, and social well-being. The PROMIS measures are useful endpoints in clinical care and in research investigations and should provide information in both instances about how different treatments affect a person's health. The PROMIS family of outcomes instruments includes adult, children, and parent-proxy reports. Several instruments are available through PROMIS, and some examples include individual tools to measure fatigue, pain, physical function, depression, peer relationships, and anger. One of the unique aspects of the PROMIS instruments is that they can be delivered through a couple of methods. For example, there are short forms consisting of 4 to 10 questions about a particular health-related dimension (eg, pain or physical function). These short forms can be predetermined through the PROMIS system, or they can be created by researchers or clinicians from the available PROMIS item banks. Alternatively, PROMIS outcome measures can be delivered through computerized adaptive testing, which is based on modern measurement theory and essentially works to decrease the burden of survey completion for the patient. Basically, computerized adaptive testing works to predict a score on a PRO instrument based on the patient's response to early questions on a survey. Thus, if there are 10 possible questions on a particular health construct (physical function) within the item-bank, the patient may only need to answer a couple of questions before the system would be confident in predicting the patient's score regarding that construct (physical function). Patient-rated outcomes developed through computerized adaptive testing require computers for administration. Either method of administration of PROMIS measures is relatively quick because the typical instrument consists of less than 10 questions. The PROMIS instruments are gaining attention and use in all areas of health care, including research, and warrant consideration when looking for a suitable instrument to address your patient's needs. To learn more about

Table 16-1.
Common Generic Patient-Rated Outcome Measure Instruments

INSTRUMENT	NUMBER OF QUESTIONS	AREAS OF EMPHASIS	WEBSITE
SF-12	12	Physical Functioning, Role Physical, Bodily Pain, General Health Perception, Vitality, Social Functioning, Role Emotional, and Mental Health	http://www.optum.com/optum-outcomes.html
DPA	16	Impairments, functional limitations, and disability	
PedsQL	23	Physical, emotional, social, and school functioning	http://www.pedsql.org/
PROMIS	Variable	Fatigue, pain, physical function, depression, peer relationships, anger, etc	http://www.nihpromis.org/measures/measureshome

Abbreviations: DPA, Disablement in the Physically Active; PedsQL, Pediatric Quality of Life Inventory; PROMIS, Patient-Reported Outcomes Measurement Information System; SF-12, Short Form 12.

the PROMIS instruments, visit their website (http://www.nihpromis.org). Table 16-1 provides a list of the common generic PRO instruments discussed in this chapter.

Common Specific Patient-Reported Outcome Instruments

Disabilities of the Arm, Shoulder and Hand

The **Disabilities of the Arm, Shoulder and Hand (DASH) questionnaire** is a 30-item PRO instrument that focuses on symptoms and disability in people with upper-extremity injuries. The DASH instructions suggest the patient consider the use of both arms (injured or healthy) when answering the questions because the instrument evaluates ability to perform an activity regardless of how it is done. Therefore, if an activity can be completed with the uninjured arm, then the patient rating may be higher than you might think it should be if the reference has been the injured arm. Another consideration with the DASH is that there is a question in the instrument that may not be appropriate for younger populations because it asks patients to rate their amount of difficulty with sexual activities. Scoring for the DASH can be completed when up to 3 questions are missed; so if this question is inappropriate for your population of interest, it is okay to remove it from the questionnaire and to treat it like a missing question. The range of scores on the DASH is from 0 (no disability and symptoms) to 100 (significant disability and symptoms), with higher scores suggestive of worse upper-extremity health. Compared with some of the other common PRO instruments, the DASH is scored with lower scores suggestive of better health than higher scores. This is a helpful reminder to always know what the low and high scores are reflective of when interpreting scores on a PRO. Scoring on the DASH is in Likert-style format, and scoring is fairly easy with a simple equation based on the number of answered questions.

The **QuickDASH** is a shortened version of the DASH questionnaire and includes 11 questions instead of the 30 questions in the original instrument. As with the DASH, the QuickDASH includes questions related to function and symptoms in people with a variety of upper-extremity conditions. Additionally, the QuickDASH produces a total score and 2 subscale scores (ie, work and sport modules), just like the DASH. The appeal of the QuickDASH compared with the DASH is that it is shorter to complete, which may be helpful when used in a busy athletic training facility. For both the QuickDASH and the DASH, it is recommended that you review their user agreements prior to use.

Pennsylvania Shoulder Score

The **Pennsylvania Shoulder Score (PSS)** is a 24-question shoulder-specific PRO instrument that evaluates pain, satisfaction, and function in people with shoulder conditions. The pain subscale consists of 3 questions that ask about pain at rest, pain during normal activities, and pain during strenuous activities. Satisfaction is a single question that asks patients to rate their satisfaction with the current level of function of their shoulder. Finally, function is measured with a subset of 20 questions that ask about the ability to complete arm movements, such as reaching overhead, activities needed for self-care, including combing hair and getting dressed, and questions related to household chores, work, and sports. Each area of emphasis is scored as an individual subscale. Response formats include visual analog scale and Likert style, with subscale scores ranging from 0 (pain, functional loss, and not satisfied) to 100 (no pain, no functional loss, and satisfied). A highlight of the PSS is that you get separate subscales for 3 areas that matter to patients. If you have a patient with a shoulder injury who has complaints of pain and issues with function, you may want to consider the PSS as part of routine patient care. One consideration for the PSS is that there are only a few questions that specifically relate to sports activities.

Functional Arm Scale for Throwers

Many of the PROs available for use are not specifically targeted toward the athletic population. As a result, some people question whether existing instruments include the types of questions that are meaningful to athletic patients. The **Functional Arm Scale for Throwers (FAST)** is a newly developed instrument for the purpose of evaluating disablement in throwing athletes, and its construction was based on disablement models. Overall, the FAST consists of 22 sport- and nonsport-related questions that combine to create 5 subscale scores related to throwing, activities of daily living, psychological effects, advancement, and pain. There is a total score, as well. The format, range of scores, and scoring of the FAST are similar to the DASH in that the response format follows a Likert style, the range of scores is from 0 to 100, and higher scores are indicative of better HRQOL. If you are managing injuries in throwing athletes, the FAST should be considered for implementation in your care process.

Kerlan-Jobe Orthopedic Clinic Overhead Athlete Shoulder and Elbow Score

Like the FAST, the **Kerlan-Jobe Orthopedic Clinic Overhead Athlete Shoulder and Elbow Score (KJOC)** is also a specific outcomes instrument targeted toward overhead athletes. The KJOC consists of 10 questions all related to upper-extremity function, athletic performance, symptoms, and interpersonal relationships, with one final total score produced. Scoring of the KJOC is through the use of a 10-cm VAS, with scores at 0 indicating lower function and scores approaching 10 indicating increasingly higher levels of function. The use of a VAS scale differs from some of the other instruments we have seen, and there would be time needed to measure and score each question. However, with only 10 items, time to score the instrument would not be that significant. There are reports that scores greater than 90 are indicative of healthy athletes, and scores less than 90 suggest that the athlete may have an injury or pain or may be functioning at less than full capacity.

Modified Oswestry

The **Modified Oswestry** is a 10-question PRO instrument designed to measure the impact of low back pain on the management of daily activities, with an emphasis on function and pain. Questions in the Modified Oswestry relate to a variety of important areas, including pain, personal care, sitting, sleeping, and social life. Each question is designed with 6 response options. Scores for all questions are summed, and a percentage ranging from 0% (no impact of back pain on daily activities) to 100% (significant impact of low back pain on daily activities) is generated. There are a number of versions of the Oswestry instrument, and care should be taken when selecting the appropriate version for your population of interest.

Lower Extremity Functional Scale

The Lower Extremity Functional Scale (LEFS) is a region-specific instrument designed to evaluate function of people with lower extremity conditions. There are 20 questions on the LEFS, and all of them relate to function, with scores ranging from 0 (lowest level of function) to 80 (highest level of function). Most of the PRO instruments we have reviewed have used a 0-to-100 range of scores, so the LEFS is a good reminder that we must be aware of score range so that we can accurately interpret the scores we obtain from patients. The LEFS, like the DASH, allows you to use the instrument for injuries within the entire extremity, so you can use the LEFS to make comparisons between people with ankle injuries and people with hip or knee injuries.

International Knee Documentations Committee Knee Score

The knee is one of the most commonly injured joints in athletics, so it is important to have a good PRO instrument to measure health changes over time for this injury. The International Knee Documentations Committee Knee Score (IKDC) is one of the more widely studied PRO instruments for the lower extremity and was designed to evaluate improvement and deterioration in symptoms, sports activities, and function in people with various knee ailments, including ligament injuries, cartilage problems, patellofemoral issues, and meniscal injuries. The IKDC consists of 19 questions that use adjectival and Likert-style response options. Scores range from 0 to 100, and higher scores are related to lower levels of symptoms as well as higher levels of function and sport activity. The inclusion of the sport subscale questions makes the IKDC appealing for athletic populations. Recently, there has been an increase in development of PRO instruments that have adult and adolescent or child versions available for use. The IKCD is one of these instruments. Recently, the pediatric version of the IKDC (Pedi-IKDC) was released, which is tailored for adolescents between the ages of 10 and 18 years. The adult and pediatric versions of the IKDC are quite similar except that there are a few more questions (22 total) in the pediatric version of the instrument. One of these questions relates to identifying whether the child completed the instrument independently or with assistance from a parent or some other adult. Additionally, the wording in the Pedi-IKDC has been simplified to align with a younger population.

Kujala Anterior Knee Pain Scale

The **Kujala Anteror Knee Pain Scale (AKPS)**, or the Kujala Patellofemoral Score (KPS), is a 13-question condition-specific PRO instrument designed to evaluate symptoms and functional limitations in people with anterior knee pain and other related conditions. There are 3 areas of emphasis in the AKPS that target symptoms, pain, and patellofemoral incongruity. Questions also target a variety of different activities, such as jumping, walking, and running, as well as impairments, such as thigh atrophy and knee range of motion. As with several of the other PRO instruments we have reviewed, scores range from 0 to 100, but in the AKPS, lower scores suggest greater disability. Scoring of the AKPS is weighted so that questions related to descending stairs, running, jumping, prolonged sitting, pain, swelling, and patellar subluxation impact the scores more than those related to walking, limping, weight bearing, squatting, thigh atrophy, and knee bending.

Knee Injury and Osteoarthritis Outcome Score

One common knee-specific instrument is the 42-item **Knee Injury and Osteoarthritis Outcome Score (KOOS)**, which is targeted to patients who have symptoms of osteoarthritis or have conditions that may lead to osteoarthritis (eg, anterior cruciate ligament injuries, meniscal injuries). However, the KOOS can be used in patient populations with a variety of knee conditions. The questions on the KOOS are related to pain, knee symptoms, function in daily living, function in sport and recreation, and quality of life. As with many of the other PRO instruments, the KOOS is designed with the response format in Likert style, with a range of scores from 0 (extreme symptoms) to 100 (no symptoms). As a result, higher scores suggest better overall health on the KOOS. The KOOS has been widely used, especially in patients following knee surgery, such as anterior cruciate ligament reconstruction. One drawback of the KOOS for use in busy athletic training facilities may be the higher number of included questions than some of the other instruments, such as the IKDC or LEFS. Like the IKDC, a version of the KOOS was developed to target younger populations and is called the KOOS-Child.

The **KOOS-Child** is a 39-question PRO instrument designed to be used in children with knee injuries who have the chance of developing osteoarthritis. Use of the KOOS-Child can be for short- (week to week) and long-term (months, years) intervals, just like most PROs. Subscales within the KOOS-Child relate to pain, symptoms, daily activities, sports and playing, and quality of life. Questions are designed with a Likert-style response format, with total scores ranging from 0 (extreme symptoms) to 100 (no symptoms). For the most part, the KOOS and the KOOS-Child are fairly similar. The general difference between the KOOS and the KOOS-Child is that the questions in the child version have been reworded for ease of understanding, and pictures have been added to some questions to facilitate understanding.

Foot and Ankle Ability Measure

The Foot and Ankle Ability Measure (FAAM) is a 29-question region-specific PRO instrument that was designed to evaluate the activities of daily living and sports activities in people with foot and ankle injuries. Questions on the FAAM are rated on Likert-style response format with score options from no difficulty with an activity to unable to do or even not applicable. Two subscales, activities of daily living and sports module, are created from the questions on the FAAM. The activities of daily living subscale ranges in scores from 0 to 84 points, and the sports module ranges in scores from 0 to 32 points. In both cases, higher scores suggest better function. Again, it is important to remember the range of scores when interpreting a PRO instrument because not all scores go from 0 to 100; such is the case with the FAAM. The FAAM sports module may be of particular interest to clinicians who treat athletes because the questions target higher level activities in which active populations may participate. For example, questions relate to jumping, landing, quickly starting and stopping, and ability to participate in sport, all of which matter to the athletic individual. The final question on the FAAM relates to a global assessment of function during sport and related activities on a 0% (inability to do typical daily activities) to 100% (performance at level prior to foot or ankle injury), which is helpful when trying to obtain a global understanding of how a patient feels about his/her health status overall.

Headache Impact Test 6

The **Headache Impact Test 6 (HIT-6)** is a 6-item PRO instrument that is condition (headache) specific and evaluates the impact of headache on HRQOL. While the HIT-6 was not designed for concussed athletes, it is relevant to this population because of the emphasis on headache. Headache is one of the most common symptoms of people with concussions, so monitoring the impact of headache on the athlete's life is valuable. Scores on the HIT-6 range from 36 to 78, with lower scores suggestive of less impact of headache on life. Questions on the HIT-6 relate to the location and severity of headache pain, impact of headache on daily activities (including school and social life), as well as the relationship of the headache to fatigue, irritability, and ability to concentrate. The developers of the HIT-6 have reported that changes in scores from one time point to another of about 5 points are clinically meaningful and changes of 3 points are noteworthy. The company that regulates the HIT-6 (Optum: http://www.optum.com/optum-outcomes.html) may require licensing to use the instrument depending on the purpose of use (eg, research vs clinical practice).

Fear Avoidance Belief Questionnaire

Fear of reinjury has received some attention in athletic health care, especially as it relates to patients with low back pain. The **Fear Avoidance Belief Questionnaire (FABQ)** was designed to measure fear avoidance in low back patients with the intent to predict those patients who have and do not have pain avoidance behavior. There are 2 subscales in the FABQ, with 1 called the physical activity subscale (questions 1 to 5) and the other called the work subscale (questions 6 to 16). The physical activity subscales are scored by summing the responses of questions 2 through 5, and the work subscale is scored by summing the responses of questions 6, 7, 9 through 12, and 15. Example questions for the physical activity subscale are, "physical activity makes my pain worse" and "physical activity might harm my back." Example questions for the work subscale are, "my work is too heavy for me" and "I should not do my normal work with my present pain." The FABQ may be of interest if you have a patient who you believe may be concerned about a return to physical activity.

Tampa Scale for Kinesiophobia

The **Tampa Scale for Kinesiophobia (TSK)** is a 17-question PRO instrument designed to evaluate kinesiophobia, or fear of movement or reinjury, in people with chronic low back pain or fibromyalgia. The response format is on a 4-point scale ranging from 1 (strongly disagree) to 4 (strongly agree). A total score is calculated by summing all of the responses. However, questions 4, 8, 12, and 16 are reversed scored. The total score for the TSK ranges from 17 to 68, with higher scores indicative of higher levels of kinesiophobia. Generally, a score higher than 37 is considered a high score. Although the TSK was originally developed for people with low back pain, it has been used successfully in other patient populations, such as those with neck pain. While there are several specific PRO instruments available, Table 16-2 provides a summary of the specific PRO instruments discussed in this chapter.

Table 16-2. Common Specific Patient-Rated Outcome Measure Instruments

INSTRUMENT	TARGET AREA/ POPULATION	NUMBER OF QUESTIONS	AREAS OF EMPHASIS	WEBSITE
DASH	Upper extremity	30	Symptoms, disability	http://www.dash.iwh.on.ca/
QuickDASH	Upper extremity	11	Symptoms, disability	http://www.dash.iwh.on.ca/
PSS	Shoulder	24	Pain, satisfaction, and function	
FAST	Throwing athlete	22	Throwing, activities of daily living, psychological effects, advancement, and pain	
KJOC	Throwing athlete	10	Upper-extremity function, athletic performance, symptoms, and interpersonal relationships	
Modified Oswestry	Low back	10	Pain and function	
LEFS	Lower extremity	20	Function	
IKDC	Knee	19	Symptoms, sports activity, function	http://www.sportsmed.org/research/IKDC_forms/
IKDC Pedi	Knee	22	Symptoms, sports activity, function	http://www.sportsmed.org/research/IKDC_forms/
AKPS	Patellofemoral pain	13	Symptoms and function	

(continued)

Table 16-2. (continued)
Common Specific Patient-Rated Outcome Measure Instruments

INSTRUMENT	TARGET AREA/ POPULATION	NUMBER OF QUESTIONS	AREAS OF EMPHASIS	WEBSITE
KOOS	Knee	42	Pain, symptoms, daily function	http://www.koos.nu/
KOOS-Child	Knee	39	Pain, symptoms, daily activities, sports and playing, quality of life	http://www.koos.nu/
FAAM	Foot and ankle	29	Activities of daily living and sports activities	
HIT-6	Head	6	Headache	http://www.optum.com/optum-outcomes.html
FABQ	Low back	16	Fear avoidance	
TSK	Low back and neck	17	Kinesiophobia	

Abbreviations: AKPS, Kujala Anterior Knee Pain Scale; DASH, Disabilities of the Arm, Shoulder and Hand Score; FAAM, Foot and Ankle Ability Measure; FABQ, Fear Avoidance Belief Questionnaire; FAST, Functional Arm Scale for Throwers; HIT-6, Headache Impact Test 6; IKDC, International Knee Documentation Committee Knee Score; IKDC Pedi, pediatric version of the IKDC; KJOC, Kerlan-Jobe Orthopedic Clinic Overhead Athlete Shoulder and Elbow Score; KOOS, Knee Injury and Osteoarthritis Outcome Score; KOOS-Child, child version of the KOOS; LEFS, Lower Extremity Functional Scale; PSS, Pennsylvania Shoulder Score; QuickDASH, shortened version of the DASH; TSK, Tampa Scale for Kinesiophobia.

Single-Item Outcome Measures

Global Ratings of Change, Function, and Disability

The **Global Rating of Change (GROC)**, **Global Rating of Function (GROF)**, and **Global Rating of Disability (GROD)** are different PRO instruments, but because they all offer global ratings, it makes sense to group them together. When a global assessment of patient change is needed, using the Global Rating of Change is a useful instrument to incorporate into patient care. The GROC is a single question that asks patients to rate the change in their health status compared with a previous point in time. This previous point in time is typically the first athletic training clinical visit or the visit before the one in which the patient is doing the rating. The response options for the GROC are in Likert style and vary in length of answer options, with as few as 5 or less to as many as 15 or more. Examples of the polar ends of the available options are "a very great deal better" to "a very great deal worse," with an option for "about the same, no change" in the middle. The GROD is similar to the GROC in that it is also a question that asks patients to globally assess their health and to perform some comparison between current health status as it relates to disability to some previous point in time. The GROD typically reads something like, "How much has your injury affected your normal daily activities in the past week?" Again, the response options for the GROD are in Likert response format and have several answer options that range from "cannot perform any of my daily activities" to "no difficulty, has not affected my daily activities." The GROF is a single-item questionnaire that asks patients to rate the level of function they have in their injured body part on a scale from 0 (no use of the injured body part) to 100 (full use of the injured body part).

Single-Item Numeric Evaluation

The **Single-Item Numeric Evaluation (SANE)** is similar to global rating measures in that patients are asked about a global aspect of health in relation to an injured body part, such as the knee. The SANE reads as follows: "If I had to give my knee a grade from 1 to 100, with 100 being the best, I would give my knee a ____." Using the SANE, the patient can grade the injured knee on a numeric linear scale, much like the GROF. However, unlike the GROF, the wording of the SANE does not explicitly target function as the context for the answer.

Satisfaction

Ratings of satisfaction have become increasingly important in health care. Satisfaction can be considered from a variety of perspectives, with 2 common purposes related to the satisfaction with current function and satisfaction with care received. For example, a single-item question about patient satisfaction reads, "How satisfied are you with the current level of function of your injured body part?" with the question scored on a scale from 0 (not satisfied) to 10 (completely satisfied). The same scale could be used to answer a question about patient satisfaction that targets care received, such as, "How satisfied are you with the care you received for your injured body part?" These 2 questions consider different aspects of satisfaction, but each may be important ratings when considering the management of health conditions and the delivery of care. There are also multi-item PROs available to measure satisfaction.

Numeric Pain Rating Scale

Pain is an important symptom to measure in patients, and athletic trainers likely do a very good job of evaluating pain routinely. Compared with other PROs, evaluation of pain most likely happens frequently and objectively. That is, clinicians may often ask patients to rate pain on a scale of 0 to 10 and then report the given value in treatment notes. The **Numeric Pain Rating Scale (NPRS)**

Table 16-3. Common Single-Item Patient-Rated Outcome Measure Instruments

INSTRUMENT	NUMBER OF QUESTIONS	AREAS OF EMPHASIS
GROC	1	Global change
GROF	1	Function
GROD	1	Disability
SANE	1	Function
Satisfaction	1	Satisfaction
NPRS	1	Pain
PSFS	1	Function

Abbreviations: GROC, Global Rating of Change; GROD, Global Rating of Disability; GROF, Global Rating of Function; NPRS, Numeric Pain Rating Scale; PSFS, Patient-Specific Functional Scale; SANE, Single-Item Numeric Evaluation.

is a single-item PRO that is focused on pain and is a formal instrument that can be used in the routine evaluation of pain. Using an 11-point scale similar to the one used for satisfaction ratings, you may ask a patient to "rate the pain associated with your injury," with a rating of "0" reflective of no pain, and a rating of "10" reflective of the worst imaginable pain. With the NPRS, the type of pain or activities causing the pain are not noted, so the context (eg, during sport activity, during rest, during daily activities) for this rating is determined by the patient. The NPRS provides a quick and easy assessment of pain and is likely very familiar to clinicians.

Patient-Specific Functional Scale

The **Patient-Specific Functional Scale (PSFS)** is an instrument that functions a little differently than the other PRO instruments we have considered thus far. Additionally, it is not in the same style that we typically think of in terms of single-item measures, but it technically consists of 1 question with the option for multiple responses. By design, the PSFS allows patients to identify functional endpoints that are important to them. An example might help to illustrate the uniqueness of the PSFS. The PSFS asks patients to identify 3 to 5 activities that they are unable to do or are having difficulty doing as a result of their primary complaint which, in athletics, most likely will be an injury. In addition to listing the items, patients also indicate the difficulty they have in performing the task on a scale that ranges from 0 (unable to perform activity) to 10 (able to perform at preinjury/condition level). Patients can complete the PSFS throughout the recovery process and are able to re-evaluate the original activities that were listed as well as identify and rate new activities as they emerge. Instead of giving patients a list of activities that have been preselected for them in a traditional PRO instrument, the PSFS allows patients to identify the activities of most interest to them. On repeated administrations (serial administration) of the PSFS, changes in those activities (eg, improvements and deteriorations) can be made. The PSFS is an important instrument to consider because it opens an opportunity to gain the patient perspective in a different way than more traditional PROs. Additionally, this instrument may be helpful in generating patient goals that are tailored to what is of most importance to the patient. Table 16-3 provides a summary of the single-item PRO instruments discussed in this chapter.

Table 16-4.
Single-Item Patient-Rated Outcome Instrument Simple Strategy

PRO	INITIAL VISIT	MID-TREATMENT	DISCHARGE/ RETURN-TO-PLAY
NPRS	X	X	X
GROC		X	X

Abbreviations: GROC, Global Rating of Change; NPRS, Numeric Pain Rating Scale; PRO, patient-rated outcome measurement.

Incorporating Patient-Rated Outcome Instruments Into Clinical Practice

Now that we have covered a variety of types of generic and specific PROs as well as multi- and single-item measures, it is time to consider how you can go about implementing these outcomes into clinical practice. Unfortunately, there is no one best way to measure patient outcomes. In collecting patient outcomes, you hope to capture meaningful changes in health status at a variety of points along the care path. For example, it may be helpful to measure changes in health status at the time of injury, at a week or 2 post injury, and then again every couple of weeks until patient discharge and/or return-to-play. It is helpful to have some basic starting point for outcomes collection, such as at an initial patient visit, so that as care progresses, you have a benchmark from which to make decisions about whether scores on the PRO instrument are improving or deteriorating from that initial assessment.

Because there is no prescription for when to administer PROs, it is helpful to consider a few strategies that have varying levels of complexity to help get you started. The simplest way to get started is to just add the most basic of PRO instruments, single-item outcome measures, into your routine patient care process. Single-item PRO instruments are a simple strategy because they apply to most types of patients and require little time to complete and score. For example, you could ask your patients to complete an NPRS at the initial and final patient care visit. If you felt comfortable with administration at the first and last visits, you might consider increasing the frequency of administration to once a week. Additionally, you could ask the patient to reflect on the change experienced by completing a GROC each week during recovery. If weekly seems too much, it is okay to decrease the frequency of administration. The point is to just get started. Table 16-4 illustrates an example of how you might set up a simple strategy using single-item PRO instruments.

While the implementation of single-item PRO instruments is the most simple approach, you may wish to use multi-item PROs because they tend to provide a more comprehensive evaluation of health status. You could follow a simple strategy by selecting one generic instrument that could be used with all of your patients, such as the DPA. For example, patients with ankle sprains, shoulder injuries, and back issues would all be asked to complete the DPA at standard time points throughout their care. Additionally, you could select a region or condition-specific PRO related to common injury sites or injuries and you would administer those instruments to the people they are related to. For example, you could select the LEFS and administer it to all people with lower-extremity injuries, regardless of the injury. Alternatively, you could select specific measures for key areas in the lower extremity, such as the IKDC for knee injuries and the FAAM for foot and ankle injuries. This strategy is simple because it does not require a lot of planning once the initial strategy is

Table 16-5.
Additional Patient-Rated Outcome Measure Instrument Administration Strategies

PRO	INITIAL VISIT	WEEK 1	WEEK 2	WEEK 3	WEEK 4	DISCHARGE/ RETURN-TO-PLAY
NPRS	X	X	X	X	X	X
DPA	X		X		X	X
FAST	X		X		X	X
GROC		X	X	X	X	X

Abbreviations: DPA, Disablement in the Physically Active; FAST, Functional Arm Scale for Throwers; GROC, Global Rating of Change; NPRS, Numeric Pain Rating Scale; PRO, patient-rated outcome measure.

mapped out. Basically, you administer the instruments that you preidentified based on a patient's general health condition or injury. While we did not discuss single-item PRO instruments with our example for this strategy, these outcomes would be easy to add and would provide a global assessment of some key areas, such as pain and perceived improvement. Just like the simple strategy, you could implement these PRO instruments at a schedule that works for you, ranging from a limited administration plan (eg, initial and final visit) to a more frequent administration plan (eg, initial visit and then weekly until return to play and/or discharge).

Finally, you may wish to implement the routine evaluation of patient outcomes in a manner that is more patient-centered in nature. Instead of focusing on the administration of single-item PRO instruments or preselecting instruments for specific injuries or injury regions, you may wish to select your PROs based on the particular concerns of the patient. For example, if you treated a lot of shoulder injuries in different types of patients (eg, some athletes and some not), you may not want to identify one PRO instrument to fit all circumstances. If you had a baseball athlete, the FAST or KJOC may be desired, but if you were treating a nonathlete who was interested in more routine daily functions, you may wish to select something more like the DASH. Of all the strategies, this patient-centered approach is the most complex because time is needed to carefully select a PRO instrument that meets the specific needs of the patient. Just like the other strategies, however, timing of administration can vary from infrequent to more frequent. Table 16-5 highlights some ideas that you could use when creating a strategy that implements single- and multi-item PRO instruments. The time points and instruments are just examples. There are limitless options that you could set up, and Table 16-5 provides some ideas to get you started.

Summary

There are a plethora of PROs available for you to utilize within your clinical practice based upon such things related to age, function, disability, kinesiophobia, and quality of life. When starting to implement PROs into routine clinical practice, perhaps the biggest piece of advice we can give is to start simple and set yourself up for success. Ultimately, it would be great to administer generic and specific outcome measures to most patients you treat, but that might not be realistic when you first start. Create a strategy that allows for success and increase your complexity as you become more comfortable with the process.

Key Points

- Respecting the unique values and needs of patients is important because what matters most to one patient may be different from what matters most to another patient, even if they have the same health condition.
- Patient-based outcomes are the clinical outcomes or endpoints that, as a clinician, you should be most interested in because they highlight the end goals that you will be focusing your treatment and intervention toward achieving.
- Health-related quality of life is not static. The variability of HRQOL makes it an important variable to routinely evaluate because decreases in HRQOL may indicate the need for a review of the treatment protocol, changes in the protocol, or referral to other health care professionals.
- Patient satisfaction typically comes from the following 2 angles: (1) the satisfaction a patient has with the recovery of his/her injured body part and (2) the satisfaction a patient has with the overall care experience.
- It is helpful to have some basic starting point for outcomes collection, such as at an initial patient visit, so that as care progresses, you have a benchmark from which to make decisions about whether scores on the PRO instrument are improving or deteriorating from that initial assessment.
- When starting to implement PROs into routine clinical practice, perhaps the biggest piece of advice we can give is to start simple and set yourself up for success.

Bibliography

Alberta FG, ElAttrache NS, Bissell S, et al. The development and validation of a functional assessment tool for the upper extremity in the overhead athlete. *Am J Sports Med.* 2010;38(5):903-911.

Bayliss MS, Batenhorst AS. *The HIT-6TM A User's Guide.* Lincoln, RI: Quality Metric Incorporated; 2002.

Beaton DE, Bombardier C, Katz JN, et al. Looking for important change/differences in studies of responsiveness. OMERACT MCID Working Group. Outcome measures in rheumatology. Minimal clinically important difference. *J Rheumatol.* 2001;28(2):400-405.

Binkley J. Measurement of functional status, progress and outcome in orthopaedic clinical practice. *Orthop Phys Ther Pract.* 1999;11:14-21.

Binkley JM, Stratford PW, Lott SA, Riddle DL. The Lower Extremity Functional Scale (LEFS): scale development, measurement properties, and clinical application. *Phys Ther.* 1999;79(4):371-383.

Blumenthal D. Part 1: quality of care—what is it? *N Engl J Med.* 1996;335(12):891-894.

Brook RH, McGlynn EA, Cleary PD. Quality of health care. Part 2: measuring quality of care. *N Engl J Med.* 1996;335(13):966-970.

Chatman AB, Hyams SP, Neel JM, et al. The Patient-Specific Functional Scale: measurement properties in patients with knee dysfunction. *Phys Ther.* 1997;77(8):820-829.

Clancy CM, Eisenberg JM. Outcomes research: measuring the end results of health care. *Science.* 1998;282(5387):245-246.

Cleland JA, Fritz JM, Whitman JM, Palmer JA. The reliability and construct validity of the Neck Disability Index and patient specific functional scale in patients with cervical radiculopathy. *Spine (Phila Pa 1976).* 2006;31(5):598-602.

Collins NJ, Misra D, Felson DT, Crossley KM, Roos EM. Measures of knee function: International Knee Documentation Committee (IKDC) Subjective Knee Evaluation Form, Knee Injury and Osteoarthritis Outcome Score (KOOS), Knee Injury and Osteoarthritis Outcome Score Physical Function Short Form (KOOS-PS), Knee Outcome Survey Activities of Daily Living Scale (KOS-ADL), Lysholm Knee Scoring Scale, Oxford Knee Score (OKS), Western Ontario and McMaster Universities Osteoarthritis Index (WOMAC), Activity Rating Scale (ARS), and Tegner Activity Score (TAS). *Arthritis Care Res (Hoboken).* 2011;63(suppl 11):S208-228.

Deyo RA. Using outcomes to improve quality of research and quality of care. *J Am Board Fam Pract.* 1998;11(6):465-473.

Evans TA, Lam KC. Clinical outcomes assessment in sport rehabilitation. *J Sport Rehabil.* 2011;20(1):8-16.

Farrar JT, Young JP Jr, LaMoreaux L, Werth JL, Poole RM. Clinical importance of changes in chronic pain intensity measured on an 11-point numerical pain rating scale. *Pain.* 2001;94(2):149-158.

Fitzpatrick R, Davey C, Buxton MJ, Jones DR. Evaluating patient-based outcome measures for use in clinical trials. *Health Technol Assess.* 1998;2(14):i-iv,1-74.

Fritz JM, Irrgang JJ. A comparison of a modified Oswestry Low Back Pain Disability Questionnaire and the Quebec Back Pain Disability Scale. *Phys Ther.* 2001;81(2):776-788.

Guyatt GH, Feeny DH, Patrick DL. Measuring health-related quality of life. *Ann Intern Med.* 1993;118(8):622-629.

Guyatt GH, Jaeschke R, Feeny DH, Patrick DL. Measurements in clinical trials: choosing the right approach. In: Spilker B, ed. *Quality of Life and Pharmacoeconomics in Clinical Trials.* 2nd ed. Philadelphia, PA: Lippincott-Raven Publishers; 1996:41-48.

Horn KK, Jennings S, Richardson G, Vliet DV, Hefford C, Abbott JH. The patient-specific functional scale: psychometrics, clinimetrics, and application as a clinical outcome measure. *J Orthop Sports Phys Ther.* 2012;42(1):30-42.

Hudak PL, Wright JG. The characteristics of patient satisfaction measures. *Spine (Phila Pa 1976).* 2000;25(24):3167-3177.

Irrgang JJ, Anderson AF, Boland AL, et al. Development and validation of the international knee documentation committee subjective knee form. *Am J Sports Med.* 2001;29(5):600-613.

Irrgang JJ, Anderson AF, Boland AL, et al. Responsiveness of the International Knee Documentation Committee Subjective Knee Form. *Am J Sports Med.* 2006;34(10):1567-1573.

Jaeschke R, Singer J, Guyatt GH. Measurement of health status. Ascertaining the minimal clinically important difference. *Control Clin Trials.* 1989;10(4):407-415.

Kamper SJ, Maher CG, Mackay G. Global rating of change scales: a review of strengths and weaknesses and considerations for design. *J Man Manip Ther.* 2009;17(3):163-170.

Kaplan SL. *Outcome Measurement & Management: First Steps for the Practicing Clinician.* Philadelphia, PA: FA Davis; 2007.

Kawata AK, Coeytaux RR, Devellis RF, Finkel AG, Mann JD, Kahn K. Psychometric properties of the HIT-6 among patients in a headache-specialty practice. *Headache.* 2005;45(6):638-643.

Kocher MS, Smith JT, Iversen MD, et al. Reliability, validity, and responsiveness of a modified International Knee Documentation Committee Subjective Knee Form (Pedi-IKDC) in children with knee disorders. *Am J Sports Med.* 2011;39(5):933-939.

Kuehl MD, Snyder AR, Erickson SE, McLeod TC. Impact of prior concussions on health-related quality of life in collegiate athletes. *Clin J Sport Med.* 2010;20(2):86-91.

Leggin BG, Michener LA, Shaffer MA, Brenneman SK, Iannotti JP, Williams GR Jr. The Penn shoulder score: reliability and validity. *J Orthop Sports Phys Ther.* 2006;36(3):138-151.

Martin RL, Irrgang JJ. A survey of self-reported outcome instruments for the foot and ankle. *J Orthop Sports Phys Ther.* 2007;37(2):72-84.

Martin RL, Irrgang JJ, Burdett RG, Conti SF, Van Swearingen JM. Evidence of validity for the Foot and Ankle Ability Measure (FAAM). *Foot Ankle Int.* 2005;26(11):968-983.

McAllister DR, Motamedi AR, Hame SL, Shapiro MS, Dorey FJ. Quality of life assessment in elite collegiate athletes. *Am J Sport Med.* 2001;29(6):806-810.

McGuine TA, Winterstein A, Carr K, Hetzel S, Scott J. Changes in self-reported knee function and health-related quality of life after knee injury in female athletes. *Clin J Sport Med.* 2012;22(4):334-340.

Michener LA. Patient- and clinician-rated outcome measures for clinical decision making in rehabilitation. *J Sport Rehabil.* 2011;20(1):37-45.

Michener LA, Leggin BG. A review of self-report scales for the assessment of functional limitation and disability of the shoulder. *J Hand Ther.* 2001;14(2):68-76.

Michener LA, Snyder AR. Evaluation of health-related quality of life in patients with shoulder pain: are we doing the best we can? *Clin Sports Med.* 2008;27(3):491-505, x.

Neuhauser D. Ernest Amory Codman MD. *Qual Saf Health Care.* 2002;11(1):104-105.

Örtqvist M, Roos EM, Broström EW, Janarv PM, Iversen MD. Development of the Knee Injury and Osteoarthritis Outcome Score for children (KOOS-Child): comprehensibility and content validity. *Acta Orthop.* 2012;83(6):666-673.

Ostelo RW, Deyo RA, Stratford P, et al. Interpreting change scores for pain and functional status in low back pain: towards international consensus regarding minimal important change. *Spine (Phila Pa 1976).* 2008;33(1):90-94.

Parsons JT, Snyder AR. Health-related quality of life as a primary clinical outcome in sport rehabilitation. *J Sport Rehabil.* 2011;20(1):17-36.

PedsQL. http://www.pedsql.org. Accessed February 14, 2014.

Piebes SK, Snyder AR, Bay RC, Valovich McLeod TC. Measurement properties of headache-specific outcomes scales in adolescent athletes. *J Sport Rehabil.* 2011;20(1):129-142.

Portney LG, Watkins MP. *Foundations of Clinical Research: Applications to Practice.* 2nd ed. Upper Saddle River, NJ: Prentice Hall Health; 2000.

PROMIS. http://www.nihpromis.org. Accessed February 19, 2014.

Quality Metric. http://www.qualitymetric.com. Accessed February 19, 2014,

Quality Metric. SF Health Surveys. http://www.qualitymetric.com/WhatWeDo/SFHealthSurveys/tabid/184/Default.aspx. Accessed April 18, 2013.

Relman AS. Assessment and accountability: the third revolution in medical care. *N Engl J Med.* 1988;319(18):1220-1222.

Roos EM, Roos HP, Lohmander LS, Ekdahl C, Beynnon BD. Knee Injury and Osteoarthritis Outcome Score (KOOS)—development of a self-administered outcome measure. *J Orthop Sports Phys Ther.* 1998;28(2):88-96.

Roos EM, Toksvig-Larsen S. Knee injury and Osteoarthritis Outcome Score (KOOS) - validation and comparison to the WOMAC in total knee replacement. *Health Qual Life Outcomes.* 2003;1:17.

Sauers EL, Dykstra DL, Bay RC, Bliven KH, Snyder AR. Upper extremity injury history, current pain rating, and health-related quality of life in female softball pitchers. *J Sport Rehabil.* 2011;20(1):100-114.

Schmitt LC, Paterno MV, Huang S. Validity and internal consistency of the international knee documentation committee subjective knee evaluation form in children and adolescents. *Am J Sports Med.* 2010;38(12):2443-2447.

Snyder AR, Martinez JC, Bay RC, Parsons JT, Sauers EL, Valovich McLeod TC. Health-related quality of life differs between adolescent athletes and adolescent nonathletes. *J Sport Rehabil.* 2010;19(3):237-248.

Snyder AR, Parsons JT, Valovich McLeod TC, Curtis Bay R, Michener LA, Sauers EL. Using disablement models and clinical outcomes assessment to enable evidence-based athletic training practice: part I - disablement models. *J Athl Train.* 2008;43(4):428-436.

Snyder AR, Valovich McLeod TC. Selecting patient-based outcome measures. *Athl Ther Today.* 2007;12(6):12-15.

Snyder AR, Valovich-McLeod TC, Sauers EL. Defining, valuing, and teaching clinical outcomes assessment in professional and post-professional athletic training education programs. *J Athl Train.* 2007;(2):31-41.

Solway S, Beaton DE, McConnell S, Bombardier C. *The DASH Outcome Measure User's Manual.* 2nd ed. Toronto, Ontario: Institute for Work and Health; 2002.

Spilker B. Introduction. In: Spilker B, ed. *Quality of Life and Pharmacoeconomics in Clinical Trials.* 2nd ed. Philadelphia, PA: Lippincott-Raven Publishers; 1996:1-10.

Spilker B, Revicki DA. Taxonomy of quality of life. In: Spilker B, ed. *Quality of Life and Pharmacoeconomics in Clinical Trials.* 2nd ed. Philadelphia, PA: Lippincott-Raven Publishers; 1996:25-31.

Stewart AL, Ware JE. *Measuring Function and Well-Being: The Medical Outcomes Study Approach.* Oxford: Oxford University Press; 1992.

Streiner DL, Norman GR. *Health Measurement Scales: A Practical Guide to Their Development and Use.* 4th ed. Oxford: Oxford University Press; 2008.

Suk M, Hanson BP, Norvell DC, Helfet DL. *Musculoskeletal Outcomes Measures and Instruments.* Vol 1. Switzerland: AO Publishing; 2009.

Testa MA, Nackley JF. Methods for quality-of-life studies. *Annu Rev Public Health.* 1994;15:535-559.

Testa MA, Simonson DC. Assessment of quality-of-life outcomes. *New Engl J Med.* 1996;334(13):835-840.

Valovich McLeod TC, Bay RC, Parsons JT, Sauers EL, Snyder AR. Recent injury and health-related quality of life in adolescent athletes. *J Athl Train.* 2009;44(6):603-610.

Valovich McLeod TC, Snyder AR, Parsons JT, Curtis Bay R, Michener LA, Sauers EL. Using disablement models and clinical outcomes assessment to enable evidence-based athletic training practice, part II - clinical outcomes assessment. *J Athl Train.* 2008;43(4):437-445.

van Meer BL, Meuffels DE, Vissers MM, et al. Knee Injury and Osteoarthritis Outcome Score or International Knee Documentation Committee Subjective Knee Form: which questionnaire is most useful to monitor patients with an anterior cruciate ligament rupture in the short term? *Arthroscopy.* 2013;29(4):701-715.

Varni JW, Seid M, Kurtin PS. PedsQL 4.0: reliability and validity of the Pediatric Quality of Life Inventory version 4.0 generic core scales in healthy and patient populations. *Med Care.* 2001;39(8):800-812.

Vela LI, Denegar C. Transient disablement in the physically active with musculoskeletal injuries, part I: a descriptive model. *J Athl Train.* 2010;45(6):615-629.

Vela LI, Denegar CR. The Disablement in the Physically Active Scale, part II: the psychometric properties of an outcomes scale for musculoskeletal injuries. *J Athl Train.* 2010;45(6):630-641.

Vlaeyen JW, Kole-Snijders AM, Boeren RG, van Eek H. Fear of movement/(re)injury in chronic low back pain and its relation to behavioral performance. *Pain.* 1995;62(3):363-372.

Von Korff M, Jensen MP, Karoly P. Assessing global pain severity by self-report in clinical and health services research. *Spine (Phila Pa 1976).* 2000;25(24):3140-3151.

Waddell G, Newton M, Henderson I, Somerville D, Main CJ. A Fear-Avoidance Beliefs Questionnaire (FABQ) and the role of fear-avoidance beliefs in chronic low back pain and disability. *Pain.* 1993;52(2):157-168.

Ware JE Jr, Kosinski M, Turner-Bowker DM, Gandek B. *User's Manual for the SF-12v2 Health Survey.* 2nd ed. Lincoln, RI: Quality Metrics Incorporated; 2007.

Ware JE, Kosinski MA, Bjorner JB, Turner-Bowker DM, Gandek B, Maruish ME. *User's Manual for the SF-36v2 Health Survey. 2nd ed.* Lincoln, RI: QualityMetric Incorporated; 2008.

Winterstein AP, McGuine TA, Carr KE, Hetzel SJ. Comparison of IKDC and SANE outcome measures following knee injury in active female patients. *Sports Health.* 2013;5(6):523-529.

17

Considerations for Selecting Patient-Rated Outcome Measures

Now that you have an understanding of the different types of patient-rated outcome (PRO) instruments available, you may be wondering how you will determine which instrument you should select for a specific patient case. With the vast number of PRO instruments available to clinicians, it is not uncommon to feel overwhelmed. As discussed in the previous chapter, there are often several PRO instruments available that focus on the same body region or generic topic (eg, health-related quality of life [HRQOL], fear of reinjury). Moreover, a new PRO instrument may be developed that upon first glance appears to be very similar to an already well-established instrument. Since there is often an abundance of possible instruments to choose from, it is vital to have a good understanding of the criteria that should be considered to help you differentiate one PRO instrument from another and to select the instrument that best fits your intended purpose.

Our ability to use PRO measurements to guide our informed decision-making process is dependent upon how well we can measure the variable in which we are interested. Therefore, before you have your patient complete a PRO instrument, it is important to ensure that the selected instrument will capture the information for which you are looking. There are several components that should be considered when selecting an appropriate PRO instrument. The focus of this chapter will be to discuss the 9 criteria that you should pay attention to when choosing a PRO instrument for your patient's case. While patient-rated outcomes can be used for a multitude of purposes (eg, research, quality improvement, patient care), we will primarily be focusing on how patient outcomes can be used to enhance your clinical decisions.

Instrument Development

The development of an instrument to assess patient outcomes is important to ensure that it was created in a systematic manner. A systematic process should entail a logical, step-by-step approach that focuses on the following 3 general phases:

1. Item generation and initial item reduction

Van Lunen BL, Hankemeier DA, Welch CE.
Evidence-Guided Practice: A Framework for Clinical Decision Making in Athletic Training (pp 227-240).

2. Item pilot testing, followed by additional item reduction
3. Establishment of instrument measurement properties

To help you understand the development process, we will discuss how the Foot and Ankle Ability Measure (FAAM) was developed. To begin, there are several ways a developer can go about generating and reducing items for a new PRO instrument, such as reviewing the literature, conducting focus groups with patients and/or content experts, and assessing previously developed PRO instruments on the topic of interest. For the FAAM, developers chose to generate potential items using the following 3 approaches: (1) conduct a thorough literature review of already published outcome measurement scales that were applicable to a variety of leg, ankle, and foot musculoskeletal disorders; (2) collect input from physical therapists who treat patients with foot and ankle disorders; and (3) collect input from patients with leg, ankle, and foot musculoskeletal conditions. Once all potential items (69 items) were generated, the developers of the FAAM accessed the American Physical Therapy Association Foot and Ankle Special Interest Group to participate in the initial item reduction. Interest group members were asked to rate each potential item on a scale of –2 (not important) to +2 (very important); items were retained if a mean score of 1 (important) was achieved.

After items for a new measurement scale have been generated and initially reduced to an acceptable number (ie, 69 potential items reduced to 34 items split into 2 scales; 26-item Activities of Daily Living subscale, 8-item Sport subscale), the developers will shift into the second phase of development: pilot testing. Once the developers of the FAAM reduced the potential items included, they recruited 1027 participants who were referred to a physical therapist to receive treatment for a musculoskeletal leg, ankle, or foot pathology. Participants were asked to complete the FAAM during their initial evaluation with the physical therapist. Following pilot testing, data analyses were conducted, and the items on the FAAM were revised for an end result of a 21-item Activities of Daily Living subscale and an 8-item Sport subscale.

The third and final phase of instrument development involves establishing the measurement properties of the new instrument. During this phase, developers will often test the instrument in the target population to establish validity, responsiveness, and reliability. However, it is also possible to continue to reduce items based on results received from this phase. For the Disabilities of the Arm, Shoulder, and Hand questionnaire, developers conducted testing in patients with leg, ankle, and foot musculoskeletal problems with the hope that analysis of the data would reveal the PRO instrument to be valid, responsive, and reliable.

Determining whether a PRO instrument was developed using a systematic process is important because it serves as the foundation for producing a valid and reliable instrument. In the upcoming sections, we discuss how to evaluate whether a PRO instrument is valid and reliable. By including patients, also referred to as **stakeholders**, and experts throughout the various stages of the development process, the instrument developers are taking the initial steps to enhance the likelihood that the instrument will capture the information it was intended for, as well as produce consistent findings. Thus, as you consider different PRO instruments for use in your clinical practice, the first step you will want to take is to determine if the instrument was developed systematically. To do so, you should conduct a simple literature search to retrieve the PRO instrument development paper. Whether an instrument has been recently developed or is well established, there is almost always a publication available that will highlight the development process. If there is a lack of information available for any aspect of the development process of a PRO instrument, you should considering using another instrument or you should be cautious with the interpretation of the information collected with this instrument.

Validity

As discussed in previous chapters, validity is necessary to ensure that a measurement actually captures the information it was designed to capture. When you begin to look at the validity of a PRO instrument, there are 3 global questions that you should consider:

1. Is the PRO instrument truly measuring what you intend to measure?
2. Is the PRO instrument truly measuring what it was designed to measure?
3. Is the PRO instrument useful for its intended purpose?

Since PRO instruments are usually developed for a specific patient population (eg, injured, adolescent, geriatric) or condition of interest (eg, patellofemoral pain, low back pain, deep vein thrombosis), it is important to ensure that the instrument is not only valid in the sense that it collects the data it was designed to collect, but that it is also a valid PRO instrument to gather the specific type of information you need to assist you and your patient during the decision-making process. More specifically, when you think about PRO instruments designed to capture information about a patient's quality of life, you want to determine the extent to which it is reasonable to conclude that the instrument really measures quality of life.

The overarching goal of evaluating the validity of PRO instruments is to ensure that the measurements you are collecting accurately reflect the patient's HRQOL or a specific construct (eg, social, physical, mental, spiritual) you are interested in capturing. While there are several types of validity that can be assessed, this section will focus on 4 types that are important to consider for PRO instruments: face validity, content validity, construct validity, and criterion validity.

If you are reading an article about the development of a PRO instrument, you will most likely notice that the author discusses face and content validity together. These 2 types of validity are related because they both address a judgment made about whether the content of the instrument fits the intended purpose; however, they assess different aspects of validity. Face validity is used to determine whether an instrument appears to measure what it is intended to measure. When assessing the face validity of a PRO instrument, it is important to carefully consider the questions in the instrument because you will be making a judgment about whether the instrument appears to address the intended subject matter. For example, in a PRO instrument that is intended to assess a patient's functional status following an ankle injury (eg, FAAM, Foot and Ankle Disability Index [FADI]), you would expect to see questions that pertain to tasks that primarily involve the lower extremity and, therefore, may be altered due to the injury. Conversely, we would not expect to see questions that ask patients to assess their functional level of the upper extremity, such as difficulty washing their hair, because that content would not be relevant to the intended purpose of the PRO instrument.

Content validity of a PRO instrument refers to how well the constructs of interest are comprehensively sampled by the questions included in the instrument. Content validity helps us to answer the question, "Do the questions included appear to capture enough information about the construct of interest?" Just like face validity, content validity is evaluated by reviewing the questions on the instrument. When questions are developed for a specific health construct, it is important to ensure that, as a whole, the questions are specific enough to collect information about the domain, yet broad enough to capture the whole picture of that construct. Consider the following example: a PRO instrument has recently been designed to assess the functional status of adolescent athletes following an ankle injury. Upon reviewing the PRO instrument, you notice that there are several questions that ask about activities of daily living, but the instrument does not include any questions about athletic tasks or recreational activities. In this instance, you would be correct to question the content validity of the instrument. Since this PRO instrument does not include questions about recreational activities, it is likely that the information collected will not capture the full spectrum of the functional level of the intended audience (ie, adolescent athletes).

Therefore, you might conclude that this PRO instrument lacks content validity for your intended use. If used, the PRO instrument may provide you with information that is not particularly useful for your clinical situation.

Face and content validity can be evaluated after a PRO instrument has been initially created, but there may be need for content validity assessments along the way. Largely, the process for evaluating face and content validity is improved if the development of the instrument was systematic in nature. Face and content validity require the basic structure of the PRO instrument to be examined to ensure that the instrument is applicable, comprehensive, and fits the intended use. Determination of these types of validity typically involves a subjective inspection of each item included in the PRO instrument, and they are usually evaluated by experts who have knowledge in PRO instrument development and/or the subject matter of the instrument. Face and content validity should also be assessed by a small pilot group of patients (ie, stakeholders) who the PRO instrument was developed to target. Even though content experts have great knowledge, they cannot replace the input and views from people who have a particular health condition. Remember, a PRO instrument that was developed in a systematic manner will help safeguard the likelihood that the instrument has good face and content validity.

The third type of validity that is important to consider for PRO instruments is **construct validity**. As a clinician, it is easy to observe whether a patient has limited range of motion, an obvious deformity, or is unable to perform a functional task. However, there are several aspects of a patient's HRQOL that are not as easily observable. For example, we often must rely on the patient to inform us about constructs that they are experiencing, such as pain, anxiety, or fear of reinjury. In an attempt to objectively capture this information, you may have your patient complete a PRO instrument that assesses these unobservable constructs. Therefore, construct validity refers to the ability of an instrument to measure a more abstract concept (ie, things that are not directly observable). Whereas face and content validity are assessed qualitatively, construct validity provides a quantitative method to assess whether a PRO instrument measures the construct it was designed to measure. There are a variety of statistical approaches that can be utilized to assess construct validity, and most of them are beyond the scope of this textbook. However, a few common methods used to evaluate construct validity warrant mention. The simplest method is to investigate the relationship or correlation of the construct of interest to other related variables. A correlation coefficient of about .60 and higher has been suggested to be evidence of construct validity. Other components that you may see to assess construct validity include convergent and discriminant validity testing or factor analyses.

Criterion validity, which often includes concurrent and predictive validity, can be described as evidence to show that a new tool is an acceptable measure because it correlates with some other previously established measurement tool, or gold standard. Unfortunately, there is no true gold standard for HRQOL instruments, so it can be challenging to determine the criterion validity of a particular PRO instrument. In the literature, you will often see that researchers get evidence for construct validity by comparing (1) a new instrument to a well-established instrument or (2) a new shorter version of an instrument to a longer version of an instrument. For example, specific PRO instruments are often correlated to generic PRO instruments, like the Short Form 12 (SF-12) or Short Form 36 (SF-36), as a means of confirming that relevant constructs in their instrument (eg, function) are actually captured. If the new scale with an emphasis on function correlates well with the SF-12 physical function subscale, then there is evidence that function was captured. Using the SF-36 as a gold standard in the development of the SF-12 is an example of the second option for construct validity evidence. The SF-36, a generic PRO instrument, was originally developed to consist of 36 items to assess various constructs of HRQOL. Since its original development, this particular PRO instrument has been shortened to a 12-item questionnaire (ie, SF-12) as well as a more condensed 8-item instrument (ie, SF-8). In both instances, criterion validity was assessed to safeguard that the questionnaires that included fewer items still captured the full spectrum of quality of life that the original 36-item version was designed to assess. These are 2 of the many ways that you may see people address criterion validity of PRO instruments. Interpreting criterion validity is relatively straightforward:

- If a PRO instrument is identified as having high criterion validity, then the agreement is acceptable between the 2 PRO instruments.
- If a PRO instrument is identified as having low criterion validity, then the agreement is poor between the 2 PRO instruments.

Of the types of validity we have considered, criterion validity is one about which you may find less information. Criterion validity assessment may not always be available for PRO instruments, partly because of the lack of a gold standard. Additionally, if a new PRO instrument correlates highly with another available PRO instrument, one might ask why there is the need for the new instrument in the first place.

Determining that an instrument is valid is essential to ensure that what is captured with an instrument is meaningful, relevant, and can be used to inform patient care decisions. Validity testing is an ongoing process that will likely never be complete. As we will also see with reliability, validity testing should be confirmed in each population with which it is used. For example, a measure with evidence of validity in one population, such as adolescent athletes, may or may not be valid for another population, such as geriatric athletes. Because routine patient-oriented outcome assessments are relatively new in athletic populations, there is an abundant amount of work that remains to be conducted to evaluate the validity of available PRO instruments for highly active populations.

Responsiveness

The responsiveness of PRO instruments rates right up at the top with instrument validity and reliability. **Responsiveness** of a PRO instrument speaks to the ability of the instrument to capture or measure meaningful change over time. It is essential for a PRO instrument to be responsive to change in health status; if it is not responsive, you would not be able to detect whether a patient gets better, stays the same, or gets worse following a particular treatment or intervention. Also, some people view responsiveness as a measure of validity because if the PRO instrument does not detect meaningful changes to patients, then it probably is not a valid tool for that population. Like validity and reliability values, it is best to refer to responsiveness values that have been determined in the population of interest (eg, athletes). To find these responsiveness values for a PRO instrument, we suggest that you consult the literature for already established values. Ideally, you want to find responsiveness values for your population of interest or for a population that most closely represents them. Responsiveness can be calculated in a variety of ways. Some of the terms you might see in the literature that indicate that an assessment of instrument responsiveness has been done are effect size, change scores, standardized response mean, Guyatt's responsiveness index, minimal important change, and **minimally clinically important difference (MCID)**. While all of these values are acceptable and speak to the responsiveness of a PRO instrument, we are going to focus on the MCID value due to its clinical applicability and ease of understanding.

The MCID is the smallest amount of change that a patient perceives as beneficial. You may hear of the MCID called a number of different things, including clinical important difference and minimal perceptible clinical improvement. In terms of PRO instruments, the MCID value is expressed as a certain number of instrument points. For example, you may see the MCID for the International Knee Documentation Committee Knee Form (IKDC) identified as 11.5 points. The IKDC is used to evaluate improvement and deterioration in symptoms, sports activities, and function in people with various knee conditions. In practice, this means that to feel confident that your patient felt improvement in knee-related health from one point in time (eg, initial treatment) to another (eg, 2 weeks post initial treatment), you would want to see an improvement in IKDC score of at least 11.5 points. Score changes of less than 11.5 points would suggest that the patient did not perceive a beneficial change in knee symptoms, sports activities, and function. While MCID is a measure of responsiveness, it is often used to interpret PRO instrument scores. Therefore, the MCID value will also be discussed in the interpretability section of this chapter.

In addition to the methods used to express responsiveness, it is also necessary to pay attention to whether a PRO instrument has a **ceiling effect** or **floor effect**. These effects can be described as the extent to which scores on a PRO instrument cluster near the more desirable (ie, ceiling) or less desirable (ie, floor) health status extreme on a measure. The problem with a PRO instrument that has reported ceiling or floor effects is that these instruments will not be able to measure improvement or deterioration in health status. For example, a PRO instrument may have a ceiling effect if athletes with significant injuries score the best score possible on the instrument. The reason it is a ceiling effect is that improvement in health (eg, getting better from the significant injury) may not be captured by the instrument because the athletes have already scored at or near the score that represents the best health. Let us consider an example. After administering the IKDC to an injured athlete, the instrument is scored at a 97; recall that the IKDC ranges from 0 to 100. A score of 97 would suggest that the athlete has fewer symptoms and good function related to daily and sport activities. The problem is that the high score was reported in someone with injury, yet because the score was so high, you likely will not be able to capture meaningful improvement. Recall that the MCID is 11.5 points and with an initial score of 97, you do not have the chance to see a change that large.

Floor effects in athletic populations may be less common because athletes are typically generally healthy. Regardless, an example may help to better illustrate how these effects work. A floor effect may be present for a PRO instrument if a very ill person scores the worst score possible on the instrument (eg, a score of 0 on the IKDC). If this very ill patient has another health event that makes his or her condition worse, the decline in health due to the new event may not be captured by the PRO instrument because he or she already scored at the poorer end of the instrument. With a floor effect, there is no room in the PRO instrument to report worse health even if health has declined.

Reliability

Along with validity and responsiveness, one of the most important instrument measurement properties is reliability. Similar to the measurement systems you use on a daily basis, you want to ensure that the PRO instrument you select accurately measures the intended constructs and that it obtains these measurements in a reliable manner. Reliability of a PRO instrument is particularly important when we consider the serial administration of PRO instruments in injured or ill populations. With serial administration, you want to ensure that each time you administer your instrument, the result is true and accurately reflects the current health status of a patient. Accurate assessment allows you to determine whether the patient's health status is changing as a result of specific treatments or interventions. Additionally, by using an unreliable instrument, you may over- or underestimate the size of benefit (ie, amount of improvement) obtained from an intervention. For example, let us say you want to know how a joint mobilization intervention affects a patient's perceived level of function. You have the patient complete the FAAM at an initial evaluation appointment as well as assess joint range of motion with a goniometer. Then, you provide the patient with 2 weeks of joint mobilization treatments. At the end of the treatment period, you have the patient complete the FAAM again, as well as reevaluate joint range of motion with a goniometer to determine whether there were any changes in the patient's perceived level of function and clinician-based assessment of function. Your hope is to find that your intervention has made improvements in both of your outcome measures (in this case a patient-based [ie, FAAM] and clinician-based measure [ie, goniometer]). In this circumstance, the ability to determine whether your intervention improved the patient's function hinges on the reliability of the instruments you used. If they were reliable, you would trust the findings obtained; on the flip side, if they were not reliable, you would not be able to make a judgment regarding patient improvement.

The concept of reliability as it relates to selecting PRO instruments may be easier to understand if we consider 2 characteristics of reliability: reproducibility and internal consistency. For a PRO instrument, **reproducibility** refers to the ability of an instrument to produce the same score when a patient completes the instrument on more than one occasion, assuming there is no change in health status. Generally, reproducibility of a PRO instrument is measured by test-retest reliability. For example, if we were going to assess a patient's pain level via the Numeric Pain Rating Scale, you would have the patient complete the single-item outcome and then ask them to complete the outcome again at a predetermined period of time later to determine whether their health status is better, the same, or worse than the first assessment. It has been suggested that a period of time between 2 and 14 days is appropriate when evaluating test-retest reliability for PRO instruments. One of the challenges with the time between administrations is that too long of a separation between time points can allow the possibility that health status has changed, which might affect scores on the instrument. Too short of a time period has limitations also, because a small amount of time between administrations may make it more likely that those who completed the instrument remember their answers. Determining the appropriate amount of time between PRO instrument administrations is dependent on a variety of factors. For each situation, it is necessary to consider the purpose of the assessment as well as what things may naturally occur between the administrations that could influence the patient's responses.

Making a decision about the reliability of a PRO instrument requires consultation with articles about the reliability of the instrument. When reading an article that discusses the reproducibility of an instrument, there are 2 common statistical tests you will likely see:

1. **Pearson product moment correlation coefficient** (ie, Pearson's *r*)
2. **Intraclass correlation coefficient (ICC)**

While it is not necessary to understand the specifics of these statistical tests at this time, we are going to cover some of the basic features of each test to help you interpret the values you may come across. To begin, it is important to highlight that these tests measure the strength of association between 2 measures. When you are looking to interpret the correlations and determine what is an acceptable value, you can use the following as a general rule of thumb:

- If you are looking at reliability over time in the same subject (within subject), an acceptable correlation is .90.
- If you are examining reliability between groups of patients, an acceptable correlation is .70.
  - You may also accept .50 to .60.

Pearson product moment correlation coefficient (ie, Pearson's *r*) is a correlational measure, meaning that it is a measure of association between 2 continuous variables (ie, interval or ratio data). The values of Pearson's *r* range from –1 to 1:

- If the Pearson's *r* value is closer to 0, then the measures have a lower correlation.
- If the Pearson's *r* value is closer to 1, then the measures have a higher positive correlation.
- If the Pearson's *r* value is closer to –1, then the measures have a higher negative correlation.

Another measure you may come across for reproducibility (ie, test-retest reliability) is the ICC. The ICC measures the strength of association between repeated variables that are measured at 2 or more repeated time points. There are 6 types of ICCs that take into consideration the purpose of the reliability study, the study design, and the type of measurement taken. A more in-depth description of the types of ICCs can be found in Chapter 8. The values for ICCs range from 0 to 1:

- If the ICC value is closer to 0, then the measures have a lower correlation.
- If the ICC value is closer to 1, then the measures have a higher correlation.

Along with reproducibility, it is also necessary to consider the internal consistency of a PRO instrument. **Internal consistency** refers to the relationship of a subset of questions to each other that are aimed at assessing the same construct or dimension (eg, physical, mental, social) of health. Often, PRO instruments include more than one question to measure a specific dimension of health because several measurements of a construct produce a more reliable estimate than a single measure. For example, if we were interested in evaluating the functional ability of someone with an upper-extremity injury, an instrument with one question related to upper-extremity function may not capture the full spectrum of the patient's functional ability. A subset or series of questions related to functional ability of the upper extremity, however, may help to capture a better overall picture of the patient's status as it relates to function. With this subset of questions in mind, it is important to note that all questions related to the same dimension should be homogenous (ie, the questions measure the same thing). For our previous example, a homogenous subset of questions should all pertain to the functional ability of the upper extremity. The SF-12 and SF-36 are great instruments to illustrate the idea of internal consistency. Both of these PRO instruments consist of 8 subscales that target various dimensions of health, including mental health, physical functioning, and social functioning, and each subscale includes at least 2 questions. To have acceptable internal consistency, you would want the questions within each subscale to be related, suggesting that they are capturing the same construct.

Internal consistency is most often measured by **Cronbach's alpha**. Generally, higher alpha values suggest higher internal consistency of the questions within a PRO instrument, with the range of possible values being from 0 (low) to 1.0 (high). Acceptable Cronbach's alpha values range from .70 to .90. With PRO instruments, you do not necessarily want the questions on the instruments to be perfectly correlated. Let us consider an example of using a generic PRO instrument that has subscales for physical and emotional health. In this example, the Cronbach's alpha value for the emotional health subscale is .98. This high value may suggest that the questions within the generic measure address a very narrow aspect of emotional health since all the questions regarding this construct have an extremely high correlation. Additionally, the high Cronbach's alpha value may suggest that some of the questions within the generic PRO instrument are redundant and, potentially, unnecessary. However, we would suspect a specific PRO instrument that measures pain for individuals with patellofemoral pain to have a relatively high Cronbach's alpha value since all items included in the scale are targeted toward the narrow focus (pain) of the condition.

As was mentioned with validity, reliability should be determined for all populations in which an instrument is intended for use. Because routine assessment of PRO instruments in athletic health care is relatively new, it is often difficult to find reliability information for instruments in athletic populations. Regardless, it is important to understand the concept of reliability when selecting a PRO instrument because if the instrument is unreliable, you will not obtain useful information for your clinical decisions.

Appropriateness

One of the most basic questions to ask yourself when you begin to review PRO instruments for use in clinical practice is whether the instrument is appropriate for its intended use. When considering appropriateness, you might think about whether the instrument meets the needs of an individual patient (eg, patient with grade II ankle sprain) or, more broadly, whether the instrument meets the needs of your target patient population, such as the types of patients who frequent your clinical practice. It would be convenient if there was one PRO instrument that met the needs of all patients and populations, but that is not the case; there is no one-size-fits-all instrument in patient-oriented outcomes assessment. In regard to individual patient care, clear identification of patient care goals is necessary so that you can match patient goals (ie, improvements in function, pain, or social health) with the type of information you will gather from the PRO instrument. If, for example, your patient's goal is to return to prior levels of function and return to participation in sport, you should aim to select an instrument that includes function as a primary focus of the instrument. If, however, pain is a common concern of your patient, you may want to narrow your search to PRO instruments that center around pain or at least include it as an emphasis of the instrument. Finally, when selecting a PRO instrument that is appropriate for your patient or patient population, it is important to consider age because there are some instruments, such as the pediatric version of the IKDC (Pedi-IKDC), that have been made for younger patients. Using a PRO instrument created for adults in younger populations may be acceptable, but questions in adult instruments should be reviewed prior to use in younger populations to ensure question relevance and appropriateness. For example, the Disabilities of the Arm, Shoulder, and Hand questionnaire includes a question related to issues with sexual function as a result of the injury. This question may be inappropriate for younger populations, such as secondary school students. When possible, instruments should be selected that meet the age range of the population of interest.

Should you be more interested in measuring outcomes in a population, such as within adolescents with musculoskeletal injury, it may be important to select instruments that are applicable to many people, such as generic PRO instruments, so that there is a common outcome measure against which to compare all people. It is possible to evaluate populations with more specific PRO instruments, but this requires selecting an instrument for body regions, such as the knee, ankle, or head. Whether your intended use is to drive individual patient care decisions or to collect patient-oriented outcomes on groups of people with similar conditions, determining the appropriateness of a PRO instrument for your intended purpose requires that you look at all of the questions in the instrument to see how well they match your aims of use. One note of caution is that there are a variety of ways to address different health constructs, so careful evaluation of the question is necessary to ensure that the way in which the questions are asked align with your purpose. Just because function may be in the title of the PRO instrument does not mean that the questions in the instrument address functions that are relevant or important to your patient or population of interest.

Precision

The **precision** of a PRO instrument refers to the types of response options included in an instrument. A precise instrument should include a good balance of questions that are simple to answer with questions that capture the full range of response options. There are several types of response options available for PRO instruments, but more often than not you will see the following 4 types of response scales in the majority of outcome instruments you select to incorporate in your patient care:

- Binary response scale
- Visual analog scale
- Adjectival scale
- Likert response scale

Binary response scales include questions that result in only 2 answer options. This type of scale produces the most straightforward response and is typically simple for the patient to complete. Examples of questions that have a binary response scale are provided in Table 17-1. In clinical practice, you use binary response scales every day during your decision-making process. Binary response scales are also common in PRO instruments. However, while binary response scales are easy for the patient to answer, depending on the type of information you are hoping to obtain from the patient, this response scale may not provide you with the full degree of a response for a question. For example, a PRO instrument may ask a patient, "Are you currently in pain?" and include a binary response scale of "yes" or "no." If a patient selects "yes," you can accurately assume that the

Table 17-1. Examples of Questions for a Binary Response Scale

QUESTION	BINARY RESPONSE SCALE	
What are the findings from the Lachman's test?	Positive	Negative
Can the patient return to play?	Return to play	No return to play
What is your sex?	Male	Female
Are you currently experiencing pain?	Yes	No

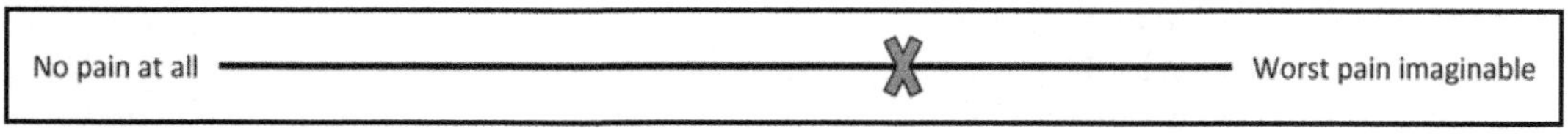

Figure 17-1. Visual analog scale.

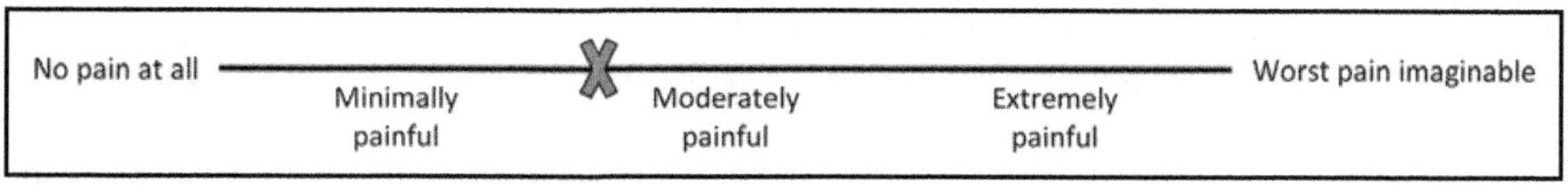

Figure 17-2. Adjectival scale continuous line.

patient is currently in pain. However, this response does not provide you with information about the severity of the pain, impact of pain on functional activities, or time of most pain (eg, during activities of daily living, rest, athletic activities). Additionally, with binary responses, you are unable to detect small, but potentially meaningful changes in health status because the information you gather tends to be more global in nature. Therefore, while a binary response scale is quick and easy to complete, its simple answer format limits the quality of the information you receive, which may also limit its usefulness.

Another response scale you may encounter on a PRO instrument is the **visual analog scale (VAS)**. The VAS is most commonly represented by a 10-cm line with phrases on either end of the line to identify the answer extremes and to indicate the direction of a response. Individuals are then asked to answer the particular question by placing an "X" or a single vertical line on the point of the line that corresponds with their answer to the question. An example of a VAS is shown in Figure 17-1. If you were trying to gauge how much pain a patient was experiencing, you may use a VAS instead of the binary response scale to gain a better understanding of the extent of the pain.

A third type of response scale you will see on PRO instruments is the **adjectival scale**. Unlike the VAS, which only uses descriptors on either end of the scale, the adjectival scale uses phrases across the continuum to measure the patient's perception. However, the adjectival scale is similar to the VAS in that responses on the scale are unipolar. A unipolar scale indicates that the responses on one end of the scale will range from none to minimum (or 0 on a VAS), while responses on the other end will range from a lot to maximum (Figure 17-2). Questions that require a response on an adjectival scale may be presented in a variety of ways, with the 2 most common mechanisms being a checkbox or a continuous line. If responses are presented with checkboxes (Figure 17-3), the patient is forced to select one of the predetermined responses. However, if the descriptors are presented with a continuous line, as displayed in Figure 17-2, the patient has the option to mark a spot on the line between 2 of the descriptors. Adjectival scales are beneficial to use on a PRO instrument because patients often have an easier time describing how they feel when descriptors are provided versus having to rely on a numeric response scale.

- ☐ No pain at all
- ☐ Minimally painful
- ☑ Moderately painful
- ☐ Extremely painful
- ☐ Worse pain imaginable

Figure 17-3. Adjectival scale checkbox.

☐ Very unsatisfied	☐ Strongly disagree
☐ unsatisfied	☐ Disagree
☑ Neutral	☐ Agree
☐ Satisfied	☐ Strongly agree
☐ Very satisfied	

Figure 17-4. Likert scale.

Finally, one of the most commonly used response scales you will encounter on a PRO instrument is the **Likert response scale**. This type of scale, developed by Dr. Rensis Likert in 1932, is a psychometric scale commonly used in surveys and PRO instruments. Likert scales are similar to adjectival scales in that this type of scale also includes a set of responses provided to an individual when answering a question. However, the primary difference from an adjectival scale is that a Likert response scale is bipolar. A bipolar scale indicates that the descriptors will go from one end of a spectrum (eg, least amount of pain), cross neutral (eg, no pain), and go to the other end of the spectrum (eg, greatest amount of pain). If you have ever completed a survey that asked you to respond to questions by selecting "strongly agree," "agree," "neutral," "disagree," or "strongly disagree," then you have completed a Likert response scale.

There are a variety of ways to set up a Likert response scale, and the number of answer choices for the scale can range from 3 choices to 13 or more choices, with the typical range between 4 to 7 selections. More answer choices included in a Likert scale item, such as the Global Rating of Change will allow for more precise information to be collected. However, there is a limit to how precisely people can assess their health status, especially if you consider specific populations, such as adolescents. An example of a Likert scale is shown in Figure 17-4. One of the benefits of using a Likert response scale is that it can provide you with more detailed information than a binary response scale. Previously, we discussed that a binary response scale only allows the patient to select "yes" or "no" to questions such as, "Has your pain changed since the initial injury?" Using a Likert response scale provides an opportunity to reformat the question to read, "How much has your pain changed since the initial injury?" with answer choices ranging from "a very great deal worse" to "a very great deal better." By using a Likert response scale, we are not only able to establish whether the patient is currently in pain, but now we can also ascertain the severity of the pain. Additionally, with the Likert style question, we have the ability to capture small, but important changes in health status that are not captured with binary scales. Thus, depending on the type of information that you are attempting to collect, a Likert response scale should be considered when more detail is wanted about specific aspects of health.

Interpretability

Along with the other selection criteria, it is important that you evaluate the **interpretability** of the PRO instrument and whether you can easily understand and explain the information obtained from the instrument. Typically, interpretation of PRO instruments is straightforward;

however, there are some things to consider that may make understanding these instruments easier. Having a patient take the time to complete a PRO instrument may be wasteful if the scores tabulated from the instrument are not reviewed and interpreted for the purpose of using them to assist patient care. Conveniently, there are guides available to help us interpret the scores on outcomes instruments. A common value suggested when considering instrument interpretability is the MCID. Since interpretability of a PRO instrument is similar to instrument responsiveness, MCID is important for both selection criteria. Remember, the MCID is the smallest difference in scores from one administration of an instrument to the next that a patient perceives as beneficial.

Let us consider another example to make sure you fully understand MCID. In this example, we will look at the MCID of the FAAM, which is 8 points for the Activities of Daily Living subscale (score range, 0 to 84 points) and 9 points for the Sports subscale (score range, 0 to 32 points). Your patient, who sustained a grade II lateral ankle sprain 3 weeks ago, completed the FAAM immediately following injury and produced a score of 52 (Activities of Daily Living) and 19 (Sport). After 2 weeks of treatment sessions, you ask the patient to complete the FAAM again. This time, the patient produced a score of 71 (Activities of Daily Living) and 25 (Sport). Remember, a higher score on the FAAM indicates a higher level of ankle-specific HRQOL. These results indicate that the patient has improved by 19 points on the Activities of Daily Living subscale and 6 points on the Sport subscale from the last time the FAAM was completed. By incorporating the MCID, we can conclude that the patient perceives their recovery has had a beneficial effect on their ankle-specific HRQOL related to activities of daily living (ie, their Activities of Daily Living subscale score increased by more than 8 points) but has not reached a minimally clinically important level of beneficial change on their ankle-specific HRQOL related to sport activities (ie, their Sport subscale score did not increase more than 9 points). This information is useful to you because now you can consider altering your treatment plan to focus on providing rehabilitation exercises that are sport specific. Thus, it is essential to ensure the PRO instrument you select produces interpretable results that can help guide you and the patient during care.

Acceptability

The **acceptability** of a PRO instrument focuses on patient friendliness (ie, will the patient accept the instrument?). An acceptable PRO instrument is one that minimizes distress to patients and, as a result, produces a high response rate from those to whom it is administered. When determining acceptability, it is important to consider the goal of the PRO instrument and whether it matches the goals of the patient. For example, a patient may be less inclined to complete a PRO instrument that measures pain if the patient does not perceive himself or herself to be in pain. It is also necessary to consider whether the number of questions included in the instrument is reasonable as well as how long it will take the patient to complete the instrument because shorter PRO instruments that can be completed relatively quickly tend to be more well received by patients than longer, more time-consuming instruments. Therefore, as you search for the best PRO instrument for your patient or patient population, you should always consider the following:

- Can the PRO instrument be completed quickly?
- Are questions within the PRO instrument clear and easy to understand?
- Are questions within the PRO instrument comfortable for patients to answer?

The attitude of the clinician is also important in ensuring that an instrument is deemed acceptable by patients. Clinicians who value the information gathered from PRO instruments are likely to have patients who find these measures more acceptable. Considering patient friendliness when selecting an appropriate PRO instrument will allow you to maximize patient response rates while simultaneously obtaining quality information that should assist with patient care decisions.

Feasibility

Feasibility is similar to acceptability except that it relates to clinician friendliness as opposed to patient friendliness. Not only is it important to consider how the patient will receive the PRO instrument, it is also essential to consider how feasible it will be for you to administer the instrument to your patients. In particular, you should consider the following:

- Can clinicians easily administer the PRO instrument to patients?
    - Is clinician training necessary for administration of the PRO instrument?
- Do patients or clinicians complete the PRO instrument?
- What costs (eg, licensing fees) are associated with administering or analyzing the PRO instrument?
- Is scoring the PRO instrument time consuming?
- How frequently should the PRO instrument be administered to the patient?

A clear assessment of feasibility is needed prior to implementation of any PRO instrument because if it is not feasible to use the instrument due to costs, training time, administration, or scoring time, then there is no value in using the instrument. There are a large number of PRO instruments that are free to use, have relatively easy scoring formulas, and do not cause burden to clinicians in terms of training, scoring, or interpreting the instrument.

Summary

Patient-rated outcome instruments are being used more within athletic training, so it is important for you to be able to determine if a particular instrument is actually the best fit. You must consider how the instrument was developed and whether validity and reliability concerns were addressed. Additionally, you must examine whether the PRO instrument is responsive enough to detect differences, if it is appropriate for the patient, if the responses are precise enough to give you the information you need, if you can interpret the information easily, and whether you and the patient can use the instrument with ease. You must ask yourself all of these things as you decide which PRO instrument to select for your patient case.

Key Points

- Instruments used to assess patient outcomes must be examined in a systematic manner for you to determine if the instrument is appropriate for a specific patient.
- Determining that an instrument is valid, reliable, reproducible, and responsive is essential to ensure that what is captured with an instrument is meaningful, relevant, and can be used to inform patient care decisions.
- One of the most basic questions to ask yourself when you begin to review PRO instruments for use in clinical practice is whether the instrument is appropriate for its intended use.
- A PRO instrument must be acceptable and feasible for widespread implementation.

Bibliography

Evans TA, Lam KC. Clinical outcomes assessment in sport rehabilitation. *J Sport Rehabil.* 2011;20(1):8-16.

Fitzpatrick R, Davey C, Buxton MJ, Jones DR. Evaluating patient-based outcome measures for use in clinical trials. *Health Technol Assess.* 1998;2(14):i-iv,1-74.

Guyatt GH, Comcardier C, Tugwell PX. Measuring disease-specific quality of life in clinical trials. *CMAJ.* 1986;134(8):889-895.

Kaplan SL. *Outcome Measurement & Management: First Steps for the Practicing Clinician.* Philadelphia, PA: FA Davis; 2007.

Martin RL, Irrgang JJ, Burdett RG, Conti SF, Van Swearingen JM. Evidence of validity for the Foot and Ankle Ability Measure (FAAM). *Foot Ankle Int.* 2005;26(11):968-983.

Poolman RW, Swiontkowski MF, Fairbank JC, Schemitsch EH, Sprague S, de Vet HC. Outcomes instruments: rational for their use. *J Bone Joint Surg Am.* 2009;91(suppl 3):41-49.

Portney LG, Watkins MP. *Foundations of Clinical Research: Applications to Practice.* 3rd ed. Upper Saddle River: Pearson Prentice Hall; 2009.

Scientific Advisory Committee of the Medical Outcomes Trust. Assessing health status and quality-of-life instruments: attributes and review criteria. *Qual Life Res.* 2002;11(3):193-205.

Snyder AR, Valovich McLeod TC. Selecting patient-based outcome measures. *Athl Ther Today.* 2007;12(6):12-15.

Streiner DL, Norman GR. *Health Measurement Scales: A Practical Guide to Their Development and Use.* 4th ed. Oxford: Oxford University Press; 2008.

Suk M, Hanson BP, Norvell DC, Helfet DL. *Musculoskeletal Outcomes Measures and Instruments.* Vol 1. Switzerland: AO Publishing; 2005.

18

Health Care Informatics

Have you ever wondered how many patient cases you manage over the course of an entire year? Or what the most common injury is that you diagnose and treat in your athletic training clinic? How about what the average time lost is from participation for patients under your care? Chances are, you have all the components you need to answer these basic but important clinical questions.

As a health care provider, you are professionally, ethically, and legally obligated to document all aspects of your patient care. Although clinicians do not often view their patient documentation as a source of information, we can learn a lot about our clinical practice (eg, patient, treatment, and value characteristics) simply by organizing, synthesizing, and analyzing the clinical data found in medical records. If you routinely, systematically, and comprehensively document your patient care, you can answer many complex and clinically meaningful questions about your clinical practice. These questions may include, "Which treatment approach is most effective in treating patients with an anterior cruciate ligament (ACL) injury?" and "Which treatment approach is most cost-efficient in treating patients with recurrent ankle inversion sprains?" While the potential benefits of patient records are apparent, clinicians often lack the necessary skills and/or tools to allow them to turn clinical data into meaningful information for patient care purposes. Due to this limitation, the study of informatics, particularly health care informatics, has recently been identified as an essential component of health care education.

The study of **informatics**, or the art and science of turning data into information, aims to improve process efficiency and productivity through the use of information technologies and information management techniques. Have you ever wondered how companies like Facebook (Facebook, Inc) provide you with advertisements in which you are inherently interested? These companies collect large amounts of data on you (eg, sex, age, what products or things you like) and target advertisements for you based on this information. For years, businesses and corporations have utilized informatics-based approaches to identify target customer populations, create personalized advertisements for individual customers, and increase overall profits. Similarly, political campaigns have utilized informatics-based approaches to predict how individuals are

Van Lunen BL, Hankemeier DA, Welch CE.
Evidence-Guided Practice: A Framework for Clinical Decision Making in Athletic Training (pp 241-250).

likely to vote so that they can identify safe areas (ie, areas that overwhelmingly support one candidate over another) and those that are swing areas (ie, areas that do not overwhelmingly support one candidate over another). This allows politicians to be more efficient and focus their campaign efforts on the swing areas since these areas will likely determine the outcome of the political race. In short, the use of informatics approaches can help groups and individuals make decisions in a more efficient and effective manner.

Although the study of informatics is not new to business and politics, it is only beginning to gain traction within the health care community. In 2003, a report by the Institute of Medicine (IOM) identified several major limitations in the health care system, including soaring health care costs (eg, unnecessary procedures, use of unproven/ineffective treatments), the lack of evidence-based decisions (eg, inability to organize and synthesize available evidence), and the inability to effectively prevent medical errors. To address these limitations, the IOM recommended that health care providers begin to facilitate the use of information technology (eg, computers, software, the Internet, mobile devices) to create an infrastructure to support quality assurance and prepare clinicians to manage the rapid accumulation of information, such as evidence from journal articles. In short, the IOM highlighted the need for informatics in the field of health care.

The use of information technologies within the health care system is often referred to as **medical informatics**. There are several fields that are captured under the umbrella of medical informatics, including clinical, imaging, and public health informatics. Each field aims to address different issues in health care and is unique in its own right. For the purposes of our discussion, we will focus on health care informatics because it relates most closely with the practicing athletic trainer. **Health care informatics** is the use of health care information technologies to support the efficient and effective delivery of patient care. Just as Facebook uses the data collected from your profile to target specific advertisements to you, you can use the clinical data you collect through your patient documentation to make better, faster, and more informed decisions for your daily clinical practice. Additionally, use of search engines and computer software can help you identify and manage information found in journal articles and textbooks to help you perform more efficiently and effectively during routine patient care. Health care informatics can take on many forms in your clinical practice, including utilizing health information technologies to form and answer clinical questions and to support evidence-based practice (EBP; eg, searching literature through online databases, organizing research articles). The following section provides you with an overview of the major components of health care informatics and highlights common considerations related to the incorporation of health care information technologies into daily clinical practice.

The Data to Wisdom Continuum

The study of informatics is nicely represented by the framework of the data to wisdom continuum (Figure 18-1), which outlines the primary steps necessary to turn data into useful information that you can use in a meaningful way. Your use of the data to wisdom continuum framework can help identify strengths and weaknesses of your clinical practice and also identify clinical questions that may help improve the quality of your patient care. We will walk through the components of the data to wisdom continuum and use an example to illustrate how this framework can be a valuable asset to your clinical practice.

The data to wisdom continuum consists of 4 primary components: data, information, knowledge, and wisdom. The first step in the data to wisdom continuum is the collection of **data**, or raw numbers or facts that are collected over time and have no inherent meaning. For example, your documentation of an ACL injury within your medical records would be considered to be data because, in and of itself, each diagnosis has no applicable meaning. However, if you were to organize and aggregate all of your injury diagnoses over the course of an entire year, you may begin to identify certain patterns within your injury data. For example, you may find that 80% of

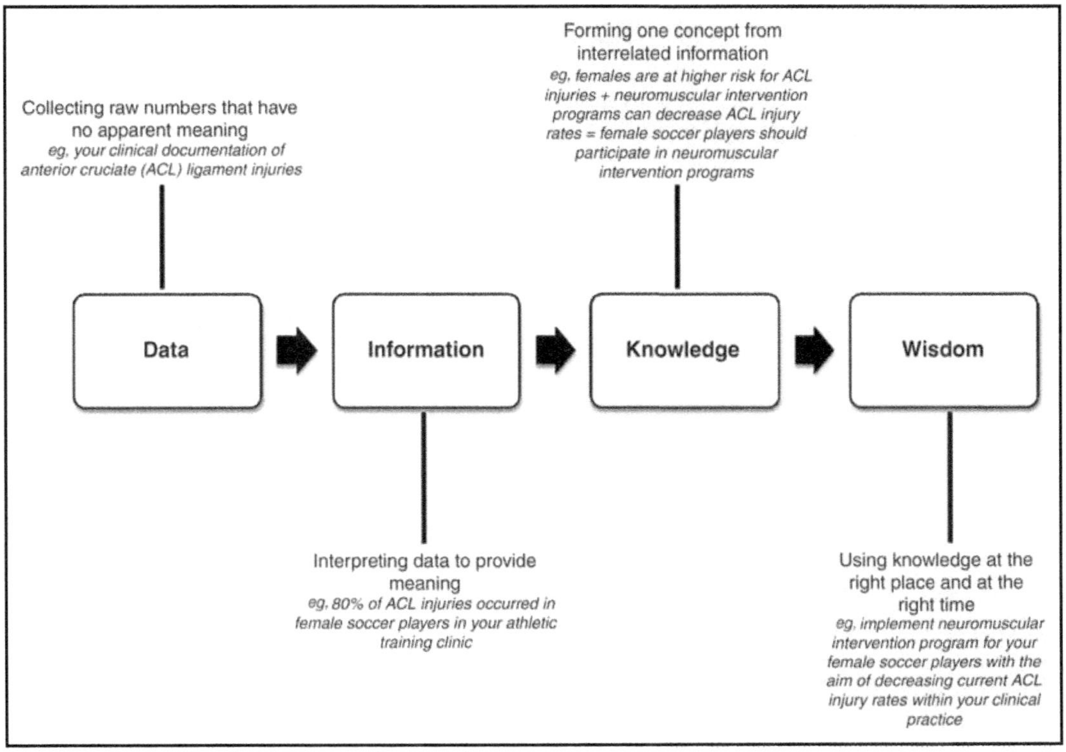

Figure 18-1. Data to wisdom continuum framework.

the ACL injuries evaluated over the course of the year were sustained by female soccer players. By organizing and interpreting your data, you have essentially turned your data into **information**, or aggregated data that possess inherent meaning that can be applied in a useful manner. With your newly created information, you can begin utilizing these findings to form clinical questions that will help inform and enhance your clinical practice. For example, based upon your data, you may formulate several foreground and background clinical questions, including the following:

- In soccer athletes, are female players at a higher risk of injury than male players?
- What is the average ACL injury rate in female soccer players?
- In female soccer players, do neuromuscular training programs decrease the incidence of ACL injuries compared with no intervention program?

As a practicing evidence-based clinician, you will utilize your clinical questions to help search the current available literature. Through your search, you might find that (1) females are at a higher risk for ACL injury, (2) your female soccer players are injuring their ACLs at a higher rate than those reported in the available literature, and (3) neuromuscular training programs can decrease injury rates by as much as 50% compared with no intervention program. Based on this information, you conclude that female soccer players should participate in neuromuscular training programs to help decrease the risk of ACL injury. Your ability to synthesize multiple interrelated pieces of information into a single concept represents turning information into **knowledge**.

The last step in the data to wisdom continuum is transforming knowledge into wisdom. **Wisdom** is knowing how and when to use knowledge to solve problems. For example, knowing that your female soccer players are injuring their ACLs at a higher rate than previously reported rates, you may implement an off-season and/or preseason neuromuscular training program with the aim of reducing the risk of injury. Your ability to recognize a problem and utilize your knowledge to solve the problem completes your informatics journey from data to wisdom.

The Clinician as a Knowledge Worker

To ensure that you remain an active participant across the data to wisdom continuum, you should act as a **knowledge worker**. As a knowledge worker, you fulfill several roles to ensure that data are transformed into information to help guide patient care decisions and improve quality of care. Specific roles of a knowledge worker include the following:

- Data gatherer
- Information user
- Knowledge user
- Knowledge builder

Perhaps the most important role you will play within the context of health care informatics is the **data gatherer**. As a data gatherer, you are responsible for collecting clinical data on all of your patients. In general, clinical data refer to the data you collect during the course of patient care, such as subject demographics (eg, age, sex, sport), clinical measurements (eg, range of motion, muscle strength) and treatment parameters (eg, duration, repetitions, sets, intensity). The good news is that clinical data are typically collected through patient care documentation and are not likely beyond the scope of your routine clinical practice. However, the documentation must be routine, systematic, and comprehensive so that the data can be aggregated effectively to produce useful and meaningful information. For example, if you are interested in understanding how certain treatment approaches impact range of motion, you should ensure that you are measuring range of motion in the same manner (eg, handheld goniometer) and at the same time points (eg, weeks 1, 2, and 3) across all of your patients. This approach will allow you to aggregate these data points more quickly and in a more meaningful manner because all of your data points will match across all patients. In contrast, if you do not take a systematic approach and instead measure range of motion using multiple methods (eg, handheld goniometer for patients A and C, electronic goniometer for patients B and D) and/or at different time points (eg, weeks 1, 2, and 3 for patients A and B and weeks 2, 4, and 6 for patients C and D) across patients, you will have a more difficult time making sense of your data because they will not represent the same types of measurements across all of your patients. As a data gatherer, it is essential that you understand what clinical data you need to collect to answer your clinical question and how to create a systematic approach by which to capture these clinical data during your daily practice.

As an **information user**, you will need to organize and interpret the collected clinical data and use the information for the decision-making process. Under this role, you should consider how the data should be stored and organized so that the process of turning data into information is streamlined. For example, many athletic trainers document patient care utilizing paper-based charts. While this approach is effective in terms of fulfilling your documentation obligations as a health care provider, it is an inefficient approach when attempting to turn clinical data into meaningful information. For example, if you documented your patient care utilizing paper-based charts and were interested in the types of injuries you treated over the course of the year, you would likely have to review each individual chart in your filing cabinet and physically count and record each injury that was documented for the year. In contrast, if you store this information electronically (eg, an electronic medical record, spreadsheet software), clinical data could be aggregated, analyzed, and interpreted more quickly.

In addition to using the information from your own clinical practice, you can also fulfill your role as an information user by finding, organizing, and managing information you extract from the current available literature. This approach is likely more familiar to you because creating a clinical question and searching the available literature for the answer is fundamental to EBP. The use of information from the available literature is often more efficient than collecting, aggregating, or analyzing patient data from your own clinical practice. However, in some cases, there may be little to no available evidence to answer your clinical question. In these instances, you will have to rely on your own patient data to answer the specific clinical question.

The last 2 roles of the knowledge worker relate to your ability to use and build knowledge. As a **knowledge user**, you can compare clinical data from an individual patient with existing knowledge. For example, you may compare the rehabilitation progress of a patient following a shoulder dislocation with findings reported in the available literature to determine how well (or how poorly) the patient is progressing. Lastly, as a **knowledge builder**, you can compile clinical data across patients to produce new knowledge. This role would require you to be competent in informatics and EBP. More specifically, after turning your clinical data into information, you should search the available literature to get a sense of how your findings compare with what has been previously reported. In our ACL example, you noticed that your injury rates are higher than those reported in the literature. In this capacity, you are fulfilling your role as a knowledge builder.

Now that we have discussed the theoretical process of informatics and the different roles you will need to fulfill to facilitate the data to wisdom continuum, we can begin to discuss the primary health care information technologies that support health care informatics. The most common health care information technologies you will encounter as a practicing AT are electronic patient records, computers, and the Internet. Due to the importance of health care information technologies in today's health care system, it is essential that you possess basic competencies (eg, using word processing and spreadsheet software, accessing the Internet, communicating through e-mail) to support your role as a knowledge worker.

Electronic Patient Records

Electronic patient records are fundamental to health care informatics because the electronic documentation of patient care supports informatics efforts in terms of turning data into useful information. The importance of electronic patient records to the future of the United States health care system is highlighted by federal initiatives aimed to increase the use of electronic patient records in hospitals and clinics. While many health care professionals often utilize the terms *electronic medical record*, *electronic health record*, and *personal health record* interchangeably, these records are distinctly different from one another. To understand the differences between these records, we must describe 5 primary characteristics of each record (Table 18-1), including the following:

- Overall purpose
- Timeline
- Ownership
- Accessibility
- Interactivity

The **electronic medical record (EMR)** is likely the most commonly recognized term in athletic training and the general health care community. The purpose of the EMR is to allow the clinician to legally record patient care documentation over the course of treatment for each episode of injury, illness, disease, or condition. In terms of timeline, the EMR typically captures the cause and course of one episode of an injury from a single entity (eg, one athletic training clinic). For example, if a patient has an ACL injury, you would record patient care documentation through your EMR from the time of injury until return to participation. Since the patient record is created in your clinic and only captures patient documentation from your clinic, the patient record is officially owned by your clinic and only accessible to the provider(s) within your work setting. While some EMRs allow the patient to view information, the patient cannot change the recorded information, and the interactivity between patient and provider is limited.

Table 18-1. Comparison of Electronic Medical Records, Electronic Health Records, and Personal Health Records

	ELECTRONIC MEDICAL RECORD	ELECTRONIC HEALTH RECORD	PERSONAL HEALTH RECORD
Overall purpose	Legal medical record created within a single entity	An aggregate of legal medical records from multiple entities	Subset of information from various encounters across multiple entities
Timeline	An episode of disease from a single entity	An episode of disease from multiple entities	Comprehensive, lifetime record of a patient's health
Ownership	Entity in which the record was created	Entity in which the record was created	Created and owned by patient
Accessibility	Restricted to providers within the single entity	Open to all appropriate medical entities	Open to patient and any appropriate medical entities with whom the patient chooses to share the record
Interactivity	Provider can view and edit information as needed; patient may be able to view the record but cannot edit information	Provider can view all information but can only edit information that he/she enters; patient may be able to view the record but cannot edit information	Both patient and provider can access and edit information

The **electronic health record (EHR)** is not as commonly recognized but is often confused with the EMR. Unlike the EMR, which is primarily restricted to the single entity, the EHR combines the legal medical records from multiple entities (eg, an AT, team physician, orthopedic surgeon, physical therapist, and sport psychologist). As such, from a timeline perspective, it captures the cause and course of one episode of an injury but from multiple entities. Referring back to the ACL example, if the patient sees the team physician, an orthopedic surgeon, a physical therapist, and a sport psychologist over the course of her recovery from injury, the EHR would aggregate all records pertaining to that specific injury from each entity and provide each clinician access to the compiled record. Each particular record would still be owned by the entity in which it was created, but it would be accessible to all appropriate providers that would need to access the record for patient care purposes. While providers can view all clinical information from the EHR, they can only change the information in the specific record that they created within their own entity. Since the EHR is a compilation of all relevant information from multiple providers for the same episode of injury, each provider can gain a complete and up-to-date perspective on the care the patient is receiving for the injury. Thus, an EHR can help streamline patient care, encourage interprofessional involvement, and improve quality of care.

The **personal health record (PHR)** is likely the least recognized term. The PHR is a subset of information from multiple encounters across multiple entities (eg, knee injury seen by an AT and team physician and high blood pressure event seen by family physician). The PHR is not a legal record of patient care but, instead, a comprehensive, lifetime record of the patient's health. Unlike the EMR and EHR, the PHR is created and owned by the patient. Providers, insurance companies, and independent companies offer patients platforms by which to create PHRs. The record is open to the patient, and the patient can grant any medical provider access to the record. The hallmark of the PHR is in its interactivity. The patient and the clinician can access, add, and/or edit the information in the record. Currently, PHRs are not very common, particularly in athletic training, because they are primarily driven by patients. However, as medical records continue to move from paper-based to electronic-based records and as global initiatives such as interdisciplinary patient care gain momentum, PHRs will likely become more common in routine patient care.

Basic Components of an Electronic Medical Record

The most commonly utilized health care information technology in support of informatics in athletic training is the EMR. When described in the context of the health care system, the basic components of an EMR include the following:

- Clinical documentation
- Data storage/repository
- Clinical messaging and email between providers and patients
- Results reporting for clinical tests
- Automated decision-making support system
- Order entry for prescription medications

In athletic training, it is likely that the EMR primarily consists of clinical documentation, data storage/repository, and clinical messaging and email. As athletic training–specific EMRs become more sophisticated, clinicians will enjoy other components, such as results reporting for clinical tests (eg, imaging results) and automated decision-making support system (eg, automated clinical recommendations based upon recorded clinical data). Despite the current limited features in athletic training–specific EMRs, clinicians can continue to reap the benefits of utilizing EMRs. These benefits include improved clinical data integrity, decreased documentation time, increased productivity, increased security, and increased access to patient records.

Patient Privacy and Confidentiality of Patient Records

As with all patient records, you must ensure that you are fulfilling legal obligations when creating, storing, and transmitting patient information through an electronic mechanism (eg, EMR). Legal considerations should be accounted for at local and national levels. Local considerations will vary depending on the state in which you are practicing as an AT. Therefore, it is your responsibility to review and comply with all appropriate state statutes or practice acts. At a national level, the 2 major federal regulations athletic trainers should consider are the **Health Insurance Portability and Accountability Act (HIPAA)** and the **Family Education Rights and Privacy Act (FERPA)**. The HIPAA is a federal law that encompasses all patient information that is collected and recorded by a health plan, health care clearinghouse, and health care provider. As a practicing health care provider, you must ensure the privacy and confidentiality of any health information recorded in any form or medium (eg, paper records, electronic records, voicemail, facsimile). In short, when considering an EMR, you should confirm that the system is compliant with HIPAA regulations to ensure that patient information remains confidential and securely stored. Other security measures may include restricting access to hardware (eg, computer), physical locks to secure hardware, authentication processes (eg, password-protected computers and software), and encryption processes, when needed. While HIPAA regulates records that are created within the context of health care, FERPA regulates records that are created within the context of an education system such as a high school or college/university, including health records. Thus, ATs providing patient care and recording patient information within an educational setting should be sure that they are complying with the standards that are set forth by HIPAA and FERPA.

Using the Computer and Internet to Support Literature Searches and Lifelong Learning

Although electronic patient records are increasing within the health care system, it is likely that you will interact with the computer and the Internet more frequently. These health care information technology tools are becoming more important to the practicing evidence-based clinician as information continues to increase and become more readily accessible. For example, it is estimated that information doubles every 3 to 10 years, and this notion is illustrated by the number of registered clinical trials over the past 2 decades. Just under 4000 clinical trials were registered at ClinicalTrials.gov in 2000, and that number surpassed 80,000 in 2010. Further, it is estimated that in 2015, 180,000 clinical trials will be registered. Attempting to sift through this vast amount of information available can hinder the efficiency of the evidence-based practicing clinician.

One of the first problems you will encounter as an evidence-based practicing clinician is sifting through the large amount of information that is available. The appropriate use of computers and the Internet can greatly enhance your ability to practice in an evidence-based manner because these health care information technologies can help you identify, manage, and store information in an efficient and effective manner. For example, the use of search engines (eg, PubMed) and electronic databases via the Internet can help you identify articles relevant to your clinical practice and/or a clinical question that you may have, while the use of bibliographic database software (eg, EndNote) can assist in organizing and managing references that you identified through your searches. The use of health care information technology tools can ensure that you are able to find the information you need and easily access that information when it is needed for your clinical practice.

In addition to literature searches, health care information technologies, such as the computer and Internet, play a vital role in lifelong learning. With an increase in information over the past several decades, practice standards are more routinely updated, thereby requiring health care professionals to stay current with the most up-to-date information and standards. As a health care professional, you must continue to improve on your skills and knowledge related to patient care. Although lifelong learning is recognized as an essential competency of a health care professional, there are barriers that can impede this process. Time, costs, and accessibility to continuing education events are examples of barriers that you will face as a practicing clinician.

Advances in technologies, computers, and the Internet provide effective platforms to support **distance education**, or education that occurs when there is physical distance between the instructor and the student. The use of technologies, such as computer-based educational management systems (eg, BlackBoard) and webinar programs, to deliver educational content from a distance is also known as **e-learning**. E-learning opportunities are often less costly, less time consuming, and more accessible because you can sit at your desk at home or work to view the educational content with no traveling or high registration fee associated with the course. Current evidence suggests that continuing education opportunities available through online approaches are just as effective as traditional approaches, which supports the use of e-Learning opportunities in support of lifelong learning.

Summary

The use of health care informatics and technologies in routine patient care is a primary component of health care delivery. Every day, you collect large amounts of clinical data about your patients that may help guide your clinical decisions and your overall practice. By applying concepts from the data to wisdom continuum and utilizing available technologies, such as electronic medical or health records, you will be able to collect clinical data in a resourceful manner and turn the data into useful information. Furthermore, as technology continues to advance and become more sophisticated, your ability to fulfill your role as a knowledge worker will be enhanced. Whether you are collecting data about your patient care and turning it into meaningful data or utilizing the Internet to search for available information to answer a clinical question, the use of health care information technologies will help you become a more efficient and effective clinician and improve patient care.

Key Points

- If you routinely, systematically, and comprehensively document your patient care and organize, synthesize, and analyze these clinical data, you can answer many complex and clinically meaningful questions about your clinical practice.
- The data to wisdom continuum outlines the primary steps necessary to turn data into useful information that you can use in a meaningful way.
- Due to the importance of health care information technologies in today's health care system, it is essential that you possess basic competencies to support your role as a knowledge worker.
- The use of an EMR provides the clinician with a database that facilitates the process of health care informatics.

Bibliography

ClinicalTrials.gov. Trends, charts, and maps. https://www.clinicaltrials.gov/ct2/resources/trends#RegisteredStudiesOverTime. Accessed November 14, 2014.

Duhigg C. How companies learn your secrets. *The New York Times*. February 16, 2012.

Hebda T, Czar P. *Handbook of Informatics for Nurses and Healthcare Professions*. 4th ed. Upper Saddle River, NJ: Pearson Prentice Hall; 2009.

Hillestad R, Bigelow J, Bower A, et al. Can electronic medical record systems transform health care? Potential health benefits, savings, and costs. *Health Aff (Millwood)*. 2005;24(5):1103-1117.

Institute of Medicine, Committee on Quality of Health Care in America. *Crossing the Quality Chasm: A New Health System for the 21st Century*. Washington, DC: National Academy Press; 2001.

Institute of Medicine, Committee on Quality of Health Care in America. *To Err Is Human: Building a Safer Health System*. Washington, DC: National Academy Press; 2000.

Jamal A, McKenzie K, Clark M. The impact of health information technology on the quality of medical and health care: a systematic review. *HIM J*. 2009;38(3):26-37.

Lobach DF. Clinical informatics: supporting the use of evidence in practice and relevance to physical therapy education. *J Phys Ther Educ*. 2004;18(3):24-34.

Pew Health Professions Commission. *Critical Challenges: Revitalizing the Health Professions for the Twenty-First Century*. San Francisco, CA: UCSF Center for the Health Professions; 1995:v.

Ruiz JG, Mintzer MJ, Leipzig RM. The impact of e-learning in medical education. *Acad Med*. 2006;81(3):207-212.

Steward M. Electronic medical records. Privacy, confidentiality, liability. *J Leg Med*. 2005;26(4):491-506.

TIGER Collaborative. Informatics competencies for every practicing nurse: recommendations from the TIGER Collaborative. http://www.thetigerinitiative.org/docs/tigerreport_informaticscompetencies.pdf. Accessed November 12, 2014.

U.S. Department of Health and Human Services. Summary of the HIPAA privacy rule. http://www.hhs.gov/ocr/privacy/hipaa/understanding/summary/privacysummary.pdf. Published May 2003. Accessed November 12, 2014.
Wright KE, Stewart J, Wright VH, Barker S. eLearning: is there a place in athletic training education? *J Athl Train.* 2002;37(4 suppl):S208-S212.

Glossary

Chapter 1

background question: A broad question used to explore issues and obtain general knowledge concerning the issue being investigated.

comparison: What you want to contrast the intervention or issue of interest against and includes things such as no intervention, placebo intervention, alternative therapies, no disease, a prognostic factor, or absence of a risk factor.

diagnosis question: Appropriate to construct when one is interested in determining whether one test is better at assessing whether an individual has a certain condition.

etiology question: Refers to the examination of the cause or causes associated with a condition and are utilized to determine which factors may be the primary elements that are associated with the greatest risk for the condition.

foreground question: A question much more specific to the case at hand that assists with identifying pieces of the clinical problem that will lead to a clinical decision particular to the patient.

intervention: Characterized by an intervention, prognosis or predictor, diagnosis or diagnostic test, etiology, or condition in which the clinician is interested.

intervention question: Assist with determining the efficacy of what is chosen for treatment to address patients' needs and lead to the determination of factors that may be important for immediate results, as well as long-term outcomes based upon the condition.

meaning-phrased question: Assists with understanding the meaning of an experience for a particular individual, group, or community and often deals with obtaining perceptual information from the patients.

outcome: Related to what the clinician is interested in examining concerning the effects of the intervention, diagnostic test, or prognosis you are seeking.

patient population: The patient population or disease of interest (eg, age range, sport played, gender, ethnicity) or targeted disorder/disease (eg, diabetes, sickle cell, anemia).

PICO: A method of clinical question construction that identifies the patient population (P), intervention (I), comparison intervention (C), and outcome of interest (O) to answer a clinical question.

PICOT: A method of clinical question construction that identifies the patient population (P), intervention (I), comparison intervention (C), outcome of interest (O), and time of interest (T) to answer a clinical question.

PIO: A method of clinical question construction that identifies the patient population (P), intervention (I), and outcome of interest (O) to answer a clinical question.

PIOT: A method of clinical question construction that identifies the patient population (P), intervention (I), outcome of interest (O), and time of interest (T) to answer a clinical question.

prognostic question: Utilized when determining the factors that may complicate the clinical plan of treatment over time and if you can then incorporate this information to better assist the patient with a favorable outcome.

time: May be appropriate in the clinical question if the outcome of interest has a specific time period of observation.

CHAPTER 2

case report: Descriptive study that conducts an in-depth examination of a patient and helps to develop and design larger studies or provide knowledge of the phenomenon to be studied further.

case series: Descriptive study that follows a group of patients who have a similar diagnosis or who are undergoing the same procedures over a certain period of time.

case study: *See* case report.

case-control study: Includes individuals who are chosen based on whether they have had the condition of interest that then seeks to identify predictors of an outcome through examination of exposures that may have contributed to one group incurring the condition of interest and the other not.

cohort study: Used to determine the incidence and after history of a condition; can be prospective or retrospective.

compilation research: The aggregation of a large pool of data from multiple studies in an attempt to answer a clinical question that may not be answerable with a single research study.

cross-sectional study design: Determines the prevalence of a condition, or the total number of cases of the condition in a given population, at a specific point in time; therefore, no causal relationships can be drawn.

descriptive study design: Examines factors at a point in time and provides information concerning the findings.

evaluative study design: Used to determine the existence and strength of a possible association between an intervention and an outcome.

***ex post facto* study design:** Examines data on subjects who already have the condition of interest and who are compared to a control group that has not had the condition.

experimental study design: The prospective investigation of groups over time, involving the manipulation of subjects; used to determine causal relationships.

meta-analysis: Compilation research that provides a quantitative assessment of the pooled statistical results from the studies that have met the inclusion criteria within the systematic review.

nonrandomized, experimental design: Involves no randomization procedures when placing individuals into groups.

observational study design: Investigators observe subjects and measure variables of interest.

prospective cohort study: Observes a group of people who do not have the condition and measures several variables that may be linked to the condition over a defined period of time. Individuals who develop the condition within the defined period of time are then compared with those that did not to determine if preexisting factors may have contributed to the condition of interest.

prospective study design: Examines the current condition and follows individuals over a designated period of time. It can also examine a group of individuals and wait until the injury of interest occurs to predict factors of contribution.

qualitative study design: Aims to develop concepts that help us to understand social phenomena in natural settings, giving emphasis to the meanings, experiences, and views of the participants.

questionnaire: An instrument utilized to gather specific data through self-reporting of a respondent's behavior, actions, and opinions related to the topic of interest.

randomized, experimental design: Subjects are randomly assigned to predetermined groupings. Inclusion of a treatment and a control group results in a randomized, controlled trial.

retrospective cohort study: Data that have been collected from other resources are used to assemble the cohort or groups to determine if risk factors for a condition exist or to clarify the outcome of an intervention.

retrospective study design: Examines data that have already been collected.

survey: Utilization of a questionnaire or interview as a methodological strategy to collect information at an identified point in time.

systematic review: Compilation research that provides a narrative of the critical evaluation of the research question during exhaustive search of the available evidence, followed by the appraisal, selection, and synthesis of many sources for a clinical question that is relevant.

time series: The observation of a participant or a group of participants over multiple time instances. Measurements are compared with prior time instances that are of interest.

CHAPTER 3

Boolean operator: A logical word or symbol that is used to connect 2 or more words or phrases in an Internet database search.

Cochrane Collaboration: An international nonprofit organization established in 1993 that aims to assist health care professionals, policy makers, and patients make informed decisions about health care. The Collaboration manages 6 databases.

controlled vocabulary or Medical Subject Heading (MeSH) searching: Terms included in the MeSH database are indexed in a controlled vocabulary hierarchy to help you become more efficient in your search when utilizing a MEDLINE affiliated database.

Cumulative Index to Nursing and Allied Health Literature (CINAHL): A collection of literature from nursing, biomedicine, health science librarianship, alternative medicine, consumer health, and numerous other health care professions, including athletic training.

database: An organized online collection of scholarly journal articles, periodicals, or books that provides a variety of information that will be helpful to you during your literature search.

exploding: During the mapping process, the search engine will retrieve not only article citations that include the keyword entered but also article citations that fall into the subheadings of the controlled vocabulary term to which the keyword is matched.

filters: Most databases also allow you to select certain limiting variables, known as filters, to help refine your literature search.

Google Scholar: A free-access Internet search engine that indexes resources from numerous scholarly publishers and is most often the top choice for clinicians searching for information.

keyword searching: Method of searching the literature through the use of simple terms from everyday vocabulary.

mapping: A feature in which the database will automatically attempt to match a keyword entered in the search box to a MeSH term that already exists.

Medical Subject Headings (MeSH): Controlled vocabulary within a hierarchy to assist with retrieving articles in a manner that goes from broad to more defined.

MEDLINE: The National Library of Medicine's bibliographical database that includes more than 19 million journal article references from numerous health fields, including medicine, dentistry, nursing, and other health care fields.

Physiotherapy Evidence Database (PEDro): A free database managed by the Centre for Evidence-Based Physiotherapy at The George Institute for Global Health in Australia. This database provides you with access to more than 22,000 randomized, controlled trials; systematic reviews; and physiotherapy clinical practice guidelines.

PubMed: A freely accessible online database maintained by the National Center for Biotechnology Information at the National Library of Medicine that provides health care professionals with free access to articles citations that are indexed in MEDLINE.

truncating: Allows you to search for all terms that are associated with a word stem. To truncate a term, you will need to enter the root of the word into the search box followed by an asterisk (*).

CHAPTER 4

***a-priori*:** The significance level is determined prior to data collection.

confidence interval: A range of values that explains how estimates of sample statistics are distributed in the population from which the sample was drawn.

construct: The idea or concept that is being measured or studied.

dependent variable: The variable that will be measured by the investigator.

descriptive statistics: Provide a summary of the main characteristics about the data collected during a study but cannot be used to draw conclusions about the hypothesis.

exhaustive: Includes all values potentially encountered.

homogeneity of variance: An assumption of parametric statistical tests that occurs when there is no discrepancy in the average dispersion of values for the dependent variable among the groups.

hypothesis: The proposed explanation of whether or why a phenomenon may occur.

independent variables: The variable that is manipulated or influenced by the researcher and may include various levels, which are determined by the research question.

inferential statistics: Statistics that are used to draw conclusions about the hypothesis posed based upon the data collected.

interval scale: Incorporates an ordinal characteristic and equal distance between adjoining data points but has no true zero point.

mutually exclusive: The subject or characteristic fits into only one category.

nominal scale: The simplest level of measurement that includes data classified into predetermined categories that are mutually exclusive and exhaustive.

nonparametric tests: Statistical tests that do not require data to have a normal distribution and that do not require the variance of the outcome variable to be equal across groups.

normal distribution: An assumption of parametric statistical tests that indicates that data are continuous and primarily cluster around a central value.

null hypothesis: Statement made by the researcher indicating there is no difference or relationship between the variables being studied.

ordinal scale: Used for data that have a rank order or hierarchy of meaning.

outliers: Data points that are numerically distant from the rest of the data.

parametric statistical tests: Statistics that are utilized to draw conclusions about particular parameters in the population from which the sample was selected via mathematical calculations and that require that assumptions are met.

power analysis: Technique that takes into consideration several components and that allows a researcher to estimate the value of one of the components provided that he or she has information for the other components.

quantitative data: An assumption of parametric statistical tests that indicates that data must have numeric values.

ratio scale: Incorporates an ordinal characteristic with equal distances between adjoining data points and has a true zero point.

research hypothesis: Directional statement made by the investigator indicating his or her expectations about the differences or relationships among the variables being investigated.

significance level: Level assigned by the investigator to represent a threshold value at which the results of the statistical test will be declared significant or nonsignificant.

skewness: The measure of the amount of asymmetry of a distribution that occurs when there are outliers.

statistical power: The ability of a statistical test to detect a significant difference if it truly exists.

type I error: Occurs when a researcher makes an incorrect decision to reject the null hypothesis when it is actually true.

type II error: Occurs when a researcher makes the incorrect decision to accept the null hypothesis.

CHAPTER 6

allocation: Refers to how a participant is placed into a group for the duration of the study.

bias: Propensity of an individual to be favorable toward one end of the spectrum; can occur in researchers and participants.

blinding: Research strategy in which either the participant, the researcher, or the clinician providing treatment are kept purposely unaware of group allocation in order to eliminate bias.

cluster sampling: Sampling method in which the researcher randomly selects a cluster of individuals who meet the inclusion criteria.

control group: Group of participants often used in clinical research as a comparison with the intervention of interest. Generally they do not participate in/receive the intervention being studied.

convenience sampling: Sampling method in which participants are recruited and selected based on convenience and accessibility.

double-blind study: Study in which the research team and the participants are unaware of the treatment groups until after the data are collected.

exclusion criteria: Characteristics that would eliminate an individual from being selected as a participant.

inclusion criteria: Characteristics and/or traits that are desired for each participant and would allow him or her to be selected for a study.

proportional stratified random sampling: Sampling method in which the researcher selects a sample with a proportion of participants that possess a particular characteristic that is equal to the proportion of the general population.

random sampling: Sampling method in which every potential participant has the same chance of being selected for inclusion in the study or for a particular treatment.

random selection: See random sampling.

single-blind study: Study in which participants cannot be blinded but the researcher or clinician is unaware of the allocation of treatment or control groups; therefore, only one aspect of the study is blinded.

stratified random sampling: Sampling method in which the researcher stratifies the total sample by the condition or variable of interest.

systematic sampling: Sampling method in which the total number of the population available for a study is divided by the number of participants needed, and selection is then performed utilizing an organizational variable or algorithm.

triple-blind study: Study in which the researchers, participants, and clinicians are unaware of the allocation to the treatment and control groups.

CHAPTER 7

compensatory equalization of treatments: A threat that occurs when a clinician or tester knows that the participant may not be getting the best treatment, so they work extra hard to help a member of the control group compensate for the lack of treatment they are receiving.

compensatory rivalry: Occurs when a participant who receives a less desirable treatment or is part of the control group tries to compensate by working harder to make up for the lack of treatment.

concurrent validity: A type of criterion-related validity that is assessed when the results of one test are compared simultaneously with the gold standard.

construct validity: The ability of an instrument or assessment to measure a more abstract concept.

content validity: The adequacy with which the particular measurement assesses all plausible constructs it is intended to measure.

criterion-related validity: The degree of effectiveness with which performance on a test or procedure predicts performance on another test or procedure; correlation between 2 tests aimed at measuring the same outcome.

diffusion: When participants of the control group and experimental group are in communication with each other.

error rate: A threat to statistical validity that occurs when the number of repeated statistical tests increases, leading to incorrect conclusions.

external validity: Aims to explain how results from a particular study can be applied to populations outside of the study.

external validity threat: Occurs when researchers draw incorrect conclusions or inferences to populations or settings other than what was originally studied.

face validity: Face validity indicates that the instrument or measurement appears to assess what it is supposed to.

gold standard: An established criterion that must be reliable, free of bias, and relevant to what you are intending to measure.

history: The unanticipated concurrent events (eg, natural disaster, change in job) that can occur outside of an experiment, which may potentially change the outcome of the study beyond the experiment.

instrumentation: The instruments and equipment used in testing procedures.

interaction of treatment and history: Occurs when the results from an experiment can only be generalized to the current experiment and should not be applied to past or future situations.

interaction of treatment and selection: The selection of participants and the inferences you can make based on the treatment.

interaction of treatment and setting: The ability of the researcher to generalize the results of the study to a setting that is different from the one where the experiment was conducted.

internal validity: Occurs when a researcher attempts to control all extraneous variables, and the only variable influencing the results of a study is the one being manipulated by the researcher. This means that the variable the researcher intended to study is the one affecting the results (cause-and-effect relationship).

internal validity threat: Includes treatments, procedures, or experiences of the participants that threaten the researcher's ability to draw accurate conclusions from the research.

matched pairs: Individuals are matched together based on a common variable, such as isotonic strength.

maturation: The changes (eg, physical, psychological, spiritual, emotional) that occur naturally to a participant over time independent of external events.

mortality: Indicates the number of participants who drop out of a research study before it is completed. Also referred to as attrition.

predictive validity: Used when you are trying to establish a predictor of a future criterion score.

regression: Occurs when unreliable testing procedures are used or when there are extreme group scores.

reliability and variance: A threat to statistical validity that occurs when conclusions are drawn from statistical analysis that are vulnerable to variations in the data that may be caused by lack of a formal collection protocol, unreliable measurements, or subjects that differ greatly.

resentful demoralization: Occurs when a participant in the control group feels devalued because he is not receiving the intervention being tested.

selection: An internal validity threat in which individuals are not randomly selected and possess a trait that may affect the outcome of the study. Also called selection bias.

statistical conclusion validity: Addresses whether there is a relationship between the dependent and independent variables.

statistical power: Addresses the ability to accurately document that there is a defined relationship between the independent and dependent variable.

testing: A threat of internal validity in which the participants become familiar with the testing procedures, and this may have an effect on the outcome measures.

validity: Whether a test or instrument measures what it is intended to measure.

validity of a measurement: Whether a particular instrument or assessment measures what it is intended to measure.

violated assumption of statistical tests: The variety of assumptions that must be met for that statistical test to be accurately applied; if an incorrect test is used, these assumptions may not be met.

CHAPTER 8

Cronbach's alpha: Statistical test utilized to measure internal consistency of measurement scales.

form: Refers to the second number within and ICC description and consists of a variety of values depending on whether the rater utilized an average of measures (k) or a single measure (1) within the reliability study.

internal consistency: A form of reliability used to assess the characteristics of a group of items that are usually within surveys or assessments to see if they are correlated with each other.

interrater reliability: The consistency of data recorded by multiple individuals who measure the same group of subjects for the same data.

intrarater reliability: The consistency of data recorded by one individual across multiple trials.

kappa statistic: Used with categorical data to assess the proportion of observed agreements as well as the agreement expected by chance.

model: Refers to the first number within an ICC description and consists of 1, 2, or 3. This value refers to a description of how the raters were chosen and assigned within a reliability study.

percent agreement: Simple form of reliability assessment that is determined by taking the sum of observed agreements divided by the number of paired scores obtained.

reliability: The consistency of a specific measurement.

test-retest reliability: Measure of reliability that assesses the stability of an instrument via testing for the same data in the same patient over a period of time.

weighted kappa statistic: Accounts for the number of categories and penalizes the disagreement in terms of seriousness.

CHAPTER 9

cutoff score: A specific score used to determine at which point the value of the test can be used to make a decision for the next course of action (ie, treatment, risk of injury increase).

false negative: The disagreement between the clinical diagnostic test and reference standard (negative clinical diagnostic finding but positive reference standard finding).

false positive: When there are positive clinical diagnostic findings but negative reference standard findings.

negative likelihood ratio: Indicates the likelihood that a negative test result was observed in a person with the condition compared to a person without the condition.

negative predictive value: An estimate of a diagnostic test to correctly determine the proportion of patients without the disease from all of the patients with negative test results.

nomogram: Figure used to plot pretest probability and likelihood ratios in order to determine posttest probability.

percent accuracy: Derived by combining the true positives and the true negatives, dividing the sum by the total number of tests performed, and then multiplying the outcome by 100 to get a percentage value.

positive likelihood ratio: Indicates that a positive test result was obtained in a person with the condition compared to a person without the condition and is expressed as a ratio.

positive predictive value: An estimate of the ability of a diagnostic test to correctly determine the proportion of patients with the disease from all of the patients with positive test results.

posttest probability: Revised probability used to be more confident in the diagnosis and improve certainty; the posttest probability is found through the use of a nomogram and entails knowing the pretest probability and likelihood ratios.

pretest probability: The odds/probability that a patient has a condition based on clinical presentation before a diagnostic test is conducted.

prevalence: The number of cases of a condition existing in a given population at any one time.

receiver operating characteristic: Uses specificity and sensitivity information from continuous data to determine a cutoff score for decision making.

reference standard: The most accurate tool (eg, radiograph to confirm a fracture, arthroscopy to confirm a ligament injury) available for assessing a current condition or determining an outcome. Sometimes called the gold standard.

sensitivity: The capability of the diagnostic test to correctly classify individuals with the condition of interest (true positives). Sensitivity can be calculated by taking all of the individuals with the condition who test positive on the clinical test and dividing that value by all of the patients who are confirmed as having the condition with the reference test and multiplying the outcome by 100 to get a percentage value.

specificity: The capability of the diagnostic test to correctly classify individuals who do not have the condition. Specificity can be calculated by taking all of the patients who had a negative diagnostic test and dividing that value by all the patients who are confirmed as not having the condition with the reference test and multiplying the outcome by 100 to get a percentage value.

true negatives: Those individuals for whom the clinical diagnostic test was negative and the reference standard was negative, indicating agreement.

true positives: Those individuals for whom the clinical diagnostic test was positive and the reference standard was positive, indicating that there was agreement.

CHAPTER 10

disease-oriented outcomes: Outcomes that include intermediate, histopathologic, physiologic, or surrogate results that may or may not reflect improvement in patient outcomes.

grade of recommendation: A letter rating system assigned to a body of evidence by comparison with a group of articles relating to the same topic.

level of evidence: The critical evaluation of a research article that rates the quality of evidence based on the research design of the study.

patient-oriented outcomes: Outcomes that matter to the patient and help them live longer or better lives.

CHAPTER 11

Appraisal of Guidelines, Research and Evaluation (AGREE) scale: A 23-item international instrument for assessing the quality of the process and reporting of clinical practice guideline development that was formulated by an international group of researchers from 13 countries in 2002.

appraisal scales: Produce numeric scores based on the incorporation of specific criteria.

Consolidated Standards of Reporting Trials (CONSORT) statement: Developed to provide guidelines and offer a standard way of reporting randomized, controlled trials. It is a 25-item checklist that includes a minimum set of recommendations for authors as they prepare randomized, controlled trials for publication.

double-blind study: A study in which neither the person administering the assessment nor the subject can identify the intervention being assessed.

Downs and Black checklist: A 27-item checklist created to 1) have a valid and reliable checklist appropriate for assessing randomized and nonrandomized studies; 2) to provide an overall score for study quality and a profile of scores not only for the quality of reporting, internal validity, and power, but also for external validity.

Grading of Recommendations Assessment, Development and Evaluation (GRADE): The GRADE working group was established in 2000 to address the need for developing a single grading system that could be used in health care. This working group was established to develop an instrument to grade quality of evidence and provide a strength of recommendation for various types of study designs.

Jadad scale: Originally developed as an appraisal tool that focused on appraisal of pain research. It is used to assess the quality of randomized, controlled trials. More specifically, this scale determines the effects of rater blinding and randomization in addition to patient withdrawals and dropouts.

Physiotherapy Evidence Database (PEDro) scale: Developed by physiotherapists to initially rate the methodological quality of randomized, controlled trials on the PEDro. The PEDro scale is an 11-item scale in which each item receives either a yes or no score.

Preferred Reporting Items for Systematic Reviews and Meta-Analyses (PRISMA): An update and expansion of the QUORUM statement. It was created to ensure that authors had a transparent and complete reporting mechanism for systematic reviews and meta-analyses through a 27-item checklist and a 4-phase diagram.

Quality Assessment of Studies of Diagnostic Accuracy included in Systematic Reviews (QUADAS) appraisal checklist: Originally developed in 2003 as an evidence-based tool to determine the methodological rigor of systematic reviews pertaining to diagnostic accuracy studies. It is a 14-item assessment tool.

Quality of Reports of Meta-Analyses of Randomized, Controlled Trials (QUORUM): The was originally created by a group of 30 individuals (including clinical epidemiologists, clinicians, statisticians, editors, and researchers) to establish specific guidelines for reviewing and reporting meta-analyses that pertain to randomized, controlled trials. It is a checklist of standards.

randomization: The allocation of subjects in which each subject is allowed the same chance of receiving the intervention and the investigators could not predict which treatment group each would be assigned to.

Standards for the Reporting of Diagnostic accuracy studies (STARD): Includes standard guidelines to improve the accuracy of reporting diagnostic research. The 25-item checklist and flow diagram are used to enhance completeness of reporting diagnostic methodology and findings, to allow readers to assess the potential for bias in the study, and to evaluate generalizability.

Strengthening in the Reporting of Observations Studies in Epidemiology (STROBE): Used for cohort, case-control, and cross-sectional studies and developed through an initiative in 2004.

STROBE provides a checklist of 22 items that should be included in observational research (ie, cohort, case-control, cross-sectional). Thus, this checklist does not evaluate research articles, but provides recommendations for standardized reporting of epidemiological studies. The fourth version of the checklist provides guidelines for observational studies in general and also provides specific information for each type of observation study being discussed.

withdrawals: Subjects who were included in the study but did not complete the entire observation period (full length of the study) or were excluded from analysis are considered to be withdrawals or dropouts.

CHAPTER 12

clinical bottom line: Summarizes how the research study relates to the clinical question.

clinical scenario: Introduction to the topic being appraised in a critically appraised topic.

critically appraised paper: Summary that focuses on appraising a single research study to help you determine if the reported results are valid, reliable, and clinically applicable.

critically appraised topic: Appraisal tool used to synthesize numerous research articles that review the same general topic of interest.

rapid critical appraisal worksheet: Worksheet with guiding questions related to validity, reliability, and clinical applicability to ensure you are collecting the necessary information to help you translate research literature into usable information.

summary of key evidence: Identifies the study design, participants, procedures, outcome measures and the results.

CHAPTER 13

clinical decision rule: When a clinical prediction rule has been validated and an impact analysis has shown to change clinical practice.

clinical prediction rules (CPRs): Decision-making tools that can be used to help clinicians determine a diagnosis, prognosis, or patient's response to a treatment.

derivation: The process in which you identify factors that have predictive value.

diagnostic CPRs: Used to help determine the probability that a patient has a particular condition of interest.

impact analysis: A study that demonstrates that the CPR has led to change in behavior, improved patient outcomes, reduced the cost of care, or improved the cost-effectiveness of treatment.

interventional CPRs: Used to determine the likelihood that a person would respond to a particular intervention or combination of interventions.

prognostic CPRs: Used to provide information about a likely outcome of patients with a specific condition.

predictor variables: Potential variables that are examined to determine their relationship to the desired outcome.

reference criterion: A well-established and accepted diagnostic test for diagnostic CPRs or a previously determined level of improvement in an interventional CPR. Also called a gold standard.

validation: Confirmation of the accuracy of the CPR in a different patient sample or different clinical setting; helps to confirm that the variables in the CPR did not result due to chance or a fluke.

CHAPTER 14

absolute risk reduction (ARR): The numerical difference in risk between an intervention group and a control group.

exposure: The opening up to the chance of an incident occurring.

incidence: The number of new injuries occurring in a sample over a defined time interval.

incidence proportion: The division of the number of athletes who sustained an injury by the total number of participants; cumulative incidence.

incidence rate: The number of new injuries that occurred during the total exposure time.

incidence rate ratio (IRR): The magnitude of an increased or decreased rate of injury between groups.

injury: As defined by the National Collegiate Athletic Association Injury Surveillance System, an injury occurs during organized intercollegiate practice or competition, requires medical attention by an athletic trainer or physician, and results in a participation restriction for at least 1 day.

numbers needed to treat to benefit (NNTB): The number of participants who need to be treated with the intervention to prevent a single injury compared to receiving no intervention.

numbers needed to treat to harm (NNTH): The number of individuals you would treat with an intervention to cause harm to one of them.

odds of being injured: The probability of an injury occurring compared to the probability of it not occurring.

odds ratio: The odds of injury for an individual who received an intervention compared to the odds of injury for an individual who did not receive the intervention.

prevalence: The segment of a group that is currently injured at a given point in time.

prevalence ratio: Utilized to examine if the injury prevalence is greater in 1 sample than another.

relative risk reduction (RRR): The percentage that injury risk is reduced in an intervention group compared to a control group.

risk ratio: A comparison of risk between 2 groups; relative risk.

sports injury epidemiology: The study of injury occurrence in athletic populations.

CHAPTER 15

active pathology: The disruption of normal cellular processes and the simultaneous homeostatic efforts of the organism to regain a normal state and is at the origin level.

activity: Execution of a specific task or action by an individual at the person level, without any social involvement.

activity limitation: A health condition that affects a patient's ability to execute a task or action.

biopsychosocial perspective: A combination of the medical and social perspectives. Biopsychosocial perspectives allow you to examine the influence of the health condition or injury on physical limitations or impairments, as well as environmental factors and social factors. This perspective is grounded in the theory that it is the interaction of the health condition or injury, limitations, impairments, and environmental and social factors that result in disablement.

body function: The physiological functions of the body systems at the organ level of the ICF disablement model.

body structure: The anatomical parts of the body at the organ level of the ICF disablement model.

disability: The inability of your patient to fulfill her necessary, desired, or expected social or personal roles and is at the societal level.

disablement: The impact of a health condition on your patient's body as well as their ability to participate in meaningful activities and to perform their desired roles in society.

disablement models: Provide the structure needed to advance the collection and dissemination of POE, thus improving evidence-guided practice in your clinical practice. These models provide consistent terminology that athletic trainers and other health care professionals can utilize when collecting, synthesizing, and disseminating POE and also when communicating across professions.

environmental factors: The physical, social, and attitudinal environments in which the patient lives and conducts their life. The subdomains of environmental factors include: alterations to the environment, technology, support and relationships, attitudes, and public services and policies.

functional limitations: Restrictions in the patient's performance specifically related to the patient's ability to complete their activities of daily living and other meaningful activities to them and is at the person level.

health condition: A disease or injury at the origin level of the ICF disablement model.

impairment: A loss or abnormality at the tissue, organ, and body system level.

International Classification of Functioning, Disability and Health (ICF): Designed to depict decreases in function on 3 health domains (body function and structure, activity, and participation) as the result of a dynamic interaction between the health condition and environmental and personal factors.

medical perspective: Views the patient's disability as a problem specific to the patient, caused by their health condition or injury, and primarily focuses on returning the patient to their normal state of health.

Nagi disablement model: The first disablement model that utilized this biopsychosocial perspective and laid the foundation for subsequent models. The Nagi disablement model describes the interaction between a health condition and your patient's environment.

organ level: Where you determine the impairment. For this level, you would use clinician-based outcome measures to assess the level of impairment, such as the weight bearing lunge test or range of motion measures with a goniometer.

origin level: Where you determine the pathology or health condition. For this level you would use diagnostic tests to confirm the pathology or health condition.

outcomes research: Evidence that is made available to you that demonstrates the final result of a treatment, most often incorporating the patient's values and experiences throughout the course of treatment and into the final outcome.

participation: Involvement in life situations at the societal level.

participation restriction: When a patient is unable to participate in life situations.

patient-oriented evidence (POE): The collection of outcomes that demonstrates the effectiveness of treatments utilized in the clinical setting from the patient's perspective.

person level: Where you assess the patient's ability to participate in meaningful activities. For this domain, you would use patient-reported outcome measures, such as the Foot and Ankle Ability Measure (FAAM), and clinician-based outcomes, such as a timed T-test, to assess the extent of the impact of the patient's health condition on the ability to participate in meaningful activities.

personal factors: The background of the patient's life, which are composed of features of the patient that are not specific to the health condition. Personal factors include sex, race, age, prior health conditions, fitness, lifestyle, habits, upbringing, coping styles, social background, and past and current experiences.

social perspective: Views society and/or the patient's environment as the creator of the person's disability and primarily focuses on what the environment or society does to promote or create your patient's disability.

societal level: Where you can assess the patient's ability to fulfill their desired role in society. Like with the person level, the societal level is evaluated through the use of patient-reported outcome measures to assess the extent of the impact of the patient's health condition on the ability to fulfill his or her role in society.

CHAPTER 16

clinician-based outcomes: Outcomes that are rated by, and of most value to, the clinician.

Disabilities of the Arm, Shoulder and Hand (DASH) questionnaire: A 30-item PRO instrument that focuses on symptoms and disability in people with upper-extremity injuries.

disability: A person's ability to fulfill necessary, desired, or expected roles in society.

Disablement in the Physically Active (DPA) scale: A 16-question instrument developed to measure disability in athletes through evaluation of 3 disablement model domains, including impairments, functional limitations, and disability.

disease-oriented evidence: Evidence related to the pathology and mechanisms of disease development and progression.

Fear Avoidance Belief Questionnaire (FABQ): A 16-question instrument designed to measure fear avoidance in low back patients with the intent to predict those patients who have and do not have pain avoidance behavior.

Foot and Ankle Ability Measure (FAAM): A 29-question region-specific PRO instrument that was designed to evaluate the activities of daily living and sports activities in people with foot and ankle injuries.

Functional Arm Scale for Throwers (FAST): A 22-question scale developed for the purpose of evaluating disablement in throwing athletes, and its construction was based on disablement models.

generic outcome measures: Ask patients to reflect on their health status from a global perspective. These measures can be used in health and ill populations and comparisons can be made between groups. They allow for a global assessment of health status.

Global Rating of Change (GROC): A single-item outcome measure that evaluates a patient's perceived change in one point in time (eg, therapy discharge) to another (eg, initial therapy visit).

Global Rating of Disability (GROD): A question that asks patients to globally assess their health and to perform some comparison between current health status as it relates to disability to some previous point in time.

Global Rating of Function (GROF): A single-item questionnaire that asks patients to rate the level of function they have in their injured body part on a numeric scale.

Headache Impact Test 6 (HIT-6): A 6-item PRO instrument that is condition (headache) specific and evaluates the impact of headache on HRQOL. While the HIT-6 was not designed for concussed athletes, it is relevant to this population because of the emphasis on headache.

health care outcomes: Meaningful results following an episode or period of intervention and can be related to the patient, clinician (or provider), and service provided.

health-related quality of life: Health-related quality of life (HRQOL) is a multidimensional construct that includes physical, psychological, social, spiritual, and economic domains of health.

instrument responsiveness: The ability of an instrument to capture small and meaningful change.

International Knee Documentations Committee (IKDC): One of the more widely studied PRO instruments for the lower extremity. It is a 19-question instrument designed to evaluate improvement and deterioration in symptoms, sports activities, and function in people with various knee ailments, including ligament injuries, cartilage problems, patellofemoral issues, and meniscal injuries.

Kerlan-Jobe Orthopedic Clinic Overhead Athlete Shoulder and Elbow Score (KJOC): A 10-question instrument, specific outcomes instrument, targeted toward overhead athletes. The KJOC consists of 10 questions that are related to upper-extremity function, athletic performance, symptoms, and interpersonal relationships, with one final total score produced.

Knee Injury and Osteoarthritis Outcome Score (KOOS): A 42-item knee-specific instrument targeted to patients who either have symptoms of osteoarthritis or have conditions that may lead to osteoarthritis (eg, ACL injuries, meniscal injuries).

KOOS-Child: A 39-question PRO instrument designed to be used in children with knee injuries who have the chance of developing osteoarthritis.

Kujala Anterior Knee Pain Scale (AKPS): A 13-question condition-specific PRO instrument designed to evaluate symptoms and functional limitations in people with anterior knee pain and other related conditions. Also called the Kujala Patellofemoral Score (KPS).

Lower Extremity Functional Scale (LEFS): A 20-question, region-specific instrument designed to evaluate function of people with lower-extremity conditions.

Modified Oswestry: A 10-question PRO instrument designed to measure the impact of low back pain on the management of daily activities, with an emphasis on function and pain.

multi-item patient-rated outcome measures (PROs): Capitalize on the limitations of single-item measures by asking patients several questions about various aspects of their health and providing a more comprehensive assessment of the construct(s) of interest.

Numeric Pain Rating Scale (NPRS): An 11-point, single-item PRO that is focused on pain and is a formal instrument that can be used in the routine evaluation of pain.

patient satisfaction: Patient satisfaction typically comes from the following: 1) the satisfaction a patient has with the recovery of his/her injured body part and 2) the satisfaction a patient has with the overall care experience.

patient-based outcomes: Patient-based outcomes, also commonly referred to as patient-rated outcomes (PRO) instruments, are surveys or questionnaires that a patient completes about his/her health status.

patient-centered care: Care that respects differences in patients and appreciates their uniqueness.

Patient-Centered Outcomes Research Institute (PCORI): The was created by the government through the 2010 Patient Protection and Affordable Care Act for the purpose of providing patients with information to make better decisions about their health and to improve the outcomes of health care services.

Patient-Reported Outcomes Measurement Information System (PROMIS) outcome measures: A family of instruments that were developed through funding from the National Institutes of Health for the purpose of creating an advanced, reliable system for measuring health outcomes from the patient perspective, with emphasis on physical, mental, and social well-being.

patient-oriented evidence that matters (POEM): The type of evidence that has the potential to impact or change clinical practice; comes from studies that ask clinical questions that are important to patients and include an emphasis on patient outcomes.

patient-rated outcome (PRO) measures: Surveys or questionnaires that patients complete about their health status; can be classified as general or specific in nature and also include single-item and multi-item options.

Patient-Specific Functional Scale (PSFS): Allows patients to identify functional end points that are important to them. The PSFS asks patients to identify 3 to 5 activities that they are unable to do or are having difficulty doing as a result of their primary complaint which, in athletics, most likely will be an injury.

Pediatric Quality of Life Inventory (PedsQL): A 23-question, generic PRO instrument tailored specifically for younger patient populations that can be used to evaluate physical, emotional, school, and social functioning.

Pennsylvania Shoulder Score (PSS): A 24-question shoulder-specific PRO instrument that evaluates pain, satisfaction, and function in people with shoulder conditions.

QuickDASH: A shortened version of the DASH questionnaire and includes 11 questions instead of the 30 questions in the original instrument. Like with the DASH, the QuickDASH includes questions related to function and symptoms in people with a variety of upper-extremity conditions.

serial administration: The repeated administration of the PRO instrument is called serial administration. Serial administration allows you to capture the peaks and valleys in HRQOL and to adjust care accordingly.

Short Form: The Medical Outcome Study Short Form (SF) family of instruments, such as the SF-12 and SF-36, are some of the most widely used generic measures of HRQOL in health care. These measures were designed for use in a wide variety of people with different conditions, injuries, and diseases and are used to calculate 8 dimensions related to HRQOL.

Single-Item Numeric Evaluation (SANE): Patients are asked about a global aspect of health in relation to an injured body part, such as the knee. Using the SANE, the patient can grade their injured body part on a numeric linear scale, much like the GROF.

single-item patient-rated outcome measures: Instruments composed of a single item, such as the global rating of change, which is a single question that asks a person to rate how much change he/she has experienced since some previous point in time (eg, the initial visit).

specific outcome measures: Specific outcome measures are narrower in scope and typically relate to specific body regions, diseases, or injuries.

Tampa Scale for Kinesiophobia (TSK): A 17-question PRO instrument designed to evaluate kinesiophobia, or fear of movement or reinjury, in people with chronic low back pain or fibromyalgia.

CHAPTER 17

acceptability: The ability of an instrument to minimize distress to patients, and as a result, produce a high response rate from those to whom it is administered.

adjectival scale: A scale that uses phrases across the continuum to measure the patient's perception.

binary response scales: Scales that include questions that result in only 2 answer options.

ceiling effect: The extent to which scores on a patient-rated outcomes instrument cluster near the more desirable health status extreme on a scale.

construct validity: The ability of an instrument to measure a more abstract concept; that is, things that are not directly observable.

criterion validity: Evidence to show that a new tool is an acceptable measure because it correlates with some other previously established measurement tool, or gold standard.

Cronbach's alpha: A standard measurement of internal consistency.

feasibility: The ability of an instrument to minimize distress to the clinician, and as such results in a more simple implementation.

floor effect: The extent to which scores on a patient-rated outcomes instrument cluster near the less desirable health status extreme on a scale.

internal consistency: The relationship of a subset of questions to each other that are aimed at assessing the same construct or dimension (eg, physical, mental, social) of health.

interpretability: The ability to easily understand and explain the information obtained from the instrument.

intraclass correlation coefficient: The measure of the strength of association between repeated variables that are measured at 2 or more repeated time points.

Likert response scale: A scale that includes a range of responses provided to an individual when answering a question that is bipolar.

minimally clinically important difference: The smallest amount of change that a patient perceives as beneficial.

Pearson product moment correlation coefficient: A correlational measure, which is a measure of association between 2 continuous variables.

precision: The types of response options included in an instrument.

reproducibility: The ability of an instrument to produce the same score when a patient completes the instrument on more than one occasion, assuming there is no change in health status.

responsiveness: The ability of the instrument to capture or measure meaningful change over time.

stakeholder: A person who has a vested interest in a given matter; in the case of patient-rated outcomes, this is the patient.

visual analog scale: A scale that is most commonly represented by a 10-cm line with phrases on either end of the line to identify the answer extremes and to indicate the direction of a response. Individuals are then asked to answer the particular question by placing an "X" or a single vertical line on the point of the line that corresponds with their answer to the question.

CHAPTER 18

data: Raw numbers or facts that are collected over time and have no inherent meaning.

data gatherer: Person responsible for collecting clinical data on all patients.

distance education: Education that occurs when there is physical distance between the instructor and the student.

e-learning: The use of technologies, such as computer-based educational management systems and webinar programs, to deliver the educational content from a distance.

electronic health record (EHR): Combines the legal medical records from multiple entities; aggregates all records pertaining to a specific injury, illness, disease, or condition from each entity and provides each clinician access to the compiled record.

electronic medical record (EMR): Allows the clinician to legally record patient care documentation over the course of treatment for each episode of injury, illness, disease, or condition.

Family Education Rights and Privacy Act (FERPA): Regulates records that are created within the context of an education system, such as a high school or college/university, including health records.

health care informatics: The use of health care information technologies to support the efficient and effective delivery of patient care.

Health Insurance Portability and Accountability Act (HIPAA): Federal law that encompasses all patient information that is collected and reported by a health plan, health clearinghouse, and health provider that ensures the privacy and confidentiality of any health information recorded in any form.

informatics: The arts and science of turning data into information. It aims to improve process efficiency and productivity through the use of information technologies and information management techniques.

information: Aggregated data that possess inherent meaning that can be applied in any useful manner.

information user: Person who organizes and interprets the collected clinical data and uses the information for the decision-making process.

knowledge: Ability to synthesize multiple interrelated pieces of information into a single concept.

knowledge builder: Person who compiles clinical data across patients to produce new knowledge.

knowledge user: Person who compares clinical data from an individual patient to existing knowledge.

knowledge worker: An active participant across the data to wisdom continuum that ensures that data are transformed into information in order to help guide patient care decisions and improve quality of care.

medical informatics: The use of information technologies within the health care system.

personal health record (PHR): A subset of information from multiple encounters across multiple entities; a comprehensive, lifetime record of the patient's health.

wisdom: Knowing how and when to use knowledge in order to solve problems.

Financial Disclosures

Dr. Dorice A. Hankemeier has no financial or proprietary interest in the materials presented herein.

Dr. Johanna Hoch has no financial or proprietary interest in the materials presented herein.

Dr. Matthew Hoch has no financial or proprietary interest in the materials presented herein.

Mr. Kenneth Lam has no financial or proprietary interest in the materials presented herein.

Dr. Jennifer McKeon has no financial or proprietary interest in the materials presented herein.

Dr. Alison Snyder Valier has no financial or proprietary interest in the materials presented herein.

Dr. Bonnie L. Van Lunen has no financial or proprietary interest in the materials presented herein.

Dr. Cailee E. Welch has no financial or proprietary interest in the materials presented herein.

For Product Safety Concerns and Information please contact our EU representative GPSR@taylorandfrancis.com Taylor & Francis Verlag GmbH, Kaufingerstraße 24, 80331 München, Germany

Batch number: 10731074

Printed by Printforce, the Netherlands